Contents

Changes in this edition   2

1. General Legal Requirements   3

1.1   Introduction   3

1.2   Medicines for human use   7
1.2.1   General sale list medicines   7
1.2.2   Pharmacy medicines   8
1.2.3   Prescription-only medicines   9
1.2.4   Wholesale dealing   16
1.2.5   Sales of medicines to exempted organisations, healthcare professionals or other persons   17
1.2.6   Labelling of medicinal products   23
1.2.7   Patient information leaflets   26
1.2.8   Use of fluted bottles   26
1.2.9   Medical devices   27
1.2.10   Restrictions on the sale of plano (zero powered) cosmetic contact lenses   27
1.2.11   Chloroform   27
1.2.12   Advertising and promotion of medicines   27
1.2.13   Handling of waste medicines   27
1.2.14   Controlled Drugs   28

1.3   Alphabetical list of medicines for human use   43
1.4   Non-medicinal poisons   75
1.5   Alphabetical list of non-medicinal poisons   79
1.6   Chemicals   82
1.7   Denatured alcohol   87
1.8   Medicines for veterinary use   91
1.9   Alphabetical list of medicines for veterinary use   97

2. Code of Ethics and Professional Standards and Guidance   103

2.1   Code of Ethics for Pharmacists and Pharmacy Technicians   103
2.2   Professional Standards and Guidance Documents   106

3. Improving Pharmacy Practice   137

3.1   Improving the quality of pharmacy practice   137
3.1.1   Clinical governance   137
3.1.2   Continuing professional development   138
3.1.3   Pharmacy support staff   140
3.1.4   Pharmacist prescribing   141

3.2   Practice guidance documents   142

3.3   Law and ethics fact sheets   146

4. References   147

4.1   Council Members and National Pharmacy Boards Members 2009-2010   147
4.2   Support for Pharmacists   148
4.3   Headquarters telephone enquiries guide   149

Index   151

Changes in this edition

The main changes in the 33rd edition of *Medicines, Ethics and Practice* are:

1. General Legal Requirements

1.1 Introduction
Minor additions and changes have been made to the list of definitions.

1.2 Medicines for Human Use
1.2.2: Pharmacy medicines (P) The section on *Personal control* includes the changes that the Medicines (Responsible Pharmacist) Regulations 2008 introduce on 1 October 2009.

A new section, *Responsible pharmacist*, has been added.

1.2.3: Prescription-only medicines (POM) The section on *Prescriptions for prescription-only medicines* has been updated to reflect that certain prescriptions may be legally valid if issued by European Economic Area (EEA), or Swiss, doctors or dentists.

A new section, *Exemptions to medicines legislation in the event of a pandemic*, has been included to provide information on recent legislation changes that will come into force in the event of a pandemic. There are four subsections: *Emergency supply, Supply of prescription-only medicines against a prescription, Conditions under which the retail sale or supply of medicines can occur* and *Labelling of certain children's medicines.*

The *Emergency supplies of prescription-only medicines* section has been updated to reflect changes in legislation. The legislation now allows dentists, and their patients, to request emergency supplies of prescription-only medicines. Emergency supplies may also be lawfully made at the request of an EEA, or Swiss, doctor or dentist, or at the request of one of their patients. The amount of a prescription-only medicine (that is not a Controlled Drug) that can now be supplied at the request of a patient has been increased from five days' to 30 days' supply.

1.2.4 to 1.2.14: Minor revisions to provide greater clarity.

1.4: Non-medicinal poisons
Minor revisions to provide greater clarity.

1.6: Chemicals
Major changes to cover new European Directives, and legislation changes, that come into force over an extended transition period.

1.7: Denatured alcohol
Minor revisions to reflect changes in legislation and to provide greater clarity.

1.8: Medicines for veterinary use
Minor revisions to reflect changes in legislation and to provide greater clarity.

2. Code of Ethics and Professional Standards and Guidance Documents

This section includes two new Professional Standards and Guidance Documents: for Continuing Professional Development and for Responsible Pharmacists.

Amendments have been made to two Professional Standards and Guidance Documents: for the Sale and Supply of Medicines, and for Internet Pharmacy Services.

3. Improving Pharmacy Practice

The following sections have been updated:
- Continuing professional development
- Pharmacy support staff
- Practice guidance documents
- Law and Ethics Fact Sheets.

Some of the information provided in *Medicines, Ethics and Practice* is updated between editions. To check for updates please see the Royal Pharmaceutical Society website, *www.rpsgb.org*. If you have queries about the content of this edition, *see* contact details pp149-150.

Published by the Royal Pharmaceutical Society of Great Britain
1 Lambeth High Street, London, SE1 7JN

New editions of *Medicines, Ethics and Practice: A Guide for Pharmacists and Pharmacy Technicians* are distributed free of charge to all practising and non-practising pharmacists and registered pharmacy technicians, to all preregistration trainees and in bulk to UK schools of pharmacy. Copies are not distributed to pharmacy premises. Additional copies are available at a cost of £29.95 each from Pharmaceutical Press, c/o MPS, The Macmillan Building, 4 Crinan Street, London N1 9XW, UK (Tel: +44 (0) 203 318 3141; Fax: +44 (0) 203 318 3139; e-mail: pharmpress@macmillansolutions.com), or you can order online at *www.pharmpress.com*

The Royal Pharmaceutical Society's Legal and Ethical Advisory Service is responsible for producing Part 1 of *Medicines, Ethics and Practice*. The content of *Medicines, Ethics and Practice* is collated and edited by Mary Snell

© Royal Pharmaceutical Society of Great Britain, 2009

All reproduction, including photocopying, rights reserved

ISBN: 978 0 85369 863 0

ISSN: 0955-4254

A catalogue record for this publication is available from the British Library

Printed in the UK by Precision Colour Printing, Haldane, Halesfield 1, Telford, Shropshire, TF7 4QQ

1: General Legal Requirements

1.1 Introduction

Part 1 of *Medicines, Ethics and Practice* is intended primarily as a practical guide to the legal restrictions on the sale or supply of medicinal products and poisons.

While every possible care has been taken in the compilation of this guide, no responsibility can be accepted for any errors or for any consequences of such errors. The aim has been to present as clear and concise a summary of the law as possible, and to interpret the various orders and regulations so as to decide the categories into which individual products should be classified. On any question of interpretation, however, it should be borne in mind that only the courts can give a legally binding decision.

Part 1 is primarily intended for the guidance of hospital and community pharmacists who are concerned with the retail sale or supply of medicines and poisons.

The Medicines Act 1968, the Poisons Act 1972 and the Veterinary Medicines Regulations 2008, together with the Misuse of Drugs Act 1971, regulate all retail and wholesale dealings in medicines and poisons. Certain non-medicinal poisons and chemicals are also subject to the labelling requirements of chemicals legislation including the Chemicals (Hazard Information and Packaging for Supply) Regulations 2002; *see* Section 1.6. It is important to appreciate at the outset that the Medicines Act 1968 applies only to substances when they are used as medicinal products or as ingredients in medicinal products. Carbon tetrachloride, for example, when administered for a medicinal purpose is a prescription-only medicine under the Medicines Act 1968, but when it is not used as a medicine it is not subject to the Medicines Act 1968. It is also important to grasp that there is no statutory list of pharmacy medicines, that is, medicines which may be sold over the counter only in registered pharmacies.

The basic principle of the Medicines Act 1968 is that all medicines may be sold or supplied by retail only from registered pharmacies except those that are included on a general sale list. The other principal statutory list is the list of prescription-only medicines which can be supplied from pharmacies, only in accordance with an appropriate practitioner's prescription.

Medicines which are not prescription-only medicines and which are not included in the general sale list are pharmacy medicines, that is, medicines which may only be sold from a registered pharmacy under the supervision of a pharmacist.

The Medicines Act 1968 applies to all medicines for human use. The Veterinary Medicines Regulations 2008 replaced the Medicines Act 1968 as far as veterinary legislation is concerned. Veterinary medicines are dealt with in Sections 1.8 and 1.9.

Similarly, there are substances used in medicines which also have non-medicinal uses. Several of these substances are included (together with other non-medicinal poisons) in the poisons list made under the Poisons Act 1972. Non-medicinal poisons are dealt with in Sections 1.4 and 1.5.

Keys to the annotations used in the list of medicines for human use (Section 1.3) and the list of medicines for veterinary use (Section 1.9) appear on the first page of each list.

1.1.1 Definitions

The following are definitions of terms used in the Medicines Act 1968 and the Misuse of Drugs Regulations 2001, as amended, or are interpretations of terms used in these sets of legislation, that are not explained in the main text of this guide:

Accountable officer is a fit, proper and suitably experienced person appointed or nominated by a designated body to ensure the safe, appropriate and effective management and use of Controlled Drugs within organisations subject to their oversight. The role and responsibilities of an accountable officer are defined under the Health Act 2006 and under The Controlled Drugs (Supervision of Management and Use) Regulations 2006.

Additional supply optometrist means a person who is registered as an optometrist, and against whose name particulars of the additional supply speciality have been entered in the relevant register (*see* p20).

Appropriate date means:

(a) in the case of a health prescription, the date on which it was signed by the appropriate practitioner giving it or a date indicated by him as being the date before which it shall not be dispensed, and

(b) in every other case, the date on which the prescription was signed by the appropriate practitioner giving it; and, where a health prescription bears both the date on which it was signed and a date indicated as being that before which it shall not be dispensed, the appropriate date is the later of those dates.

Appropriate non-proprietary name means, briefly:

(a) any name, or abbreviation, or suitable inversion of such name, at the head of a monograph in a "specified publication" (see below); or

(b) where the product is not described in a monograph, the British approved name; or

(c) where there is no monograph name or British approved name, the international non-proprietary name (INN); or

(d) where there is no monograph name, British approved name or INN, the accepted scientific name or any other name descriptive of the true nature of the product.

Appropriate practitioner *See* p11, under "Prescriptions for prescription-only medicines".

Appropriate quantitative particulars means, briefly, the quantity of each active ingredient (or that part of the active molecule responsible for the therapeutic or pharmacological activity) identified by its appropriate non-proprietary name and expressed in terms of weight, volume, capacity or, for certain products, in units of activity or as a percentage.

The quantity to be shown is:

(a) the quantity in each dosage unit (for pastilles and lozenges only it can be shown as a percentage), or

(b) if there is no dosage unit, the quantity of each active ingredient in the container, or

(c) if the product contains any active ingredient which cannot be definitively characterised, the quantity of the ingredient present in the highest proportion (diluents, excipient, etc, need not be stated).

The quantity of antimicrobial preservative added to a biological medicinal product must be stated. This applies to antigens, toxins, antitoxins, sera, antisera and vaccines.

The quantity can be expressed in terms of the dilution of the unit preparation for a homoeopathic product (ie, a product prepared in accordance with the methods of homoeopathic medicine or similar system which is sold or supplied as a homoeopathic product and is so described by the person who sells or supplies it).

Care home in relation to:

(a) England and Wales has the same meaning as in the Care Standards Act 2000; and

(b) Scotland means the accommodation provided by a care home service.

Care home service has the same meaning as in the Regulation of Care (Scotland) Act 2001.

Clinical management plan means a written plan (which may be amended from time to time) relating to the treatment of an individual patient agreed by:

(a) the patient to whom the plan relates,

(b) the doctor or dentist who is a party to the plan, and

(c) any supplementary prescriber who is to prescribe, give directions for administration or administer under the plan.

Common name in relation to a relevant medicinal product means the international non-proprietary name, or, if one does not exist, the usual common name.

Community practitioner nurse prescriber means a person:

(a) who is a registered nurse or a registered midwife, and

(b) against whose name is recorded in the professional register an annotation signifying that he is qualified to order drugs, medicines and appliances from the Nurse Prescribers' Formulary for Community Practitioners in the current edition of the *British National Formulary*.

Container means, briefly, the inner receptacle which holds the medicinal product. A package is every other outer receptacle.

Cosmetic means any substance or preparation intended to be applied to the various surfaces of the human body including epidermis, pilary system and hair, nails, lips and external genital organs, or the teeth and buccal mucosa wholly or mainly for the purpose of perfuming them, cleansing them, protecting them, caring for them or keeping them in condition, modifying their appearance (whether for aesthetic purposes or otherwise) or combating body odours or normal body perspiration.

Dispensed medicinal product includes a medicinal product prepared or dispensed by a practitioner (doctor, dentist or veterinarian) or prepared or dispensed in accordance with a prescription given by a practitioner and a medicinal product prepared or dispensed in a registered pharmacy by or under the supervision of a pharmacist, either in accordance with a specification furnished by the purchaser (for example, a customer's recipe) or in accordance with the pharmacist's own judgement as to the treatment required for a person present in the pharmacy (ie, counter-prescribing).

Dosage unit means:

(a) where a medicinal product is in the form of a tablet or capsule or is an article in some other similar pharmaceutical form, that tablet, capsule or other article, or

(b) where a medicinal product is not in any such form as aforesaid, the unit of measurement which is used as the unit by reference to which the dose of the medicinal product is measured.

EEA healthcare professional means:

(a) a doctor who is lawfully engaged in medical practice in a relevant European state, or

(b) a dentist who is lawfully engaged in dental practice in a relevant European state (including a person whose formal qualifications as a doctor are recognised for the purposes of the pursuit of the professional activities of a dental practitioner under Article 37 of the European Directive 2005/36/EC)

where "relevant European state" means an EEA state, other than the United Kingdom, or Switzerland.

Effervescent in relation to a tablet, means containing not less than 75 per cent, by weight of the tablet, of ingredients included wholly or mainly for the purpose of releasing carbon dioxide when the tablet is dissolved or dispersed in water.

100 5784111

Expiry date means the date after which, or the month and year after the end of which, the medicinal product should not be used, or the date before which or the month and year before the beginning of which, the medicinal product should be used.

External use means application to the skin, hair, teeth, mucosa of the mouth, throat, nose, ear, eye, vagina or anal canal when a local action only is intended and extensive systemic absorption is unlikely to occur; and references to medicinal products for external use shall be read accordingly except that such references shall not include throat sprays, throat pastilles, throat lozenges, throat tablets, nasal drops, nasal sprays, nasal inhalations or teething preparations.

Food includes beverages, confectionery, articles and substances used as ingredients in the preparation of food, and includes any manufactured substance to which there has been added any vitamin and which is advertised as available and for sale to the general public as a dietary supplement.

General Sale List medicine means a medicine for which all active ingredients are listed in the Medicines (Products Other Than Veterinary Drugs) (General Sale List) Order 1984 or are so classified in their marketing authorisation.

Health prescription means a prescription issued by a doctor, a dentist, a supplementary prescriber, a community practitioner nurse prescriber, a nurse independent prescriber or a pharmacist independent prescriber under or by virtue of:
(a) in England and Wales, the National Health Service Act 1977,
(b) in Scotland, the National Health Service (Scotland) Act 1978, and
(c) in Northern Ireland, the Health and Personal Social Services (Northern Ireland) Order 1972.

IRME practitioner means, in relation to a medical exposure, a practitioner for the purposes of the Ionising Radiation (Medical Exposure) Regulations 2000.

Maximum daily dose (mdd) means the maximum quantity of a substance contained in the amount of a medicinal product which it is recommended should be taken or administered in any period of 24 hours.

Maximum dose (md) means the maximum quantity of a substance contained in the amount of a medicinal product which it is recommended should be taken or administered at any one time.

Maximum strength (ms) means either:
(i) the maximum quantity of a substance by weight or volume contained in a dosage unit of a medicinal product; or
(ii) the maximum percentage of a substance contained in a medicinal product calculated in terms of weight in weight (w/w), weight in volume (w/v), volume in weight (v/w) or volume in volume (v/v) as appropriate; or
(iii) if the maximum percentage calculated in those ways differs, the higher or highest such percentage.

Medicinal product means any substance or article (not being an instrument, apparatus or appliance) which is manufactured, sold, supplied, imported or exported for use wholly or mainly in either or both of the following ways, that is to say:
(a) use by being administered to one or more human beings for a medicinal purpose;

(b) use as an ingredient in the preparation of a substance or article which is to be administered to one or more human beings for a medicinal purpose.

Medicinal purpose means any one or more of the following purposes, that is to say:
(a) treating or preventing disease;
(b) diagnosing disease or ascertaining the existence, degree or extent of a physiological condition;
(c) contraception;
(d) inducing anaesthesia;
(e) otherwise preventing or interfering with the normal operation of a physiological function, whether permanently or temporarily, and whether by way of terminating, reducing or postponing, or increasing or accelerating, the operation of that function or in any other way.

Nurse independent prescriber means a person:
(a) who is a registered nurse or a registered midwife, and
(b) against whose name is recorded in the professional register an annotation signifying that he is qualified to order drugs, medicines and appliances as a nurse independent prescriber or a nurse independent/supplementary prescriber.

Operating department practitioner means a person who is registered under the Health Professions Order 2001 as an operating department practitioner.

Optometrist independent prescriber means a person:
(a) who is a registered optometrist, and
(b) against whose name is recorded in the relevant register an annotation signifying that he is qualified to order drugs, medicines and appliances as an optometrist independent prescriber.

Parenteral administration means administration by breach of the skin or mucous membrane.

Pharmacist independent prescriber means a person:
(a) who is a pharmacist, and
(b) against whose name is recorded in the relevant register an annotation signifying that he is qualified to order drugs, medicines and appliances as a pharmacist independent prescriber.

Prescriber identification number means the number recorded against a person's name by the relevant National Health Service agency for the purposes of that person's private prescribing.

Prescription-only medicine means a medicinal product of a description or falling within a class specified in Article 3 of the Prescription Only Medicines (Human Use) Order 1997.

Private prescribing means issuing prescriptions other than health prescriptions.

Professional register means the register maintained by the Nursing and Midwifery Council under Article 5 of the Nursing and Midwifery Order 2001.

Professional registration number means the number recorded against a person's name in the register of any body that licenses or regulates any profession of which that person is a member.

Radioactive medicinal product means a medicinal product which is, which contains or which generates a radioactive substance and which is, contains or generates that substance in order, when administered, to utilise the radiation emitted therefrom.

Radiopharmaceutical means a medicinal product which, when ready for use, contains one or more radionuclides included for a medicinal purpose.

Registered chiropodist means a person who is registered in Part 2 of the register maintained by the Health Professions Council under Article 5 of the Health Professions Order 2001.

Registered dietitian means a person who is registered in Part 4 of the register maintained by the Health Professions Council under Article 5 of the Health Professions Order 2001.

Registered midwife means a person registered in the Midwives' Part of the professional register.

Registered nurse means a person registered in the Nurses' Part or Specialist Community Public Health Nurses' Part of the professional register.

Registered occupational therapist means a person who is registered in Part 6 of the register maintained by the Health Professions Council under Article 5 of the Health Professions Order 2001.

Registered optometrist means a person whose name is registered in the register of optometrists maintained under Section 7(a) of the Opticians Act 1989, or in the register of visiting optometrists from relevant European States maintained under Section 8B(1)(a) of the Act.

Registered orthoptist means a person who is registered in Part 7 of the register maintained by the Health Professions Council under Article 5 of the Health Professions Order 2001.

Registered orthotist and prosthetist means a person who is registered in Part 10 of the register maintained by the Health Professions Council under Article 5 of the Health Professions Order 2001.

Registered paramedic means a person who is registered in Part 8 of the register maintained by the Health Professions Council under Article 5 of the Health Professions Order 2001.

Registered pharmacy means premises for the time being entered in the register required to be kept under the Medicines Act 1968 by the Registrar of the Royal Pharmaceutical Society of Great Britain (or of Northern Ireland, as appropriate).

Registered physiotherapist means a person who is registered in Part 9 of the register maintained by the Health Professions Council under Article 5 of the Health Professions Order 2001.

Registered radiographer means a person who is registered in Part 11 of the register maintained by the Health Professions Council under Article 5 of the Health Professions Order 2001.

Registered speech and language therapist means a person who is registered in Part 12 of the register maintained by the Health Professions Council under Article 5 of the Health Professions Order 2001.

Relevant medicinal product means, except in Regulation 3A and paragraph 1A of Schedule 3 (of the Medicines for Human Use [Marketing Authorisations Etc.] Regulations 1994, as amended) a medicinal product for human use to which the provisions of the 2001/83/EC Directive apply other than:
(a) a traditional herbal medicinal product, or (b) a homoeopathic medicinal product that fulfils the conditions laid down in Article 14(1) of the 2001 Directive.
(This definition is taken from the Medicines for Human Use (Marketing Authorisations Etc.) Regulations 1994, as amended.)

Repeatable prescription means a prescription which contains a direction that it may be dispensed more than once.

Retail pharmacy business means a business (not being a professional practice carried on by a practitioner) which consists of or includes the retail sale of medicinal products other than medicinal products on a general sale list (whether medicinal products on such a list are sold in the course of that business or not).

Specified publication means the European Pharmacopoeia, the British Pharmacopoeia, the British Pharmaceutical Codex, the International Pharmacopoeia, the Cumulative List of Recommended International Nonproprietary Names, the British National Formulary, the Dental Practitioners' Formulary (or other official compendia which may in the future be produced under the Medicines Act 1968, Section 99) and the list of names prepared and published under Section 100 of the Medicines Act 1968.

Strength in relation to a relevant medicinal product means the content of active ingredient in that product expressed quantitatively per dosage unit, per unit volume or by weight, according to the dosage form.

Supplementary prescriber means:
(a) a registered nurse, (b) a pharmacist, (c) a registered midwife, or
(d) a person whose name is registered in the part of the register maintained by the Health Professions Council in pursuance of Article 5 of the Health Professions Order 2001 relating to:
(i) chiropodists and podiatrists; (ii) physiotherapists;
(iii) radiographers: diagnostic or therapeutic; or (e) a registered optometrist
against whose name is recorded in the relevant register an annotation or entry signifying that he is qualified to order drugs, medicines and appliances as a supplementary prescriber or, in the case of a nurse or midwife, as a nurse independent/supplementary prescriber.

Unit preparation means a preparation, including a mother tincture, prepared by a process of solution, extraction or trituration with a view to being diluted tenfold or one hundredfold, either once or repeatedly, in an inert diluent and then used either in this diluted form or, where applicable, by impregnating tablets, granules, powders or other inert substances.

Veterinary medicinal product means:
(a) any substance or combination of substances presented as having properties for treating or preventing disease in animals; or
(b) any substance or combination of substances that may be used in, or administered to, animals with a view either to restoring, correcting or modifying physiological functions by exerting a pharmacological, immunological or metabolic action, or to making a medical diagnosis.

Veterinary requisition means a requisition which states, in accordance with Article 14 paragraph (2)(ii) of the Misuse of Drugs Regulations 2001, as amended, that the recipient is a veterinary surgeon or veterinary practitioner.

1.2 Medicines for human use

Section 1.2 covers the following:

General sale list medicines (1.2.1)
Pharmacy medicines (1.2.2)
Prescription-only medicines (1.2.3)
Wholesale dealing (1.2.4)
Sales of medicines to exempted organisations, healthcare professionals or other persons (1.2.5)
Labelling of medicinal products (1.2.6)
Patient information leaflets (1.2.7)
Use of fluted bottles (1.2.8)
Medical devices (1.2.9)
Plano (zero powered) cosmetic contact lenses (1.2.10)
Chloroform: sale and supply (1.2.11)
Advertising and promotion of medicines (1.2.12)
Handling of waste medicines (1.2.13)
Controlled Drugs (1.2.14)

Classes of medicinal products

There are three classes of products under the Medicines Act 1968, namely:
(1) General sale list medicines (GSL)
(2) Pharmacy medicines (P)
(3) Prescription-only medicines (POM).

The legal requirements which apply to the sale, supply, dispensing and labelling of each class are dealt with separately below.

Meaning of "retail sale" and "wholesale dealing"

The selling of a medicinal product constitutes "wholesale dealing" if it is sold to a person for the purpose of:

(a) selling or supplying it, or
(b) administering it, or causing it to be administered to one or more human beings;
the sale, supply or administration being in the course of a business carried on by the purchaser.

Any sale which does not fall within this definition of "wholesale dealing" is a retail sale. The restrictions on the retail sale of medicinal products also apply to supply and to supplying "in circumstances corresponding to retail sale," which includes the dispensing of prescriptions under the National Health Service.

1.2.1 General sale list medicines (GSL)

GSL medicines are those medicinal products which in the opinion of the appropriate Ministers can, with reasonable safety, be sold or supplied otherwise than by or under the supervision of a pharmacist. These are listed in the Medicines (Products Other than Veterinary Drugs) (General Sale List) Order 1984 (GSL Order). GSL medicines can also be classified as such as a result of their marketing authorisation.

All GSL medicines, except those that have been designated as foods or cosmetics, must be licensed products (it should be noted that a medicinal product made up in a pharmacy for sale from that pharmacy without a marketing authorisation, is classified as a pharmacy medicine even though all its ingredients are in the GSL Order).

Products not on general sale

Part of the GSL Order specifies certain classes of medicinal products for human use which shall not be available on general sale. They are medicinal products promoted, recommended or marketed:

(a) for use as anthelmintics,
(b) for parenteral administration,
(c) for use as eye drops,
(d) for use as eye ointments,
(e) for use as enemas,
(f) for use wholly or mainly for irrigation of wounds or of the bladder, vagina or rectum, or,
(g) for adminstration wholly or mainly to children being a preparation of aloxiprin or aspirin.

Foods and cosmetics

Medicinal products which are for sale or supply either for oral administration as a food or for external use as a cosmetic are general sale list medicines. This does not include products which are prescription-only medicines, eye drops or eye ointments, or any product that contains either:

(a) vitamin A, vitamin A acetate or vitamin A palmitate with a maximum daily dose equivalent to more than 7,500 international units of vitamin A or 2,250 micrograms of retinol; or
(b) vitamin D with a maximum daily dose of more than 400 units of antirachitic activity.

Retail sale of GSL medicines

Medicinal products on a general sale list may only be sold by retail, offered or exposed for sale by retail, or supplied in circumstances corresponding to retail sale either at registered pharmacies, or in circumstances where the following conditions are fulfilled:

(a) The place at which the medicinal product is sold, offered, exposed for sale or supplied, must be premises at which the person carrying on the business is the occupier and which he is able to close so as to exclude the public. Sales from automatic machines should only be made from machines located in premises which the occupier is able to close so as to exclude the public.
(b) The medicinal product must have been made up for sale in a container elsewhere and not have been opened since the product was made up for sale in it.

Pharmacy Only (PO)

A PO medicine is a product that is licensed as a GSL medicine, but is restricted to sale through pharmacies only. PO medicines do not need to be sold under the supervision of a pharmacist, however the premises must be under the personal control of a pharmacist which is a requirement for pharmacy premises to be lawfully trading. These medicines may be available for self-selection by members of the public.

1.2.2 Pharmacy medicines (P)

A pharmacy medicine means a medicinal product which:

(1) is not a prescription-only medicine or a medicinal product on a general sale list; or,

(2) is a product referred to and presented for sale in the manner described below:

(a) Products for human use containing aloxiprin, aspirin or paracetamol which are offered or exposed for sale by retail in packs containing:

(i) in the case of effervescent tablets, (a) which do not contain aspirin, or where the amount of aspirin in each tablet does not exceed 325mg, more than 30 tablets; (b) where the amount of aspirin in each tablet exceeds 325mg, but does not exceed 500mg, more than 20 tablets;

(ii) in the case of tablets that are not effervescent, where they are enteric-coated tablets, containing more than 75mg aspirin only, more than 28 tablets, or where they contain aloxiprin, or aspirin or paracetamol or a combination of any or all of those substances, more than 16 tablets;

(iii) in the case of powder or granules, more than 10 sachets;

(iv) in the case of capsules, where they contain aloxiprin, aspirin or paracetamol or a combination of any or all of those substances, more than 16 capsules.

(v) in the case of liquid preparations of paracetamol, intended for persons aged 12 years and over, more than 160ml; intended for persons less than 12 years, individual doses of more than 5ml each, or more than 20 unit doses.

(b) Tablets for human use containing bisacodyl which are offered or exposed for sale by retail in a container or package containing more than 40 tablets.

(c) Products for human use containing ibuprofen which are offered or exposed for sale by retail in containers or packages containing:

(i) in the case of tablets, more than 16 tablets;

(ii) in the case of capsules, more than 16 capsules;

(iii) in the case of powders or granules, more than 12 sachets;

(iv) in the case of a product for topical use, more than 2.5g of ibuprofen;

(v) in the case of liquid preparations, individual unit doses of more than 5mls each, or more than 20 unit doses.

(d) Products for topical human use containing clotrimazole which are offered or exposed for sale by retail in a container or package containing more than 500mg of clotrimazole.

(e) Products for human use containing sodium picosulphate in a container or package of more than 60ml of the product.

(f) Products for human use containing loperamide hydrochloride in a container or package of more than 6 tablets or capsules.

(g) Products for human use containing cetirizine hydrochloride in a container or package of more than 7 tablets.

(h) Products for human use containing loratidine in a container or package of more than 7 tablets.

(i) Products for human use containing ranitidine hydrochloride in a container or package of more than 12 tablets.

(j) Products for human use containing famotidine in a container or package of more than 12 tablets.

(k)) Products for human use containing heparinoid in a container or package of more than 20g of the product.

(l) Products for human use containing mepyramine maleate in a container or package of more than 20g of the product.

(m) Products for human use containing ibuprofen lysine in a container or package containing more than 16 tablets.

The classification of an individual product will be dependent upon the conditions of that product's marketing authorisation.

Changes in the event of a pandemic *See* p13 for changes to this legislation in the event of a pandemic.

Retail sale of pharmacy medicines

Pharmacy medicines may not be sold, offered or exposed for sale by retail, or supplied in circumstances corresponding to retail sale in the course of a business carried on by any person, unless:

(a) that person is, in respect of that business, a person lawfully conducting a retail pharmacy business;

(b) the product is sold, offered or exposed for sale, or supplied on premises which are a registered pharmacy; and

(c) that person, or, if the transaction is carried out on his behalf by another person, then that other person is, or acts under the supervision of, a pharmacist.

A retail pharmacy business must be under the personal control of a pharmacist so far as it concerns the sale of all medicinal products, including products on a general sale list.

From 1 October 2009, the requirement to have a pharmacist in personal control will be replaced by the legal requirement to have a responsible pharmacist at each registered pharmacy premises so far as concerns the sale and supply of all medicinal products, including those on the general sale list (*see* p9).

Medicines sales

Sales of non-prescribed medicines from pharmacies should comply with the Code of Ethics and the supporting Professional Standards and Guidance Documents. This includes the requirements that all staff whose work regularly includes the sale of pharmacy medicines must be competent, and that assistants must be trained to know when the pharmacist should be consulted.

Personal control

NB: The requirement to have a pharmacist in personal control of registered pharmacy premises in relation to the sale and supply of medicines will be replaced with the requirement to have a responsible pharmacist from 1 October 2009.

Personal control is a requirement of the Medicines Act 1968 and there is limited case law on the matter. A number of cases have been considered by the Statutory Committee, and while each case is viewed on its merits, the following advice is offered to pharmacists.

All supplies of prescription-only medicines (POMs) and pharmacy (P) medicines from registered retail pharmacy premises must be made by or under the supervision of a pharmacist. Sales of general sale list (GSL) medicines do not require supervision, but do require a pharmacist to be in personal control of the premises. Thus, if a pharmacist is not in personal control, for instance because he or she is not on the registered pharmacy premises, no sales of any medicines can be made, and this includes GSL medicines.

If a pharmacist was not in personal control, the premises could remain open for trading as long as nothing requiring the presence of a pharmacist (ie, POMs, Ps and GSLs) is sold. If a decision is made to close the pharmacy while the pharmacist is not in personal control and the pharmacy has a contract with the primary care organisation (PCO) to dispense NHS prescriptions, the PCO should be contacted as to close the pharmacy may be in breach of that contract.

Pharmacists who registered with the Society by virtue of a qualification in pharmacy awarded in a relevant European State, are not able to be the pharmacist in personal control of premises in Great Britain that have been registered as a pharmacy for less than three years.

Responsible pharmacist

From 1 October 2009, the requirement to have a pharmacist in personal control of registered pharmacy premises is replaced with the need to have a responsible pharmacist. Every registered pharmacy will be required to have a responsible pharmacist appointed, who has a legal duty to ensure the safe and effective running of the pharmacy in relation to the sale and supply of medicines. Pharmacists should refer to the professional standards and guidance for responsible pharmacists on p134.

Under Sections 70 and 71 of the Medicines Act 1968, a notice will have to be conspicuously displayed in the registered pharmacy. The notice must detail the name of the responsible pharmacist, their registration number and the fact that they are for the time being in charge of business at those premises.

The requirements relating to the responsible pharmacist are set out in the Medicines (Pharmacies) (Responsible Pharmacist) Regulations 2008 which come into force on 1 October 2009. The responsible pharmacist will be required to establish (if not already established), maintain and review pharmacy procedures that must cover certain matters as required by the Regulations. These include arrangements for the safe and effective running of the pharmacy in relation to the sale and supply of medicines. The responsible pharmacist will also be required to make a pharmacy record which includes details on who the responsible pharmacist for the pharmacy is on any particular day and time. The pharmacy record must be kept for five years under the Regulations. Failure to complete the pharmacy record, or to keep it, is a criminal offence. The Regulations allow pharmacy procedures and records to be kept electronically and/or as a hard paper copy. Both the pharmacy procedures and records must be available at the premises for inspection. Pharmacists should refer to the professional standards and guidance for responsible pharmacists on p134 which detail the information the pharmacy procedures and records must contain by law.

The Regulations enable the responsible pharmacist to be absent from the pharmacy for a maximum of two hours, during the operational hours of the pharmacy between midnight and midnight. The total period of absence allowed for all the responsible pharmacists during one 24 hour period must not exceed two hours. The responsible pharmacist is responsible for the safe and effective running of the pharmacy during all times they are appointed, including during periods of absence. The Regulations state that in order for a responsible pharmacist to be absent, there must be arrangements in place to ensure that the responsible pharmacist is contactable and able to return with reasonable promptness. If the responsible pharmacist cannot remain contactable or cannot return with reasonable promptness, arrangements must be put in place for another pharmacist to be contactable and available to provide advice.

Where a responsible pharmacist has been appointed, GSL medicines can continue to be sold over-the-counter in the absence of the responsible pharmacist, providing the responsible pharmacist is absent in accordance with the conditions detailed in the Regulations.

However, the supervision requirements for the sale and supply of P and POM medicines have not been changed and still remain a requirement under the Medicines Act 1968. The sale and supply of P and POM medicines must not occur in the absence of the responsible pharmacist, unless a second pharmacist is present to supervise the sale and supply of P and POM medicines. The government will be considering changes to the supervision requirements at a later date.

Where the pharmacy is operating without an appointed responsible pharmacist, the sale and supply of medicines would be unlawful. If there is more than one pharmacist working in the pharmacy, only one may be the responsible pharmacist at any one time.

Further information can be found on the Society's website, *www.rpsgb.org* or at *www.responsiblepharmacist.org*

Collection and delivery arrangements from central points

Article 2 of the Medicines (Collection and Delivery Arrangements-Exemption) Order 1978, which came into operation on 30 October 1978, states that the restrictions imposed by Section 52 and 53 of the Medicines Act 1968 shall not apply to the supply of any medicinal product for human use on premises which are not a registered pharmacy, where such a supply is in accordance with a prescription given by a doctor or dentist, and forms part of a collection and delivery arrangement used by a person who lawfully conducts a retail pharmacy business.

Essentially this enables pharmacists to make arrangements for patients to drop off prescriptions issued by a doctor or dentist and collect the dispensed medicines from a general point that is not a pharmacy.

Further guidance on setting up these schemes is available on the Society's website, *www.rpsgb.org*.

1.2.3 Prescription-only medicines (POM)

Prescription-only medicines are those medicinal products described as such in the POM Order.

The main classes of prescription-only medicines are as follows:

(1) Medicinal products in respect of which a marketing authorisation has been granted, which in the marketing authorisation are classified as being prescription-only medicines;

(2) Medicinal products in respect of which no marketing authorisation has been granted consisting of or containing a substance listed in column 1 of Schedule 1;

(3) Medicinal products that are for parenteral administration;

(4) Medicinal products that are Controlled Drugs unless a marketing authorisation has been granted in respect of that medicinal product in which the product is classified as being a pharmacy or general sale list medicine;

(5) Cyanogenetic substances, other than preparations for external use;

(6) Medicinal products that on administration emit radiation, or contain or generate any substance which emits radiation, in order that radiation may be used;

(7) Medicinal products in respect of which marketing authorisation has been granted consisting of or containing aloxiprin, aspirin or paracetamol in the form of non-effervescent tablets or capsules which in the marketing authorisation are classified as being pharmacy only or general sale list medicines.

(8) Medicinal products in respect of which a marketing authorisation has been granted consisting of or containing pseudoephedrine salts or ephedrine base or salts in all pharmaceutical forms which in the marketing authorisation are classified as being pharmacy only medicines.

Exemptions from prescription-only medicine status

There are a number of exemptions from prescription-only control, and pharmacists should refer to the alphabetical list of medicines for human use (Section 1.3) to determine the category of medicine, and whether any particular exemption applies.

Some medicines are exempt from prescription-only control, only when in the form of particular licensed medicines. For example, hydrocortisone is a prescription-only medicine, but when in the form of a licensed product, for which the indications fall within the terms specified for an exemption, the product is licensed as a pharmacy medicine. No other hydrocortisone products can be sold without prescription, and the licensed products must only be sold within the terms of their licence (they cannot, for example, be mixed with other medicinal products, even where they are pharmacy only or even general sale list medicines). For examples, refer to the alphabetical list of medicines for human use (Section 1.3).

Some medicinal products are exempted from prescription-only status when sold or supplied for the treatment of specified conditions, and at dosages not exceeding stated maxima. However, the labelling of such products is complex, and pharmacists are advised to sell or supply only licensed products specially packed for over the counter sale.

Exemption for products consisting of or containing pseudoephedrine salts or ephedrine base or salts

It is unlawful to sell or supply a product or products containing more than 720mg of pseudoephedrine salts or more than 180mg ephedrine base (or salts) to a person at any one time (ie, in one transaction) except in accordance with a prescription.

A sale or supply without a prescription may be made of more than one product containing only one of these substances, provided that the total amount sold does not exceed the above limit. However, it is unlawful to sell or supply a pseudoephedrine-containing product at the same time as an ephedrine-containing product in one transaction

Administration of prescription-only medicines

The legislation provides that no one may administer a parenteral prescription-only medicine otherwise than to himself, unless he is an appropriate practitioner or is acting in accordance with the directions of an appropriate practitioner.

Administration of parenteral medicines for the purpose of saving a life in an emergency

The legislation provides that no-one may administer a parenteral prescription-only medicine otherwise than to himself, unless he is an appropriate practitioner or is acting in accordance with the directions of an appropriate practitioner.

The following list of medicines for use by parenteral administration, are exempt from this restriction when administered for the purpose of saving life in an emergency.

Adrenaline injection 1 in 1000 (1mg in 1ml)
Atropine sulphate injection
Atropine sulphate and obidoxime chloride injection
Atropine sulphate and pralidoxime chloride injection
Atropine sulphate, pralidoxime mesilate and
  avizafone injection
Chlorphenamine injection
Dicobalt edetate injection
Glucagon injection
Glucose injection 50%
Hydrocortisone injection
Naloxone hydrochloride
Pralidoxime chloride injection
Pralidoxime mesilate injection
Promethazine hydrochloride injection
Snake venom antiserum
Sodium nitrite injection
Sodium thiosulphate injection
Sterile pralidoxime

Administration of smallpox vaccine

The legislation provides that no one may administer a parenteral prescription-only medicine otherwise than to himself, unless he is an appropriate practitioner or is acting in accordance with the directions of an appropriate practitioner. Smallpox vaccine for parenteral administration to human beings is exempt from this restriction where either:

1. (a) the vaccine has been supplied by, or on behalf of, or under arrangements made by:
(i) the Secretary of State,
(ii) the Scottish Ministers,
(iii) the National Assembly for Wales,
(iv) the Department of Health, Social Services and Public Safety,
(v) an NHS body; and
(b) the vaccine is administered for the purpose of providing protection against smallpox virus in the event of a suspected or confirmed case of smallpox in the United Kingdom, OR:

2. (a) the vaccine has been supplied by, or on behalf of, or under arrangements made by Her Majesty's Forces;
(b) the vaccine is administered for the purpose of providing protection against smallpox virus to:
(i) members of Her Majesty's Forces; or
(ii) other persons employed or engaged by those Forces.

For the purposes of this section, "NHS body" means:
(a) the Common Services Agency,

(b) a Strategic Health Authority, Health Authority or Special Health Authority,

(c) a Primary Care Trust,

(d) a Local Health Board, or

(e) an NHS Trust or NHS foundation trust.

Administration by operators

The legislation provides that no-one may administer a parenteral prescription-only medicine otherwise than to himself, unless he is an appropriate practitioner or is acting in accordance with the directions of an appropriate practitioner. This restriction does not apply to:

1. a radioactive medicinal product, administration of which results in a medical exposure; or,

2. any other prescription only medicine if it is being administered in connection with a medical exposure.

The following conditions must be satisfied:

(a) The radioactive medicinal product or other prescription only medicine is administered by an operator acting in accordance with the procedures and protocols referred to in regulation 4(1) and 4(2) of the Ionising Radiation (Medical Exposure) Regulations 2000;

(b) The medical exposure has been authorised by an IRME practitioner or, where this is not practicable, by an operator acting in accordance with written guidelines issued by an IRME practitioner;

(c) The IRME practitioner is the holder of a certificate granted under the Medicines (Administration of Radioactive Substances) Regulations 1978;

(d) The radioactive medicinal product or other prescription only medicine is not a Controlled Drug; and

(e) In the case of a prescription only medicine which is not a radioactive medicinal product, it is specified in the protocols (as referred to in subsection [a]) in connection with a medical exposure.

Administration of prescription-only medicines in hospital

The Medicines Act 1968 does not specify that the directions of an appropriate practitioner need be in writing, in order to authorise administration. Nevertheless, it is good practice to ensure that whenever a prescription-only medicine is administered it has been authorised in writing by an appropriate practitioner before administration takes place.

Some hospitals have formulated policies to permit administration in an emergency on the telephoned or verbal request of an appropriate practitioner, usually involving two nurses checking one another. Some hospitals have also formulated policies for the routine administration of prescription-only (and pharmacy and general sale list) medicines. Such a policy should be carefully considered and agreed by medical, nursing and pharmaceutical staff, to ensure that patients are not put at risk. If in doubt, the Department of Health should be consulted, where the hospital is in England, along with the legal advisors of the hospital. Hospitals in Scotland should contact the Scottish Executive and hospitals in Wales should contact the Department of Health and Social Services.

Prescriptions for prescription-only medicines

A prescription-only medicine may be sold or supplied by retail only in accordance with a prescription given by an appropriate practitioner (*see* p13 for changes to this legislation in the event of a pandemic).

Appropriate practitioners include United Kingdom registered doctors, dentists, nurse independent prescribers, pharmacist independent prescribers, veterinary surgeons and veterinary practitioners, supplementary prescribers, EEA or Swiss doctors and EEA or Swiss dentists (*see below*).

Supplementary prescribers can issue prescriptions for any prescription-only medicine when acting in accordance with a clinical management plan (*see* p14).

Until additional changes to the Misuse of Drugs Regulations 2001 take place, pharmacist independent prescribers will not be able to prescribe Controlled Drugs, and nurse independent prescribers will continue to be limited to the range of Controlled Drugs they can currently prescribe for particular indications. Optometrist independent prescribers are appropriate practitioners in relation to the descriptions and classes of medicinal products specified in Article 3 of the POM Order, other than medicinal products that are Controlled Drugs or for parenteral administration or both. Community practitioner nurse prescribers are appropriate practitioners for descriptions and classes of prescription-only medicines specified in Schedule 3 of the POM Order.

Following a change in legislation on 3 November 2008, a prescription issued by an EEA or Swiss healthcare professional is legally valid in the UK. EEA healthcare professional refers only to doctors or dentists who are registered to practise in an EEA country or in Switzerland. UK registered doctors and dentists are excluded as they are already covered by current medicines legislation. EEA or Swiss healthcare professionals are not permitted to issue prescriptions for Schedule 1-5 Controlled Drugs and medicines that do not have a UK marketing authorisation.

Further information on dispensing prescriptions issued by EEA or Swiss healthcare professionals can be found on the Society website, *www.rpsgb.org*.

Pharmacists can telephone the General Medical Council (0845 357 3456) to confirm that a doctor is registered, and the General Dental Council (020 7887 3800) to confirm that a dentist is registered.

Pharmacists can telephone the Nursing and Midwifery Council (020 7333 9333) to confirm a nurse's registration status.

Pharmacists can telephone the Society's Registration Department (020 7572 2532) to confirm a pharmacist's registration status.

Supplementary prescriber or independent prescriber status can be checked against the relevant register held by the appropriate professional or regulatory body. Contact details for medical and dental regulatory authorities in EEA states and Switzerland can be found on the Society's website (*www.rpsgb.org*).

To be valid, a prescription issued by an appropriate practitioner:

(a) shall be signed in ink with his own name by the appropriate practitioner giving it;

(b) shall be written in indelible ink (this includes typewriting and computer generated prescriptions). A health prescription, which is not for a Controlled Drug specified in Schedule 1, 2 or 3 to the Misuse of Drugs Regulations, can be written by means of carbon paper or similar material but must be signed in indelible ink by the practitioner giving it;

(c) shall contain the following particulars:

(i) the address of the appropriate practitioner giving it,

(ii) the appropriate date,

(iii) such particulars as indicate whether the appropriate practitioner giving it is a doctor, dentist, supplementary prescriber, community practitioner nurse prescriber, nurse independent prescriber, optometrist independent prescriber, pharmacist independent prescriber, EEA or Swiss doctor or an EEA or Swiss dentist,

(iv) where the appropriate practitioner giving it is a doctor, dentist, supplementary prescriber, community practitioner nurse prescriber, nurse independent prescriber, optometrist independent prescriber, pharmacist independent prescriber, EEA or Swiss doctor or an EEA or Swiss dentist, the name, address and the age, if under 12, of the person for whose treatment it is given;

(d) shall not be dispensed after the end of the period of six months from the appropriate date, unless it is a repeatable prescription in which case it shall not be dispensed for the first time after the end of that period nor otherwise than in accordance with the direction contained in the repeatable prescription;

(e) in the case of a repeatable prescription that does not specify the number of times it may be dispensed, shall not be repeated on more than one occasion unless it is a prescription for oral contraceptives in which case it may be dispensed a total of six times (ie, five repeats) before the end of the period of six months from the appropriate date.

A private prescription must be retained for two years from the date on which the prescription only medicine was sold or supplied, or, for a repeat prescription, the date on which the medicine was supplied for the last time.

A prescription, other than a prescription for a Controlled Drug listed in Schedule 1,2 or 3 of the Misuse of Drugs Regulations 2001, may still be valid where it is created in an electronic form, is signed with an advanced electronic signature of the person prescribing it, and is sent to the person who is dispensing it as an electronic communication.

Advanced electronic signature means an electronic signature which is uniquely linked to the signatory, capable of identifying the signatory, created using means that the signatory can maintain under their sole control and which is linked to the data to which it relates in such a manner that any subsequent change of data is detectable. Signatory means the appropriate practitioner issuing the prescription.

When a prescription-only medicine is also a Controlled Drug listed in Schedule 2 or 3 of the Misuse of Drugs Regulations 2001, a prescription must also be written in accordance with the requirements of those Regulations. Note: repeat prescriptions are not permitted for Schedule 2 and 3 Controlled Drug prescriptions (*see* Section 1.2.14).

Validity of dental prescriptions

A dentist is an appropriate practitioner for the purpose of prescribing prescription-only medicines. A prescription written by a dentist is valid under the Medicines Act 1968 even where the item prescribed is not in the Dental Practitioners' Formulary. Under the terms of service, an FP10(D) prescription written by a dentist is valid only if the medicinal products ordered are in the Dental Practitioners' Formulary, but a private prescription can order any prescription-only (or pharmacy or general sale list) medicine. A pharmacy will be reimbursed for any drug that is on an FP10(SS) prescription form

unless that drug is not prescribable on the NHS. This is regardless of who has written it, eg, hospital doctor or hospital dentist. Dentists are required by their registration body to restrict their prescribing to areas in which they are competent, and this would therefore mean that a dentist should generally prescribe only medicines which have uses in dentistry.

Facsimile transmission of prescriptions

A "fax" of a prescription does not fall within the definition of a legally valid prescription (see above), because it is not written in indelible ink, and has not been signed by an appropriate practitioner. A fax can, however, confirm that at the time of receipt, a valid prescription is in existence.

Any pharmacist who decides to dispense a prescription-only medicine against a fax, without sight of the original prescription, must ensure that adequate safeguards exist to ensure that the integrity of the original prescription is maintained, and that the prescription will be in his possession within a short time. Any doubt as to the content of the original prescription, caused by poor reproduction, must be overcome before the medicine is supplied. As it is possible to fax a prescription many times, the pharmacist is advised to ensure that no dispensing against a fax takes place unless the system used for the sending or receipt of faxes is secure. Under no circumstances can medicines listed in Schedules 2 or 3 of the Misuse of Drugs Regulations 2001 be dispensed against a fax.

Forged prescriptions

It can be extremely difficult to detect a forged prescription, but every pharmacist should be alert to the possibility that any prescription calling for a product liable to misuse could be a forgery. In many instances, the forger may make a fundamental error in writing the prescription or the pharmacist may get an instinctive feeling that the prescription is not genuine because of the way the patient behaves.

If the prescriber's signature is known, but the patient has not previously visited the pharmacy, or is not known to be suffering from a condition which requires the medicinal product prescribed, the signature should be scrutinised and, if possible, checked against an example on another prescription known to be genuine. Large doses or quantities should be checked with the prescriber in order to detect alterations to previously valid prescriptions.

If the prescriber's signature is not known, the prescriber must be contacted and asked to confirm that the prescription is genuine. The prescriber's telephone number must be obtained from the telephone directory, or from directory enquiries, not from the headed notepaper, as forgers may use false letter headings.

A list of matters which should alert a pharmacist to making further checks is given below. This list is not exhaustive.

(1) Unknown prescriber.

(2) New patient.

(3) Excessive quantities.

(4) Uncharacteristic prescribing or method of writing prescription by a known doctor.

(5) Dr before or after prescriber's signature.

These precautions should be applied to all prescriptions for drugs liable to misuse and not only for Controlled Drugs. The dispensing of a forged prescription for a Controlled Drug or prescription-only medicine can constitute a criminal offence.

Exemptions to medicines legislation in the event of a pandemic

The Department of Health will announce when a pandemic situation is imminent or has arisen, at which time the following provisions will apply.

Emergency supply

In the event of a pandemic, or in anticipation of a disease being imminently pandemic which poses a serious or potentially serious risk to human health, the conditions for making an emergency supply at the request of a patient are relaxed in that the pharmacist will not need to interview the person who requests the medicine.

The pharmacist will still be required to satisfy himself/ herself that the treatment had been prescribed on a previous occasion by an appropriate practitioner and that the dose is appropriate for the person to be treated to take.

Currently, a dentist is not included as being an appropriate practitioner for this particular change to emergency supply legislation. In the event of a pandemic, or a disease being imminently pandemic, the legislation does not remove the requirement to interview the person requesting the medicine, if the patient was originally prescribed the medicine by a dentist. However, it is important to remember that in normal circumstances an emergency supply can be made at the request of a patient if the medicine was originally prescribed by a dentist. This is an anomaly in the legislation and the Medicines and Healthcare products Regulatory Agency (MHRA) does intend to amend the legislation so that this relaxation will also apply at the request of a patient previously prescribed a medicine by a dentist in the future. The MHRA and the Home Office are also considering whether an expanded range of Controlled Drugs should be available via the emergency supply provisions during a pandemic. Further guidance will be issued in the pharmaceutical press to inform pharmacists of any changes. Also *see* Emergency supplies of prescription-only medicines (pp15-16).

Supply of prescription-only medicines against a prescription

In the event, or in anticipation, of pandemic disease, the requirement whereby prescription-only medicines are only sold or supplied (in circumstances corresponding to retail sale) in accordance with a prescription given by an appropriate practitioner, will not apply.

This change will only apply when a disease is pandemic, or in anticipation of a disease being imminently pandemic, and a serious or potentially serious risk to human health. In such an event, supplies will be made from designated collection points in accordance with a specific protocol. In England, the Department of Health will announce when supplies under such a protocol can be made. In Scotland and Wales the relevant government departments will make the announcements.

The protocol must be approved by Ministers, an NHS body or the Health Protection Agency.

The protocol must contain criteria as to:
(i) symptoms of, and treatment for, that disease;
(ii) the recording of the name of the person who supplies the prescription only medicine to the person to be treated (or to a person acting on that person's behalf) and of the evidence that the medicine was supplied to the person to be treated (or to a person acting on that person's behalf).

Further guidance will be issued on protocols when more information is available.

Conditions under which the retail sale or supply of medicines can occur

In the event, or in anticipation, of a pandemic disease, the requirement for prescription-only medicines and pharmacy medicines to be sold or supplied from registered pharmacy premises, and the requirement that such transactions are made by or under the supervision of pharmacist, will not apply. This change will only apply while a disease is, or in anticipation of, a disease being imminently pandemic and a serious risk, or potentially serious risk, to human health and is in accordance with a specific protocol. The requirements for the protocol are the same as described above.

Labelling of certain children's medicines

The MHRA has temporarily authorised the distribution of unlicensed oseltamivir powder and an unlicensed oral liquid formulation of oseltamivir for administration to infants under one year of age in the prevention or treatment of influenza. The oral solution will be prepared in designated licensed NHS manufacturing units.

Linked to this authorisation, in the event of a disease being imminently pandemic or pandemic and a serious or potentially serious risk to human health, the labelling requirements for antiviral medicines in the form of a solution intended for the treatment of a child under the age of one year, will be simplified. Under such circumstances the container of the product only needs to be labelled with the following:
(i) the name of the person to whom the medicine is to be administered;
(ii) the date on which the medicine is dispensed; and
(iii) the necessary and usual instructions for proper use.

Written directions to supply (in hospitals)

The legislation allows a hospital to sell or supply a prescription-only medicine in the course of its business, against a patient specific "written direction" of a person (other than a veterinary surgeon or veterinary practitioner) who is an appropriate practitioner in relation to that medicine, instead of a prescription. The written direction does not need to comply with the requirements specified for prescriptions, but does need to relate to a specific patient. The intention is to permit the sale or supply of medicines against the patient's bed card or patient notes.

Most entries on a patient's bed card are directions to administer. However, providing the wording is clear, the entry can be taken as authority to make a supply, for example as take home medication. Providing the entry fulfils the requirements the details can be transposed onto an order form, to be used in pharmacy to prepare the take home medication. It is good practice for the transposition to be carried out by a pharmacist. By carrying out this transcription the pharmacist is not prescribing, as the original written direction to supply was made by a practitioner.

Patient group directions

The legislation also permits the supply of prescription-only medicines under a patient group direction (PGD).

A PGD is a written direction relating to supply and/or administration of a prescription-only medicine to persons generally (subject to specified exclusions), and is signed by a doctor or a dentist, and by a pharmacist.

The following is a list of the persons who are permitted under the Regulations to supply or administer under a PGD:

Registered paramedics or individuals who hold a certificate of proficiency in ambulance paramedic skills issued by, or with the approval of, the Secretary of State;

Pharmacists;

Registered dietitians;

Registered midwives;

Registered nurses;

Registered occupational therapists;

Registered optometrists;

Registered orthotists and prosthetists;

Registered speech and language therapists;

Registered chiropodists;

Registered orthoptists;

Registered physiotherapists;

Registered radiographers.

There are three main types of PGD. The first category allows authorised healthcare professionals to supply medicines on behalf of an NHS body. The second circumstance in which PGDs are permissible is to assist a doctor or dentist providing primary care NHS services. The third type is where an NHS body authorises a PGD for the supply and/or administration of a POM by a named person lawfully conducting a retail pharmacy business. In addition, supply and/or administration of POMs under a PGD can be made on behalf of an independent clinic/hospital or medical agency, a prison service, the armed forces or a police force. For the circumstances in which certain Controlled Drugs may be supplied or administered under a PGD, *see* p38.

The Royal Pharmaceutical Society has produced a fact sheet (*Patient Group Directions: A Resource Pack For Pharmacists*) containing comprehensive information to support pharmacists involved in any way with PGDs. The fact sheet can be downloaded as a PDF file from the Society's website (*www.rpsgb.org*), or copies can be obtained by sending a C4 stamped (72p) addressed envelope to the Legal and Ethical Advisory Service

Pharmacist prescribers

Pharmacist supplementary prescribers can, in accordance with the terms of a clinical management plan, prescribe prescription-only medicines, or if the product is for parenteral administration, either administer it or give directions for its administration. The clinical management plan must relate to the patient for whom the product is prescribed or is to be administered and the plan must be in effect at the time the prescription is given or the product is administered.

A clinical management plan must state the following:

(a) the name of the patient to whom the plan relates;

(b) the illnesses or conditions which may be treated by the supplementary prescriber;

(c) the date the plan takes effect and when it is to be reviewed by the doctor or dentist who is a party to the plan;

(d) reference to the class or description of medicinal product which can be prescribed or administered under the plan;

(e) any restrictions or limitations as to the strength or dose or period of use of any product which may be prescribed or administered under the plan;

(f) relevant warnings about known sensitivities or difficulties of the patient with particular medicinal products;

(g) arrangements for notifying suspected or known adverse reactions to any medicinal product prescribed or administered under the plan and to any medicinal product taken at the same time as a medicinal product prescribed or administered under the plan; and

(h) circumstances in which the supplementary prescriber should refer to, or seek the advice of the doctor or dentist who is a party to the plan.

Supplementary prescribers must have access to the same health records of the patient to whom the plan relates as the doctor or dentist who is party to the clinical management plan. For the circumstances in which Controlled Drugs may be prescribed by a supplementary prescriber, *see* p37.

For further information on supplementary prescribing by pharmacists, *see* p141.

Pharmacist independent prescribers can prescribe any medicine, with the exception of unlicensed medicines and Controlled Drugs (this may be subject to change in the near future), for any clinical condition but they must only prescribe within their professional and clinical competence.

Until changes are made to the Misuse of Drugs Regulations 2001, pharmacist independent prescribers will not be able to prescribe any controlled drugs. Pharmacists will be informed of any changes when these occur via the pharmaceutical press and further guidance will be issued as necessary.

Community practitioner nurse prescribers and nurse independent prescribers

Community practitioner nurse prescribers are able to prescribe medicines included in the nurse prescribers' formulary for community practitioners (refer to part XVIIB(i) of the Drug Tariff). Pharmacists should refer to the current Drug Tariff for the up to date list.

Nurse independent prescribers can prescribe any licensed medicine for any medical condition that the nurse prescriber is competent to treat. Nurse independent prescribers can only prescribe certain controlled drugs for certain indications (*see* p37).

Prescription records

Every person lawfully conducting a registered retail pharmacy business or a registered pharmacy within a hospital is required to keep a record in respect of every sale or supply of a prescription-only medicine, unless

(a) it is a sale or supply in pursuance of a "health prescription" or a prescription for an oral contraceptive; or

(b) a separate record of the sale or supply is made in the Controlled Drugs register; or

(c) the sale is by way of wholesale dealing and the order or invoice (or copies) relating to the sale is retained for two years.

As an alternative to a bound book, pharmacists may elect to keep their records electronically, but should note that all the particulars below must be recorded, adequate backups must be made and arrangements made so that the Society's Inspectors can examine the records during visits with minimal disruption to the dispensing process.

The particulars to be recorded in the case of a sale or supply of a prescription-only medicine in pursuance of a prescription are:

(a) the date on which the medicine was sold or supplied;
(b) the name, quantity and, except where it is apparent from the name, the pharmaceutical form and strength of the medicine sold or supplied;
(c) the date on the prescription;
(d) the name and address of the practitioner, supplementary prescriber, community practitioner nurse prescriber, nurse independent prescriber, optometrist independent prescriber, pharmacist independent prescriber or EEA or Swiss doctor or dentist giving the prescription;
(e) the name and address of the person for whom the medicine was prescribed.

For second and subsequent supplies made on a repeat prescription it is sufficient to record the date of supply and a reference to the entry in the record relating to the first supply.

The entry must be made on the day the sale or supply takes place or, if that is not reasonably practicable, on the next following day. The prescription-only record must be preserved by the owner of the retail pharmacy business for a period of two years from the date of the last entry in the register.

Even where exempt from the strict legal requirement to make an entry in the prescription-only medicine register (for example when a separate entry has been made in the Controlled Drugs register or for certain wholesale transactions), it is still good practice to keep such records. Hospital pharmacies need to keep such records only if the supply of the prescription-only medicine required registration as a pharmacy (no records are required under the Medicines Act for medicines supplied in the course of the business of the hospital). If any concerns arise, the Society's Legal and Ethical Advisory Service should be contacted for clarification.

Emergency supplies of prescription-only medicines

In an emergency a person lawfully conducting a retail pharmacy business can sell or supply a prescription-only medicine if and so long as certain conditions are satisfied. There are two kinds of emergency supply - those made at the request of a doctor, dentist, supplementary prescriber, community practitioner nurse prescriber, nurse independent prescriber, optometrist independent prescriber, pharmacist independent prescriber, EEA or Swiss doctor or an EEA or Swiss dentist and those made at the request of a patient. Different conditions apply to each type. Note: An emergency supply at the request of an EEA or Swiss doctor or EEA or Swiss dentist, or one of their patients, cannot lawfully be made for a Schedule 1, 2, 3, 4 or 5 Controlled Drug or for medicines that do not have a UK marketing authorisation.

Supply made at the request of a doctor, dentist, supplementary prescriber, community practitioner nurse prescriber, nurse independent prescriber, optometrist independent prescriber, pharmacist independent prescriber, EEA or Swiss doctor or an EEA or Swiss dentist

The conditions that apply are:
(a) that the pharmacist by or under whose supervision the prescription-only medicine is to be sold or supplied is satisfied that the sale or supply has been requested by a doctor, dentist, supplementary prescriber, community practitioner nurse prescriber, nurse independent prescriber, optometrist independent prescriber, pharmacist independent prescriber, EEA or Swiss doctor or an EEA or Swiss dentist who by reason of some emergency is unable to furnish a prescription immediately;

(b) that the doctor, dentist, supplementary prescriber, community practitioner nurse prescriber, nurse independent prescriber, optometrist independent prescriber, pharmacist independent prescriber, EEA or Swiss doctor or an EEA or Swiss dentist has undertaken to furnish the person lawfully conducting the retail pharmacy business with a prescription within 72 hours;
(c) that the prescription-only medicine in question is sold or supplied in accordance with the directions of the doctor, dentist, supplementary prescriber, community practitioner nurse prescriber, nurse independent prescriber, optometrist independent prescriber, pharmacist independent prescriber, EEA or Swiss doctor or an EEA or Swiss dentist requesting it;
(d) that the prescription-only medicine is not a Controlled Drug specified in Schedule 1, 2 or 3 to the Misuse of Drugs Regulations (an emergency sale or supply of phenobarbitone or phenobarbitone sodium is permitted, at the request of the doctor, dentist or supplementary prescriber, provided that it is for use in the treatment of epilepsy and does not contain any of the other substances in Schedules 1, 2, or 3 to the Misuse of Drugs Regulations 2001); where the request is made by an EEA or Swiss doctor or an EEA or Swiss dentist, the prescription-only medicine is not a Controlled Drug specified in Schedule 1,2,3,4 or 5 of the Misuse of Drugs Regulations 2001;
(e) that an entry is made in the prescription-only register on the day of the supply or, if impracticable, the next day following, stating:
(i) the date on which the medicine was sold or supplied,
(ii) the name, quantity and, except where it is apparent from the name, the pharmaceutical form and strength of the medicine,
(iii) the name and address of the practitioner, supplementary prescriber, community practitioner nurse prescriber, nurse independent prescriber, optometrist independent prescriber, pharmacist independent prescriber, EEA or Swiss doctor or an EEA or Swiss dentist requesting the emergency supply,
(iv) the name and address of the person for whom the prescription-only medicine was prescribed,
(v) the date on the prescription, and
(vi) when the prescription is received, the entry should be amended to include the date on which the prescription is received.

Supply made at the request of a patient

The conditions that apply to supplies made at the request of a patient are:
(a) that the pharmacist by or under whose supervision the prescription-only medicine is to be sold or supplied has interviewed the person requesting the medicine and has satisfied himself:
(i) that there is an immediate need for the prescription-only medicine requested to be sold or supplied and that it is impracticable in the circumstances to obtain a prescription without undue delay;
(ii) that treatment with the prescription-only medicine requested has on a previous occasion been prescribed by a doctor, dentist, supplementary prescriber, community practitioner nurse prescriber, nurse independent prescriber, optometrist independent prescriber, pharmacist independent prescriber, EEA or Swiss doctor or an EEA or Swiss dentist for the person requesting it, and;
(iii) as to the dose which in the circumstances it would be appropriate for that person to take;
(b) that no greater quantity of the prescription-only medicine in question than will provide five days' treatment in the case of a Controlled Drug (ie, phenobarbitone, phenobarbitone sodium or a Schedule 4 or 5 Controlled Drug) or 30 days for other prescription-only medicines, is sold or supplied, except that there may be sold or supplied where the medicine in question is:

(i) a preparation of insulin, an ointment, a cream or an aerosol for the relief of asthma, which has been made up for sale in a container elsewhere than at the place of sale or supply, the smallest pack that the pharmacist has available may be sold or supplied ("aerosol" means a product which is dispersed from its container by a propellant gas or liquid),

(ii) an oral contraceptive, a quantity sufficient for a full treatment cycle may be sold or supplied;

(iii) an antibiotic in liquid form for oral administration, the smallest quantity that will provide a full course of treatment may be sold or supplied;

(c) that the pharmacist by or under whose supervision the medicine is sold or supplied makes an entry in the prescription-only register on the day of the supply, or if impracticable, the next day following, stating:

(i) the date on which the prescription-only medicine was sold or supplied;

(ii) the name, quantity and, except where it is apparent from the name, the pharmaceutical form and strength of the medicine;

(iii) the name and address of the person requiring the prescription only medicine;

(iv) the nature of the emergency (ie, why the patient requires the prescription-only medicine, and the reason why a prescription cannot be obtained);

(d) that the container or package must be labelled to show:

(i) the date of supply;

(ii) the name, quantity and, where appropriate, the pharmaceutical form and strength;

(iii) the name of the person requesting the prescription only medicine;

(iv) the name and address of the pharmacy;

(v) the words "Emergency Supply;"

(vi) the words "Keep out of the reach of children" (or similar warning);

(e) that the prescription-only medicine is not a Controlled Drug specified in Schedule 1, 2 or 3 to the Misuse of Drugs Regulations (an emergency sale or supply of phenobarbitone or phenobarbitone sodium is permitted, at the request of the patient, provided that it is for use in the treatment of epilepsy and does not contain any of the other substances in Schedules 1, 2, or 3 to the Misuse of Drugs Regulations 2001) and does not consist of or contain a substance in the following list:

Ammonium bromide
Calcium bromide
Calcium bromidolactobionate
Embutramide
Fencamfamin hydrochloride
Fluanisone
Hexobarbitone
Hexobarbitone sodium
Hydrobromic acid
Meclofenoxate hydrochloride
Methohexitone sodium
Pemoline
Piracetam
Potassium bromide
Prolintane hydrochloride
Sodium bromide
Strychnine hydrochloride
Tacrine hydrochloride
Thiopentone sodium

Note: The patient of an EEA or Swiss doctor or EEA or Swiss dentist is not permitted to obtain Schedule 1-5 Controlled

Drugs or medicines that do not have a UK marketing authorisation as an emergency supply.

Changes in the event of a pandemic *See* p13 for changes to this legislation in the event of a pandemic.

1.2.4 Wholesale dealing

The Medicines Act 1968 requires most persons who engage in wholesale dealing to possess a licence. Persons lawfully conducting a retail pharmacy business may sell by wholesale provided the sale constitutes no more than an inconsiderable part of the business.

Although the term inconsiderable has not been the subject of judicial interpretation, it is likely that a pharmacy which wholesales no more than five per cent of its total medicines trade, will fall within this exemption. In any cases of doubt, the Medicines and Healthcare products Regulatory Agency (MHRA) should be consulted.

The wholesale of pharmacy or prescription-only medicines may only take place if the purchaser is authorised to sell or supply or to administer the medicines to human beings in the course of their business. Therefore a registered pharmacy can wholesale medicines to:

(a) practitioners (in other words, a doctor, dentist or veterinary practitioner entitled to practice in this country);

(b) any person lawfully conducting a retail pharmacy business (ie, another registered retail pharmacy);

(c) authorities or persons carrying on the business of:

(i) an independent hospital, independent clinic or independent medical agency, or

(ii) a hospital or health centre that is not an independent hospital or independent clinic

(d) any person who may sell by retail or supply in circumstances corresponding to retail sale by virtue of an exemption (see "Sales of medicines to exempted organisations, healthcare professionals or other persons" below) but only in respect of the medicinal products covered by the exemption;

(e) a Health and Social Services trust established under Article 10 of the Health and Personal Social Services (Northern Ireland) Order 1991;

(f) a National Health Service trust established under Section 5 of the National Health Service and Community Care Act 1990 or Section 12A of the National Health Service (Scotland) Act 1978 or a NHS foundation trust within the meaning of Section 1(1) of the Health and Social Care (Community Health and Standards) Act 2003;

(g) the Common Services Agency for the Scottish Health Service established under Section 10 of the National Health Service (Scotland) Act 1978;

(h) a Health Authority or Special Health Authority;

(i) a Primary Care Trust;

(j) a person other than an excepted person who carries on a business consisting (wholly or partly) of supplying medicinal products in circumstances corresponding to retail sale, or if administering such products, pursuant to an arrangement made with:

(i) the Common Services Agency, as referred to above;

(ii) a Health Authority or Special Health Authority;

(iii) a Health and Social Services trust, a National Health Service trust or an NHS foundation trust, as referred to above; or

(iv) a Primary Care Trust.

(k) A person, other than an excepted person who carries on a business consisting (wholly or partly) of the supply or administration of medicinal products for the purpose of assisting the provision of health care by or on behalf of, or under arrangements made by:

(i) a police force in England, Wales or Scotland

(ii) the Police Service of Northern Ireland

(iii) a prison service

(iv) Her Majesty's Forces

(l) Ministers of the Crown and Government departments and officers thereof.

Pharmacists must not wholesale medicines to holders of wholesale dealer's licences. The holder of a wholesale dealer's licence may only obtain supplies of medicines from either:

(i) a manufacturer's licence holder or a wholesale dealer's licence holder; or

(ii) a person authorised by another EEA State to manufacture or distribute medicines by way of wholesale dealing.

Therefore, this prevents a wholesaler dealer buying medicines, by way of wholesale, from a registered pharmacy.

Where a wholesale transaction occurs, only whole packs can be supplied and the pharmacy should not label the medicines.

Pharmacists will be aware that non-pharmacy outlets cannot sell pharmacy medicines. Pharmacists should therefore be alert to any requests for multiple packs of pharmacy medicines which could be being purchased for onward sale.

Records of wholesale supplies of prescription-only medicines

An entry must be made in the prescription-only register when a registered pharmacy makes a wholesale supply of a prescription-only medicine (unless the pharmacist maintains a copy of the order or invoice – see below). This record may be written or alternatively recorded electronically. The details that must be recorded include:

(a) the date on which the prescription-only medicine was sold or supplied;

(b) the name, quantity and, except where it is apparent from the name, the pharmaceutical form and strength of the medicine sold or supplied;

(c) the name and address, trade, business or profession of the person to whom the medicine is sold or supplied;

(d) the purpose for which it is sold or supplied.

If a copy of the order or invoice requesting the supply is retained by the owner of the retail pharmacy business there is no legal requirement for an entry to be made in the prescription-only register when the supply is made by way of wholesale dealing or where a separate record of the sale or supply is made in accordance with the Misuse of Drugs Regulations 2001.

It is good practice to record the wholesale supply in the prescription-only register and to maintain a copy of the order or invoice requesting the supply. By doing this the pharmacist will readily be able to account for all stocks which have left the pharmacy, without the dangers associated with the loss of the copy of an invoice or order.

All orders or invoices must be kept for two years from the date of the sale or supply.

1.2.5 Sales of medicines to exempted organisations, healthcare professionals or other persons

Legislation restricts the retail sale, supply and administration of medicines (general sale list, pharmacy and prescription-only medicines) *see* pp7-14. There are certain exemptions from these restrictions. This means that particular people and organisations are exempt from the conditions (eg, the need to have a valid prescription) in specific circumstances. This section of *Medicines, Ethics and Practice* will list the people and organisations that are exempt from the controls that apply and what conditions (if any) there are on that person or organisation when they sell, supply or administer those medicines to an individual.

In order to sell, supply or administer these medicines the people and/or organisations must first be able to obtain them. These medicines can be obtained from a registered pharmacy. When a registered pharmacy supplies these medicines to the individual or organisation this is a wholesale transaction (*see* Section 1.2.4). Pharmacists must keep a record in the prescription-only register of the wholesale supply of any prescription-only medicines, or keep a copy of the order for prescription-only medicines provided by the individual or organisation requesting the medicines for two years. It is good practice to make a record in the prescription-only register and keep the order for two years. Pharmacists can only supply original and complete packs when making a wholesale supply and must not label the product in any way.

In the case of Controlled Drugs additional restrictions will apply. Any pharmacist who is asked for advice, or who wishes to check on the legality of wholesaling medicines to such persons or organisations should contact the Society's Legal and Ethical Advisory Service for advice.

Hospitals and health centres

The restrictions on sale or supply of prescription-only medicines do not apply to the sale or supply of any such medicine in the course of the business of a hospital where the medicine is sold or supplied for the purpose of being administered (whether in the hospital or elsewhere) to a particular person in accordance with the written directions of a person (other than a veterinary surgeon or veterinary practitioner) who is an appropriate practitioner in relation to that medicine.

The restrictions on the sale, offer for sale, or supply of any other medicinal product (not being a prescription-only medicine) do not apply when the sale, offer for sale, or supply is in the course of the business of a hospital, or health centre for the purpose of being administered (whether in the hospital or health centre or elsewhere) to a particular person in accordance with the written directions of a nurse prescriber, pharmacist independent prescriber or supplementary prescriber.

The written directions need not satisfy the requirements for a prescription given in the POM Order but must relate to the particular person to whom the medicine is to be administered (*see* p13).

The restrictions on sale or supply of prescription-only medicines, pharmacy medicines and general sale list medicines do not apply when the sale, offer for sale, or supply is in the course of the business of a hospital, or health centre for the purpose of being administered (whether in the hospital or health centre or elsewhere) in accordance with the directions of a doctor or dentist (*see* Administration of prescription-only medicines in hospital, p11).

Practitioners

The restrictions on sale or supply of prescription-only medicines, pharmacy medicines and general sale list medicines do not apply to the sale, offer for sale or supply of any such medicinal product by a doctor or dentist to a patient of his, or to a person under whose care such a patient is.

Midwives

The wholesale of medicines to a midwife from a registered pharmacy for the midwife to SELL OR SUPPLY to their patients

Registered midwives can sell or supply the following medicines. Therefore, they can obtain these medicines by wholesale from a registered pharmacy:
(a) all general sale list medicines;
(b) all pharmacy medicines;
(c) prescription-only medicines containing any of the following substances:
    Chloral hydrate
    Ergometrine maleate (only when contained in a medicinal product which is not for parenteral administration)
    Pentazocine hydrochloride
    Phytomenadione
    Triclofos sodium

A midwife can only sell or supply these medicinal products, under certain conditions. These conditions are:
(i) the sale or supply shall be only in the course of their professional practice;
(ii) in the case of ergometrine maleate they can only sell or supply a medicinal product that is not for parenteral administration.

A supply made by a registered pharmacy to a midwife under this exemption is a wholesale transaction. For the requirements concerned with wholesale transactions *see* Section 1.2.4.

The wholesale of medicines to a midwife from a registered pharmacy for the midwife to ADMINISTER to their patients

Registered midwives can administer the following parenteral medicines. Therefore, they can obtain these medicines by wholesale from a registered pharmacy:
    Diamorphine
    Ergometrine maleate
    Lignocaine (lidocaine)
    Lignocaine hydrochloride (lidocaine hydrochloride)
    Morphine
    Naloxone hydrochloride
    Oxytocins (natural and synthetic)
    Pentazocine lactate
    Pethidine hydrochloride
    Phytomenadione
    Promazine hydrochloride

A midwife can only administer the above parenteral medicines under certain conditions. These conditions are:
(i) the administration is in the course of their professional practice.
(ii) in the case of promazine hydrochloride, lignocaine and lignocaine hydrochloride it shall only be administered while attending on a woman in childbirth.

A supply made by a registered pharmacy to a midwife under this exemption is a wholesale transaction. For the requirements concerned with wholesale transactions *see*

Section 1.2.4. Any pharmacist who is asked for advice or wishes to check on the legality of supplying any of the Controlled Drugs listed above, ie, diamorphine, morphine, pethidine or pentazocine to a midwife should contact the Society's Legal and Ethical Advisory Service for advice.

Chiropodists

The wholesale of medicines to a chiropodist from a registered pharmacy for the chiropodist to SELL OR SUPPLY to their patients

Registered chiropodists can obtain these medicines by wholesale from a registered pharmacy:
(a) General sale list medicines which are for external use;
(b) Any of the following pharmacy medicines for external use:
(i) potassium permanganate crystals or solution;
(ii) ointment of heparinoid and hyaluronidase; and
(iii) products containing as their only active ingredients, any of the following substances, not exceeding the strength specified in each case:
    Borotannic complex 9.0%
    Buclosamide 10.0%
    Chlorquinaldol 3.0%
    Clotrimazole 1.0%
    Crotamiton 10.0%
    Diamthazole hydrochloride 5.0%
    Econazole nitrate 1.0%
    Fenticlor 1.0%
    Glutaraldehyde 10.0%
    Griseofulvin 1.0%
    Hydrargaphen 0.4%
    Mepyramine maleate 2.0%
    Miconazole nitrate 2.0%
    Phenoxypropan-2-ol 2.0%
    Podophyllum resin 20.0%
    Polynoxylin 10.0%
    Pyrogallol 70.0%
    Salicylic acid 70.0%
    Terbinafine 1.0%
    Thiomersal 0.1%

The registered chiropodist can only sell or supply these medicinal products, under certain conditions. These conditions are:
(i) the sale or supply shall be only in the course of their professional practice;
(ii) the medicinal product has been made up for sale and supply in a container elsewhere than at the place at which it is sold or supplied.

Registered chiropodists who have the relevant annotation in the Health Professions Council register signifying that they are qualified to use the medicines specified below, can obtain these medicines by wholesale from a registered pharmacy:
(a) Any of the following prescription-only medicines:
(i) Co-dydramol 10/500 tablets;
(ii) Amorolfine hydrochloride cream where the maximum strength of the amorolfine in the cream does not exceed 0.25 per cent by weight in weight;
(iii) Amorolfine hydrochloride lacquer where the maximum strength of the amorolfine in the lacquer does not exceed 5 per cent by weight in volume;
(iv) Topical hydrocortisone where the maximum strength of the hydrocortisone in the medicinal product does not exceed 1 per cent by weight in weight;

(v) Amoxicillin;

(vi) Erythromycin;

(vii) Flucoxacillin;

(viii) Tioconazole 28%;

(ix) Silver sulfadiazine;

(b) Preparations which are not prescription-only medicines:

(i) Ibuprofen.

The chiropodist can only sell or supply these medicinal products under certain conditions. These conditions are:

(i) the sale or supply shall be only in the course of their professional practice;

(ii) the medicinal product has been made up for sale and supply in a container elsewhere than at the place at which it is sold or supplied;

(iii) in the case of co-dydramol 10/500 tablets the quantity sold or supplied to a person at any one time shall not exceed the amount sufficient for 3 days' treatment to a maximum of 24 tablets; and

(iv) in the case of ibuprofen the maximum dose is 400mg, the maximum daily dose is 1,200mg and the maximum pack size is 3,600mg for 3 days treatment.

A supply made by a registered pharmacy to a registered chiropodist under this exemption is a wholesale transaction. For the requirements concerned with wholesale transactions *see* Section 1.2.4.

Pharmacists can only supply original and complete packs to chiropodists as this is a wholesale transaction. Pharmacists should therefore consider which pack size they wholesale to chiropodists especially in the case of co-dydramol and ibuprofen as chiropodists are limited to the quantity they can supply to their patients and are unable to alter the pack size once it has been supplied to them from the pharmacy.

The wholesale of medicines to a chiropodist from a registered pharmacy for the chiropodist to ADMINISTER to their patients

Registered chiropodists, who have the relevant annotation in the Health Professions Council register signifying that they are qualified to use the medicines specified below, can obtain these medicines by wholesale from a registered pharmacy:

Adrenaline

Bupivacaine hydrochloride

Bupivacaine hydrochloride with adrenaline where the maximum strength of the adrenaline does not exceed 1mg in 200ml of bupivacaine hydrochloride

Levobupivacaine hydrochloride

Lignocaine (Lidocaine) hydrochloride

Lignocaine (Lidocaine) hydrochloride with adrenaline where the maximum strength of the adrenaline does not exceed 1mg in 200ml of lignocaine (lidocaine) hydrochloride

Mepivacaine hydrochloride

Methylprednisolone

Prilocaine hydrochloride

Ropivacaine hydrochloride

A chiropodist can only administer the above parenteral prescription only medicines if the administration is in the course of their professional practice.

A supply made by a registered pharmacy to a registered chiropodist under this exemption is a wholesale transaction. For the requirements concerned with wholesale transactions *see* Section 1.2.4.

Optometrists

The wholesale of medicines to a registered optometrist from a registered pharmacy for the optometrist to SELL OR SUPPLY to their patients

Registered optometrists can sell or supply the following medicines. Therefore, they can obtain these medicines by wholesale from a registered pharmacy:

(a) all general sale list medicines;

(b) all pharmacy medicines.

(c) Certain prescription-only medicines which are not for parenteral administration. These medicines include:

Eye drops or eye ointments that are prescription-only medicines by reason only that they contain:

(i) mafenide propionate, or

(ii) not more that 30% sulphacetamide sodium, or

(iii) sulphafurazole diethanolamine equivalent to not more than 4% sulphafurazole, or

Eye drops that are prescription-only medicines by reason only that they contain no more than 0.5% chloramphenicol.

Eye ointments that are prescription-only medicines by reason only that they contain no more than 1% chloramphenicol.

Prescription-only medicines because they contain any of the following substances:

Cyclopentolate hydrochloride

Fusidic acid

Tropicamide

A registered optometrist can only sell or supply these medicinal products, under certain conditions. These conditions are:

(i) In the case of general sale list medicines and pharmacy medicines the sale or supply must be in the course of their professional practice.

(ii) In the case of prescription-only medicines the sale or supply must be in the course of their professional practice and in an emergency.

A supply made by a registered pharmacy to a registered optometrist under this exemption is a wholesale transaction. For the requirements concerned with wholesale transactions *see* Section 1.2.4.

The sale or supply of the above prescription only medicines requires the pharmacist to be presented with an order signed by the registered optometrist. The signed order allows the pharmacist to make a supply directly to a patient under the care of an optometrist. It is not, however, a prescription, as a prescription is an authority to supply prescription-only medicines issued by an appropriate practitioner, and an optometrist does not come under this definition.

In making such a supply, pharmacists must ensure that they comply with the professional requirements of the Code of Ethics, in that the product supplied must be labelled accordingly, a patient information leaflet must be provided and the sale or supply must be recorded in the prescription-only register. The pharmacist must also be satisfied that the optometrist has provided sufficient information and advice to enable safe and effective use of the medicine and has made a follow-up appointment where necessary.

The wholesale of medicines to a registered optometrist from a registered pharmacy for the optometrist to ADMINISTER to their patients

Registered optometrists can also obtain the following medicines by wholesale from a registered pharmacy:

Amethocaine hydrochloride
Lignocaine (Lidocaine) hydrochloride
Oxybuprocaine hydrochloride
Proxymetacaine hydrochloride

A supply made by a registered pharmacy to a registered optometrist under this exemption is a wholesale transaction. For the requirements concerned with wholesale transactions see Section 1.2.4.

Additional supply optometrists

The wholesale of medicines to a registered additional supply optometrist from a registered pharmacy for the additional supply optometrist to SELL OR SUPPLY to their patients

Registered additional supply optometrists can sell or supply the following medicines so long as they are not for parenteral administration. Therefore, they can obtain these medicines by wholesale from a registered pharmacy:

(i) Acetylcysteine
(ii) Atropine sulphate
(iii) Azelastine hydrochloride
(iv) Diclofenac sodium
(v) Emedastine
(vi) Homotropine hydrobromide
(vii) Ketotifen
(viii) Levocabastine
(ix) Lodoxamide
(x) Nedocromil sodium
(xi) Olopatadine
(xii) Pilocarpine hydrochloride
(xiii) Pilocarpine nitrate
(xiv) Polymyxin B/ bacitracin
(xv) Polymixin B/ trimethoprim
(xvi) Sodium cromoglycate

A registered additional supply optometrist can only sell or supply these medicinal products, under certain conditions. The condition is that:

(i) In the case of prescription only medicines the sale or supply must be in the course of their professional practice and in an emergency.

A pharmacist may supply the prescription only medicines (listed above [i] to [xvi]) directly to a patient under the care of a registered additional supply optometrist on presentation of a signed order issued by the additional supply optometrist. The signed order is not, however, a prescription, as a prescription is an authority to supply prescription-only medicines issued by an appropriate practitioner, and an additional supply optometrist does not come under this definition.

In making such a supply, pharmacists must ensure that they comply with the professional requirements of the Code of Ethics, in that the product supplied must be labelled accordingly, a patient information leaflet must be provided and the sale or supply must be recorded in the prescription-only register. The pharmacist must also be satisfied that the additional supply optometrist has provided sufficient information and advice to enable safe and effective use of the medicine and has made a follow-up appointment where necessary.

Registered additional supply optometrists can also obtain the following medicines by wholesale from a registered pharmacy:

(i) Thymoxamine hydrochloride

A supply made by a registered pharmacy to a registered additional supply optometrist under this exemption is a wholesale transaction. For the requirements concerned with wholesale transactions see Section 1.2.4.

Drug treatment services

The wholesale of medicines to persons employed or engaged in the provision of lawful drug treatment services from a registered pharmacy for the drug treatment service to SUPPLY (BUT NOT SELL) to their patients

A person employed or engaged in the provision of lawful drug treatment service may supply the following medicinal product. Therefore, they can obtain this medicinal product by wholesale from a registered pharmacy:

Ampoules of sterile water for injection containing not more than 2 ml of sterile water.

A person employed or engaged in the provision of lawful drug treatment service can only supply these medicinal products, under certain conditions. The condition is that:

(i) The supply shall be only in the course of provision of lawful drug treatment services.

A supply made by a registered pharmacy to a person employed or engaged in the provision of a lawful drug treatment service under this exemption is a wholesale transaction. For the requirements concerned with wholesale transactions see Section 1.2.4.

Shipping personnel

The wholesale of medicines to the owner or the master of a ship (including masters of foreign ships) which does not carry a doctor on board from a registered pharmacy for the SUPPLY (BUT NOT SALE) to persons on the ship.

The owner or master of a ship (which does not carry a doctor on board) may supply the following medicines. Therefore, they can obtain these medicines by wholesale from a registered pharmacy:

(a) all general sale list medicines;
(b) all pharmacy medicines;
(c) all prescription-only medicines (including Controlled Drugs (see p31).

The owner or master of a ship (which does not carry a doctor on board) can only supply these medicinal products, under certain conditions. The condition is that:

(i) The supply is necessary for the treatment of persons on the ship.

A supply made by a registered pharmacy to a owner or master of a ship under this exemption is a wholesale transaction. For the requirements concerned with wholesale transactions see Section 1.2.4.

The wholesale of medicines to the owner or the master of a ship which does not carry a doctor on board from a registered pharmacy for the ADMINISTRATION to persons on the ship

The owner or master of a ship (which does not carry a doctor on board) may administer the following medicines. Therefore, they can obtain these medicines by wholesale from a registered pharmacy:

(a) All prescription only medicines that are for parenteral administration.

The owner or master of a ship (which does not carry a doctor on board) can only administer these medicinal products, under certain conditions. The condition is that:

(i) That the supply is necessary for the treatment of persons on the ship.

A supply made by a registered pharmacy to a owner or master of a ship under this exemption is a wholesale transaction. For the requirements concerned with wholesale transactions *see* Section 1.2.4. Pharmacists who receive a request for a supply of medicines from the owner of master of a ship would then need to establish the identity of the owner or master of the ship and ensure that the request is genuine. The company owning the ship could be contacted for confirmation or the Lloyds Register of Shipping could be checked. The pharmacist should also check that the prescription only medicines which have been requested are appropriate for the category of ship by contacting the Maritime and Coastguard Agency (MCA) on 0870 600 6505.

Royal National Lifeboat Institution

The wholesale of medicines to the Royal National Lifeboat Institution and certified first aiders of the Institution from a registered pharmacy for the SUPPLY (BUT NOT SALE) to sick and injured persons.

The Royal National Lifeboat Institution and certified first aiders of the Institution may supply the following medicines. Therefore, they can obtain these medicines by wholesale from a registered pharmacy:

(a) all general sale list medicines;
(b) all pharmacy medicines;
(c) all prescription-only medicines.

The Royal National Lifeboat Institution and certified first aiders of the Institution can only supply these medicinal products, under certain conditions. These conditions are:

(i) In the case of general sale list medicines and pharmacy medicines the supply is necessary for the treatment of sick and injured persons.

(ii) In the case of prescription-only medicines the supply is necessary for the treatment of sick or injured persons in the exercise of the functions of the Institution.

A supply made by a registered pharmacy to Royal National Lifeboat Institution and certified first aiders of the Institution under this exemption is a wholesale transaction. For the requirements concerned with wholesale transactions *see* Section 1.2.4.

First aid organisations

The wholesale of medicines to the British Red Cross Society, St John Ambulance Association and Brigade, St Andrew's Ambulance Association and the Order of Malta Ambulance Corps from a registered pharmacy for the SUPPLY (BUT NOT SALE) to sick and injured persons

The British Red Cross Society, St John Ambulance Association and Brigade, St Andrew's Ambulance Association and the Order of Malta Ambulance Corps may supply the following medicines. Therefore, they can obtain these medicines by wholesale from a registered pharmacy:

(a) all general sale list medicines;
(b) all pharmacy medicines;

The British Red Cross Society, St John Ambulance Association and Brigade, St Andrew's Ambulance Association and the Order of Malta Ambulance Corps can only supply these medicinal products, under certain conditions. These condition is that:

(i) The supply is necessary for the treatment of sick and injured persons.

A supply made by a registered pharmacy to these first aid organisations under this exemption is a wholesale transaction. For the requirements concerned with wholesale transactions *see* Section 1.2.4.

Occupational health schemes (OHSs)

The wholesale of medicines from a registered pharmacy to a person operating an OHS for the SUPPLY (BUT NOT SALE) in the course of the OHS

The person operating an OHS may supply the following medicines. Therefore, they can obtain these medicines by wholesale from a registered pharmacy:

(a) all general sale list medicines;
(b) all pharmacy medicines;
(c) all prescription-only medicines.

The person operating an OHS can only supply these medicinal products, under certain conditions. These conditions are:

(i) That the supply shall be in the course of the OHS;

(ii) That the individual supplying the prescription-only medicine, if not a doctor, shall be a registered nurse acting in accordance with the written instructions of a doctor as to the circumstances in which prescription-only medicines of the description in question are to be used in the course of the OHS.

In the case of prescription-only medicines the pharmacist must have an order in writing signed by a registered doctor or a registered nurse.

A supply made by a registered pharmacy to an OHS under this exemption is a wholesale transaction. For the requirements concerned with wholesale transactions *see* Section 1.2.4.

The wholesale of medicines from a registered pharmacy to a person operating an OHS for the ADMINISTRATION in the course of the OHS

The person operating an OHS may administer the following medicines. Therefore, they can obtain these medicines by wholesale from a registered pharmacy:

(a) All prescription-only medicines that are for parenteral administration.

The person operating an OHS can only administer these parenteral medicinal products, under certain conditions. These conditions are:

(i) That the administration is in the course of the occupational health scheme;

(ii) That the individual administering the prescription-only medicine, if neither a doctor nor acting in accordance with the directions of a doctor, is a registered nurse acting in accordance with the written instructions of a doctor as to the circumstances in which prescription-only medicines of the description in question are to be used in the course of the OHS.

The pharmacist must have an order in writing signed by a registered doctor or a registered nurse.

A supply made by a registered pharmacy to an OHS under this exemption is a wholesale transaction. For the requirements concerned with wholesale transactions *see* Section 1.2.4.

Offshore installations - First aid personnel

The wholesale of medicines to the person employed as the qualified first-aider on offshore installations for the SUPPLY (BUT NOT SALE) to persons on the installation

The person employed as the qualified first-aider on offshore installations may supply the following medicines. Therefore, they can obtain these medicines by wholesale from a registered pharmacy:

(a) all general sale list medicines;

(b) all pharmacy medicines;

(c) all prescription-only medicines.

The person employed as the qualified first-aider on off-shore installations can only supply these medicinal products, under certain conditions. The condition is that:

(i) The supply shall be only so far as is necessary for the treatment of persons on the installation.

A supply made by a registered pharmacy to a person employed as the qualified first-aider on offshore installations under this exemption is a wholesale transaction. For the requirements concerned with wholesale transactions *see* Section 1.2.4.

The wholesale of medicines to the person employed as the qualified first-aider on offshore installations for the ADMINISTRATION to persons on the installation

The person employed as the qualified first-aider on off-shore installations may administer the following medicines. Therefore, they can obtain these medicines by wholesale from a registered pharmacy:

(a) all prescription-only medicines that are for parenteral administration.

The person employed as the qualified first-aider on off-shore installations can only administer these medicinal products, under certain conditions. The condition is that:

(i) The administration shall be only so far as is necessary for the treatment of persons on the installation.

A supply made by a registered pharmacy to a person employed as the qualified first-aider on offshore installations under this exemption is a wholesale transaction. For the requirements concerned with wholesale transactions *see* Section 1.2.4.

Paramedics

The wholesale of medicines to persons who hold a certificate of proficiency in ambulance paramedic skills issued by, or with the approval of, the Secretary of State or persons who are registered paramedics to be ADMINISTERED to sick or injured persons

A registered paramedic may administer the following parenteral medicines. Therefore, they can obtain these parenteral medicines by wholesale from a registered pharmacy:

(a) diazepam;

(b) succinylated modified fluid gelatin 4 per cent intravenous infusion;

(c) medicines containing the substances ergometrine maleate 500mcg per ml with oxytocin 5iu per ml, but no other active ingredient;

(d) prescription-only medicines for parenteral administration containing one or more of the following substances but no other active ingredients:

Adrenaline acid tartrate
Amiodarone
Anhydrous glucose
Benzylpenicillin
Bretylium tosylate
Compound sodium lactate intravenous infusion (Hartmann's solution)
Ergometrine maleate
Frusemide
Glucose
Heparin sodium
Lignocaine (Lidocaine) hydrochloride
Metoclopramide
Morphine sulphate (injection to a maximum strength of 20mg)
Morphine sulphate (oral)
Nalbuphine hydrochloride
Naloxone hydrochloride
Polygeline
Reteplase
Sodium bicarbonate
Sodium chloride
Streptokinase
Tenecteplase

The registered paramedic can only administer these medicinal products, under certain conditions. These conditions are:

(i) That the administration shall be only for the immediate, necessary treatment of sick or injured persons;

(ii) In the case of a prescription-only medicine containing heparin sodium shall be only for the purpose of cannula flushing.

This applies to both NHS paramedics and privately employed (including self-employed) paramedics.

A supply made by a registered pharmacy to a registered paramedic under this exemption is a wholesale transaction. For the requirements concerned with wholesale transactions *see* Section 1.2.4.

Any pharmacist who is asked for advice or wishes to check on the legality of supplying any of the Controlled Drugs listed above, ie, diazepam or morphine sulphate to a registered paramedic should contact the Society's Legal and Ethical Advisory Service for advice.

Other exempted persons and organisations

The following persons or organisations have exemptions from restrictions of the retail sale and/or supply of certain medicinal products in relation to certain specified purposes:

Dental schemes
The operator or commander of an aircraft
Unorthodox practitioners
Marketing authorisation holders and holders of manufacturers' licences
Group authorities and licences
Persons selling or supplying to universities, institutions concerned with higher education or institutions concerned with research
Persons selling or supplying to public analysts / sampling officers / NHS drug testing / British Standards Institution
Prison officers
Health authorities or primary care trusts

Persons holding a certificate in first aid from the Mountain Rescue Council of England and Wales, or from the Northern Ireland Mountain Rescue Co-ordinating Committee
Persons carrying on the business of a school providing full-time education

A pharmacist who is approached to make a sale or supply to any of the above can check with the Society's Legal and Ethical Advisory Service if any doubts exist as to the extent of the purchasers' authority.

1.2.6 Labelling of medicinal products

This section outlines what must appear on the container of relevant medicinal products that are general sale list medicines, pharmacy medicines and prescription only medicines.

This section also details the information that must appear of the dispensing label when relevant medicinal products are dispensed.

The legislation that underpins the labelling of medicines is the Medicines for Human Use (Marketing Authorisations Etc.) Regulations 1994, the Medicines (Labelling) Regulations 1976 and European Directives. Those medicinal products that are controlled drugs must also be labelled in accordance with the Misuse of Drugs Regulations 2001.

For a definition of "relevant medicinal product" *see* p6. Effectively this refers to a licensed medicinal product.

Changes in the event of a pandemic *See* p13 for changes to this legislation in the event of a pandemic.

1.2.6.1 Labelling of dispensed relevant medicinal products

A dispensed relevant medicinal product, so far as a pharmacist is concerned, is defined as a relevant medicinal product prepared or dispensed in accordance with a prescription given by a practitioner.

The following must appear on the label when relevant medicinal products are dispensed:
(a) the name of the person to whom the medicine is to be administered;
(b) the name and address of the person who sells or supplies the medicinal product;
(c) the date on which dispensed;
(d) where the medicinal product has been prescribed by a practitioner the following particulars as s/he may request;
(i) the name of the product or its common name,
(ii) directions for use, and
(iii) precautions relating to the use of the product.
If the professional opinion of the pharmacist is that any of those particulars (d (i), (ii), (iii)) are inappropriate and having taken necessary steps to consult with the practitioner, s/he is unable to do so, s/he may substitute other particulars of the same kind;
(e) the words "Keep out of the reach of children" or words of direction bearing a similar meaning.

NB: The Society would strongly advise that pharmacists place the phrase "Keep out of the reach and sight of children" on dispensing labels as good practice, to be in line with the requirements of manufacturers. This is a good practice requirement and not mandatory.

Where the container of a dispensed medicinal product is enclosed in a package immediately enclosing that container, the particulars required under (a), (b), (c) and (d) may be omitted from the label on the container if they appear on the label on the package.

Where several containers of medicinal products of the same description are supplied in a package, the particulars required under (d) need only appear on the label on the package containing all the products, or may appear on only one of the label of the individual containers or packages. All the remaining containers must, however, be labelled with all the other particulars.

Other information may be added if the pharmacist considers it to be necessary. For other/additional labelling requirements *see* pp23-26.

1.2.6.2 Labelling of dispensed non-relevant medicinal products

A non-relevant medicinal product is essentially an unlicensed medicine, for example a medicine extemporaneously prepared by a pharmacist under Section 10 of the Medicines Act 1968 against a prescription.

The requirements for the dispensing label for non-relevant medicinal products are the same as the requirements for the dispensing label of a relevant medicinal product (*see* Section 1.2.6.1). The only exemption to this is when a pharmacist extemporaneously prepares a product in accordance with a specification furnished by the person to whom the product will be sold or supplied, under Section 10(3)(a) of the Medicines Act 1968. In this case the "directions for use" may be omitted from the dispensing label.

1.2.6.3 Labelling of assembled (prepacked) medicines

Some pharmacists assemble medicines by breaking down bulk containers into quantities more appropriate for use against prescriptions. This, technically, falls within the definition of assembly, and all medicines should be properly labelled. Medicines repackaged in this way can only be sold or supplied from that pharmacy or from another pharmacy under the same ownership. Prepacking at the request of medical practitioners or for a separate legal entity is not permitted without an assembly licence.

The particulars which are required are:
(a) the name of the medicinal product;
(b) the appropriate quantitative particulars of the medicinal product (the ingredients);
(c) the quantity of the medicinal product in the container;
(d) any special requirements for the handling and storage of the medicinal product;
(e) the expiry date;
(f) the batch reference, preceded by the letters "BN" or "LOT" or other letters indicating a batch reference.

All medicines assembled in such a way must be relabelled before being supplied to a patient as a dispensed medicinal product.

1.2.6.4 Labelling of chemists' nostrums

The following requirements apply to medicinal products which are prepared in a registered pharmacy for retail sale from that pharmacy and which are not advertised (such products are familiarly known as "chemists' nostrums"). The preparation and the sale or supply must be carried out by or under the supervision of a pharmacist.

The label of the container of such a medicinal product and any package immediately enclosing it must show the following standard labelling particulars:

(a) name of the product;
(b) pharmaceutical form;
(c) appropriate quantitative particulars;
(d) quantity;
(e) directions for use;
(f) handling and storage requirements (if any);
(g) expiry date;
(h) the words "Keep out of the reach of children" or words of a similar meaning;
(i) where appropriate, the words "Warning. Do not exceed the stated dose," in a rectangle in which there is no other matter (this would be necessary where one or more of the ingredients are prescription-only medicines, incorporated in such a way as to exempt it from prescription-only control);
(j) the name and address of the seller;
(k) the letter P in a rectangle.

1.2.6.5 Manufacturers' labelling requirements for relevant medicinal products

The regulations covering labelling and patient information leaflets are set out in Title V of Council Directive 2001/83/EC which was amended by Council Directive 2004/27/EC. The information below is from the updated regulation as amended by Council Directive 2004/27/EC. However, pharmacists should note that although the amendments made by Council Directive 2004/27/EC have been implemented into UK legislation and affect all new applications submitted to the MHRA from 30 October 2005, existing marketing authorisations have until 30 October 2010 to comply.

The following particulars must appear on the outer packaging of medicinal products or, where there is no outer packaging, on the immediate packaging.

(a) the name of the medicinal product followed by its strength and pharmaceutical form, and, if appropriate, whether it is intended for babies, children or adults; where the product contains up to three active substances, the international non-proprietary name (INN) shall be included, or, if one does not exist, the common name;
(b) a statement of the active substances expressed qualitatively and quantitatively per dosage unit or according to the form of administration for a given volume or weight, using their common names;
(c) the pharmaceutical form and the contents by weight, by volume or by number of doses of the product;
(d) a list of those excipients known to have a recognized action or effect and included in the detailed guidance published pursuant to Article 65. However, if the product is injectable, or a topical or eye preparation, all excipients must be stated;
(e) the method of administration and, if necessary, the route of administration. Space shall be provided for the prescribed dose to be indicated;
(f) a special warning that the medicinal product must be stored out of the reach and sight of children;
(g) a special warning, if this is necessary for the medicinal product;
(h) the expiry date in clear terms (month/year);

(i) special storage precautions, if any;
(j) specific precautions relating to the disposal of unused medicinal products or waste derived from medicinal products, where appropriate, as well as reference to any appropriate collection system in place;
(k) the name and address of the marketing authorisation holder and, where applicable, the name of the representative appointed by the holder to represent him;
(l) the number of the authorisation for placing the medicinal product on the market;
(m) the manufacturer's batch number;
(n) in the case of non-prescription medicinal products, instructions for use.

All labelling of containers and packages of relevant medicinal products shall be:
(i) legible;
(ii) indelible;
(iii) clearly comprehensible; and
(iv) either in the English language only or in English and in one or more other languages provided that the same particulars appear in all languages used.

Containers and packages of relevant medicinal products may be labelled to show:
(1) a symbol or pictogram designed to clarify the above particulars;
(2) other information compatible with the summary of product characteristics which is useful for health education.

There must not be any labelling of a promotional nature.

The requirement for a container or package of a relevant medicinal product to be labelled to show its name is not met by the container or package being labelled to show an invented name which is liable to be confused with the common name.

1.2.6.6 Warnings and other special labelling requirements

For dispensed medicines *see* Sections 1.2.6.1 and 1.2.6.2 for the labelling of dispensed medicinal products (p23). In addition to the labelling particulars shown for chemists' nostrums and relevant medicinal products above, there are certain other particulars, warnings and phrases which must be shown on the labels of containers and packages of certain medicinal products. Different requirements apply to general sale list products, pharmacy medicines and prescription-only medicines.

1.2.6.7 Manufacturers' labelling requirements for general sale list products

When a relevant medicinal product, on a general sale list is sold or supplied by retail (but not as a dispensed relevant medicinal product), in addition to the appropriate particulars listed in section 1.2.6.5 it must be also labelled to show the following:

(a) if the product contains aloxiprin, aspirin or paracetamol, the words "If symptoms persist consult your doctor" and, except where the product is for external use only, the recommended dosage;

(b) if the product contains aloxiprin, the words "Contains an aspirin derivative";

(c) if the product contains aspirin, except where the product is for external use only or where the name of the product includes the word "aspirin" and appears on the container or package, the words "Contains aspirin";

(d) if the product contains paracetamol, except where the name of the product includes the word "paracetamol" and appears on the container or package, the words "Contains paracetamol";

(e) if the product contains paracetamol, the words "Do not exceed the stated dose" (this should appear adjacent to the directions for use/recommended dosage where this appear on the container or package);

(f) if the product contains paracetamol, unless it is wholly or mainly intended for children who are twelve years old or younger, the words "Do not take with any other paracetamol-containing products", and

(i) if a package leaflet accompanying the product displays the words "Immediate medical advice should be sought in the event of an overdose, even if you feel well, because of the risk of delayed, serious liver damage", the words "Immediate medical advice should be sought in the event of an overdose, even if you feel well", or

(ii) if no package leaflet accompanies the product or the package leaflet does not display the words "Immediate medical advice should be sought in the event of an overdose, even if you feel well, because of the risk of delayed, serious liver damage", the words "Immediate medical advice should be sought in the event of an overdose, even if you feel well, because of the risk of delayed, serious liver damage";

(g) if the product contains paracetamol and is wholly or mainly intended for children who are twelve years old or younger, the words "Do not give with any other paracetamol-containing products"; and

(i) if a package leaflet accompanying the product displays the words "Immediate medical advice should be sought in the event of an overdose, even if the child seems well, because of the risk of delayed, serious liver damage", the words "Immediate medical advice should be sought in the [event] of an overdose, even if the child seems well", or

(ii) if no package leaflet accompanies the product or the package leaflet does not display the words "Immediate medical advice should be sought in the event of an overdose, even if the child seems well, because of the risk of delayed, serious liver damage", the words "Immediate medical advice should be sought in the event of an overdose, even if the child seems well, because of the risk of delayed, serious liver damage";

(h) if the product contains aspirin or aloxiprin, the words "Do not give to children aged under 16 years, unless on the advice of a doctor".

NB: Where the words set out in more than one of the paragraphs above (ie, [b], [c] and [d]) are required, there may be substituted for those words other words showing that the product contains more than one of the substances aloxiprin, aspirin and paracetamol and naming the substances so contained, except that in the case of aloxiprin the words "aspirin derivative" shall appear and the word "aloxiprin" need not appear.

Where the words set out in one or more of paragraphs (b) to (g) above are required, such words must appear in a prominent position and be within a rectangle within which there is no other matter, except where word set out in more than one of those paragraphs appear on the container or package then

any of them may appear together within a rectangle within which there must be no other matter of any kind.

1.2.6.8 Labelling of products for pharmacy sale only

Medicinal products, including relevant medicinal products, for pharmacy sale only, when sold or supplied by retail in addition to appropriate particulars above, must be labelled as follows:

(1) With the capital letter "P" in a rectangle containing no other matter. (That also applies to sales by wholesale.)

(2) If containing aspirin, aloxiprin or paracetamol, in the manner described above for medicinal products on a general sale list.

(3) If exempt from prescription-only control by reason of the proportion or level in the product of the prescription-only substance, with the words "Warning. Do not exceed the stated dose." (This does not apply to products for external use or products containing any of the substances set out in 5 below.)

(4) If for the treatment of asthma or other conditions associated with bronchial spasm or if they contain ephedrine or any of its salts, with the words "Warning. Asthmatics should consult their doctor before using this product." (This does not apply to products for external use.)

(5) If the product contains an antihistamine or similar substances or any of their salts or molecular compounds with the words "Warning. May cause drowsiness. If affected do not drive or operate machinery. Avoid alcoholic drink." (This does not apply to products for external use or where the product is for external use only or where the marketing authorisation contains no warning relating to the sedatating effect of the product in use.)

(6) If the product is an embrocation, liniment, lotion, liquid antiseptic or other liquid preparation or gel and is for external application, with the words "For external use only."

(7) If the product contains hexachlorophane, either with the words "Not to be used for babies" or a warning that the product is not to be administered to a child under two years except on medical advice.

The relevant warning phrase or phrases described under "Labelling of general sale list products" and "Labelling of products for pharmacy sale only" above must be in a rectangle within which there is no other matter. That does not apply to the phrases "Do not exceed the stated dose" or "If symptoms persist consult your doctor" on the labels of products required to be labelled because of their aspirin, aloxiprin or paracetamol content.

Where more than one of the phrases (1) to (7) in this section ("Labelling of products for pharmacy sale only") is applicable to a particular product, the phrases may be together within a rectangle although the wording must not be altered or combined except that the word "Warning" need only appear once.

1.2.6.9 Manufacturer's labelling requirements for prescription-only medicines

In addition to appropriate particulars above, the container and package of every relevant medicinal product which is a prescription-only medicine must be labelled:

(a) to show the letters "POM" in capitals within a rectangle within which there shall be no other matter of any kind (except in the case of a dispensed medicine);

(b) if the product is an embrocation, liniment, lotion, liquid antiseptic, or other liquid preparation or gel and is for external application, with the words "For external use only;"

(c) if the product contains hexachlorophane, either with the words "Not to be used for babies" or a warning that the product is not to be administered to a child under two years except on medical advice.

The phrases described above must be within a rectangle within which there is no other matter of any kind.

1.2.7 Patient information leaflets

Each time a relevant medicinal product is supplied a patient information leaflet must also be supplied.

1.2.8 Use of fluted bottles

The Medicines (Fluted Bottles) Regulations 1978, as amended, require liquid medicinal products for external use to be sold or supplied in a bottle the outer surface of which is fluted vertically with ribs or grooves recognisable by touch if, and only if, the product contains any of the substances listed in the following Schedule:

Aconite; alkaloids of

Adrenaline; its salts

Amino-alcohols esterified with benzoic acid, phenylacetic acid, phenylpropionic acid, cinnamic acid or the derivatives of these acids; their salts

p-Aminobenzenesulphonamide; its salts; derivatives of p-aminobenzenesulphonamide having any of the hydrogen atoms of the p-amino group or of the sulphonamide group substituted by another radical; their salts

p-Aminobenzoic acid; esters of; their salts

Ammonia except in medicinal products containing less than 5% weight in weight of ammonia

Arsenical substances, the following: arsenic sulphides; arsenates; arsenites; halides of arsenic; oxides of arsenic; organic compounds of arsenic

Atropine; its salts

Cantharidin; cantharidates

Carbachol

Chloral; its addition and its condensation products other than alphachloralose; their molecular compounds

Chloroform except in medicinal products containing less than 1% volume in volume of chloroform

Cocaine; its salts

Creosote obtained from wood except in medicinal products containing less than 50% volume in volume of creosote obtained from wood

Croton, oil of

Demecarium bromide

Dyflos

Ecothiopate iodide

Ephedrine; its salts except in medicinal products containing less than the equivalent of 1% weight in volume of ephedrine

Ethylmorphine; its salts

Homatropine; its salts

Hydrofluoric acid; alkali metal bifluorides; potassium fluoride; sodium fluoride; sodium silicofluoride except in mouth washes containing not more than 0.05% weight in volume of sodium fluoride

Hyoscine; its salts

Hyoscyamine; its salts

Lead acetates except in medicinal products containing lead acetates equivalent to not more than 2.2% weight in volume of lead calculated as elemental lead

Mercury, oxides of; nitrates of mercury; mercuric ammonium chloride; mercuric chloride; mercuric iodide; potassium mercuric iodide; organic compounds of mercury; mercuric oxycyanide; mercuric thiocyanate except in medicinal products containing not more than 0.01% weight in volume of phenylmercuric salts or 0.01% weight in volume of sodium ethyl mercurithiosalicylate as a preservative

Nitric acid except in medicinal products containing less than 9% weight in weight of nitric acid

Opium

Phenols (any member of the series of phenols of which the first member is phenol and of which the molecular composition varies from member to member by one atom of carbon and two atoms of hydrogen); compounds of phenol with a metal except in:

(a) medicinal products containing one or more of the following:

Butylated hydroxytoluene

Carvacrol

Creosote obtained from coal tar

Essential oils in which phenols occur naturally

Tar (coal or wood), crude or refined

tert-Butylcresol

p-tert-Butylphenol

p-tert-Pentylphenol

p-(1,1,3,3-tetramethylbutyl) phenol

Thymol

(b) mouth washes containing less than 2.5% weight in volume of phenols;

(c) any liquid disinfectant or antiseptics not containing phenol and containing less than 2.5% weight in volume of other phenols;

(d) other medicinal products containing less than 1% weight in volume of phenols

Physostigmine; its salts

Picric acid except in medicinal products containing less than 5% weight in volume of picric acid

Pilocarpine; its salts except in medicinal products containing less than the equivalent of 0.025% weight in volume of pilocarpine

Podophyllum resin except in medicinal products containing not more than 1.5% weight in weight of podophyllum resin

Solanaceous alkaloids not otherwise included in this Schedule

Some exceptions to fluted bottle requirements

The fluted bottle requirements do not apply where:

(a) medicinal products are contained in bottles with a capacity greater than 1.14 litres;

(b) medicinal products are packed for export for use solely outside the UK;

(c) medicinal products are sold or supplied solely for the purpose of scientific education, research or analysis;

(d) eye or ear drops are sold or supplied in a plastic container;

(e) where the product licence, marketing authorisation or any variation of any such licence or authorisation, enables medicinal products to be contained in a bottle otherwise than in accordance with the requirements;

(f) where the clinical trial certificate otherwise provides;

(g) where a substance listed above is contained in a medicinal product which is classified as being on prescription only, unless sold or supplied by retail sale or in accordance with a prescription given by a practitioner.

1.2.9 Medical devices

The Medical Devices Regulations 2002, as amended, have implemented international law, European Devices Directives which provide for mandatory CE Marking of all medical devices covered by them. This includes some dressings, blood pressure monitors, contact lens care products, glucose meters, test kits e.g. cholesterol and screening tests.

The CE Marking means that a manufacturer claims that his device is safe within a benefit risk analysis, performs as claimed and is fit for its intended purpose. For all except the simplest devices, this CE Marking is checked by a certification organisation known as a notified body, of which there are over 80 across Europe, each designated by their national competent authority.

Nowadays many medical devices are being used or sold by pharmacists. There are a number of considerations that all pharmacists and pharmacists staff should know about such devices when deciding to recommend, sell, stock, or employ within a supplied pharmacy service. Principals of appropriate procurement, safe use, maintenance and repair and guidance on reporting device related adverse events are set out as a series of practical check lists in 'Devices in Practice' available from the Medicines and Healthcare products Regulatory Agency website (*www.mhra.gov.uk*).

Emphasis is placed on post market surveillance which includes the mandatory reporting of all serious adverse events by the manufacturer. Further information can be obtained from the Society's Legal and Ethical Advisory Service or directly from the Medicines and Healthcare and products Regulatory Agency (*www.mhra.gov.uk*).

1.2.10 Restrictions on the sale of plano (zero powered) cosmetic contact lenses

Pharmacists are advised that they must not sell plano (zero powered) cosmetic contact lenses unless they are sold under the supervision of a registered optician, dispensing optician or doctor.

Pharmacists wishing to sell zero powered contact lenses must do so in accordance with the relevant legal requirements contained within The Opticians Act 1989, and the subsequent Rules and Regulations. Failure to do so could result in action being taken for breach of the legislation. For further information on these legal requirements, the General Optical Council should be consulted on 020 7580 3898 (*www.optical.org*; e-mail: *goc@optical.org*).

1.2.11 Chloroform: sale and supply

The Medicines (Chloroform Prohibition) Order 1979, as amended, prohibits the sale or supply of any medicinal product consisting of or containing chloroform, which is for human use, except in the following circumstances.

A sale or supply may be made:

(1) (a) by a doctor or dentist to a patient of his, where the medicinal product has been specially prepared by that doctor or dentist for administration to that particular patient, or

(b) by a doctor or dentist who has specially prepared the medicinal product at the request of another doctor or dentist for administration to a particular patient of that other doctor or dentist, or

(c) from a registered pharmacy, hospital or by a doctor or dentist where the medicinal product has been specially prepared, in accordance with a prescription given by a doctor or dentist for a particular patient of his, in a registered pharmacy, hospital or by a doctor or dentist

(2) (a) to a hospital, doctor or dentist either solely for use as an anaesthetic or solely for use as an ingredient in the preparation of a substance to be used as an anaesthetic, or both

(b) to a person who buys or obtains it for the purpose of selling or supplying it to a hospital, doctor or dentist either solely for use as an anaesthetic or solely for use as an ingredient in the preparation of a substance or article to be used as an anaesthetic, or both, or

(3) (a) where the medicinal product contains chloroform in a proportion of not more than 0.5% (w/w) or (v/v), or

(b) where the medicinal product is solely for use in dental surgery, or

(c) where the medicinal product is solely for use by being applied to the external surface of the body which for the purpose of this Order does not include any part of the mouth, teeth or mucous membranes, or

(4) where the medicinal product is for export, or

(5) where the medicinal product is sold for use as an ingredient in the preparation of a substance or article in a registered pharmacy, a hospital or by a doctor or dentist.

See also "Substances restricted to professional users" (p86).

1.2.12 Advertising and promotion of medicines: Acceptance of gifts and inducements to prescribe or supply

The Medicines (Advertising) Regulations 1994 govern the supply, offer or promise of gifts to healthcare professionals, including pharmacists, by drug manufacturers and distributors. Pharmacists accepting items such as gift vouchers, bonus points, discount holidays, sports equipment, etc, would be in breach of Regulation 21. Pharmacists are, therefore, advised not to participate in such offers.

1.2.13 Handling of waste medicines

England and Wales

The Hazardous Waste (England and Wales) Regulations 2005 only allow community pharmacists in England and Wales to accept waste which is classified as household waste. This includes patient returned medication from patients or individuals. Where a patient has produced waste medicines in their own home, these can be returned to any pharmacy, (which has registered an exemption). The exemption does not restrict who may return the waste medicines from the household to the pharmacy. Waste from other sources requires a licence or registered exemption.

Community pharmacists would have to determine if the waste to be returned was classified as household waste, or not, before accepting it. Household waste (including waste medication) that can be accepted back to a community pharmacy is waste from:

(a) a domestic property;

(b) a caravan;

(c) a residential care home providing residential care only (NOT nursing care); or

(d) a moored vessel used wholly for the purposes of living accommodation.

Waste from a home providing nursing care (previously a nursing home) or unwanted/expired stock returned from a doctor, dentist, vet, midwife or nurse would be classed as industrial waste and would require licences from the Environment Agency (08708 506506) for its storage and treatment (destruction or deblistering). It should also be noted that the carriage of waste requires a licence from the Environment Agency.

The removal of individual tablets or capsules from a blister strip or the decanting of liquids from bottles should be avoided as this falls within the definition of waste treatment, which is a licensable activity. The Environment Agency has confirmed that the removal of a blister strip from other inert packaging, so that the blister strip can be placed in the waste container and the outer packaging can be recycled, would not be regulated as a licensable waste treatment.

Scotland

In Scotland, the Waste Management Licensing Amendment (Scotland) Regulations 2006 allow registered pharmacies to accept patient returned medication from patients or individuals. The Regulations have enabled certain waste to be returned to pharmacies from care services, including all care homes (irrespective of whether or not they employ nurses). "Care services" for the purposes on the above Regulations has the same meaning as in Section 2 of the Regulation of Care (Scotland) Act 2001. By way of clarification the care services defined as those from which pharmacies in Scotland may accept returned waste include the following:

(a) a support service; (b) a care home service; (c) a school care accommodation service; (d) an independent health care service; (e) a nurse agency; (f) a child care agency; (g) a secure accommodation service; (h) an offender accommodation service; (i) an adoption service; (j) a fostering service; (k) an adult placement service; (l) child minding; (m) day care of children; and (n) a housing support service.

The Scottish Environment Protection Agency can be contacted on 01786 457700.

Deblistering is allowed only in the case of Controlled Drugs where it is necessary to remove the solid dosage form from the blister strip or tablet bottle in order to denature the drug and render it irretrievable. (*See* p39-42 for further information on the denaturing of Controlled Drugs.)

1.2.14 Controlled Drugs

The Misuse of Drugs Act 1971 controls "dangerous or otherwise harmful drugs" which are designated as "Controlled Drugs." The primary purpose of the Misuse of Drugs Act is to prevent the misuse of Controlled Drugs. It does that by imposing a total prohibition on the possession, supply, manufacture, import or export of Controlled Drugs except as allowed by regulations or by licence from the Secretary of State. The use of Controlled Drugs in medicine is permitted by the Misuse of Drugs Regulations 2001, as amended. Other regulations deal with the safe custody of Controlled Drugs and with the notification of and supply of drugs to misusers.

The classes to the Act are of no practical importance to pharmacists and practitioners. In the Misuse of Drugs Regulations, the drugs are classified in five schedules according to different levels of control. It is those classifications that are described in the following paragraphs. In the main alphabetical list of medicines for human use in this book they are marked CD Lic, CD POM, CD No Register POM, CD Benz POM, CD Anab POM, or CD Inv. P or POM, according to the controls (detailed below) which apply to each drug.

Schedule 1 drugs (CD Lic)

Schedule 1 includes the hallucinogenic drugs (for example LSD), the ecstasy-type substances and cannabis, which have virtually no therapeutic use. Production, possession and supply of drugs in this Schedule are limited, in the public interest, to purposes of research or other special purposes. A licence from the Home Office is needed for any of these purposes, and, apart from licence holders, the class of persons who may lawfully possess them is very limited. It does not include practitioners and pharmacists except under licence. There is an exception to the prohibition on the possession of a Schedule 1 Controlled Drug under certain conditions for specific purposes in the case of a fungus that contains psilocin or an ester of psilocin.

Some pharmacists, particularly those working within hospital, may be asked to deal with substances removed from patients on admission, which may be Schedule 1 products (for example cannabis). As a licence is required to possess Schedule 1 products, the pharmacist cannot take possession of the product other than in the two cases where exemptions are granted. The first exemption, is where a person takes possession of a Controlled Drug for the purpose of destruction, and the second, for the purpose of handing over to a police officer. Guidance should be sought from the Home Office regarding destruction of Schedule 1 Controlled Drugs.

The patient's confidentiality should normally be maintained, and the police should be called in on the understanding that there will be no identification of the source. If, however, the quantity is so large that the drug could not be purely for personal use, the pharmacist may decide that the greater interests of the public require identification of the source. Such a decision should not be taken without first discussing with the other health professionals involved in the patient's care, and the hospital's legal adviser.

In theory, the patient should give authority for the removal and destruction of the drug. If the patient refuses, then the hospital may feel that it has no alternative other than to call in the police. Under no circumstances can a Schedule 1 drug be handed back to a patient at discharge, as the person doing so could be guilty of an offence of unlawful supply of a Controlled Drug. The penalties for this type of offence are high, and often involve a custodial sentence.

Schedule 2 drugs (CD POM)

Schedule 2 includes the opiates (such as diamorphine, morphine and methadone), the major stimulants (such as the amphetamines) and quinalbarbitone. A licence is needed to import or export drugs in this Schedule, but they may be manufactured or compounded by a licence holder, a practitioner, a pharmacist, or a person lawfully conducting a retail pharmacy business acting in his capacity as such. A pharmacist may supply them to a patient only on the authority of a prescription in the required form (see below) issued by an appropriate practitioner.

The drugs may be administered to a patient by a doctor or dentist, a nurse independent prescriber (who may administer certain Controlled Drugs under certain circumstances, see p37), a supplementary prescriber in accordance with a clinical management plan, or by any person acting in accordance with the directions of a doctor, dentist, nurse independent prescriber or a supplementary prescriber in accordance with a clinical management plan.

Requirements for safe custody in pharmacies apply to all Schedule 2 Controlled Drugs except quinalbarbitone. The requirement for safe custody of Schedule 2 drugs also applies to patient returned Schedule 2 drugs, until such time as they are denatured for disposal. Restrictions concerning the destruction of stock (requiring an authorised witness to be present) applies to these drugs, and the provisions relating to the marking of containers and the keeping of records must also be observed.

Schedule 3 drugs (CD No Register POM)

Schedule 3 includes a small number of minor stimulant drugs such as benzphetamine, and other drugs (such as buprenorphine, midazolam, phenobarbitone and temazepam) which are not thought so likely to be misused as the drugs in Schedule 2, nor to be so harmful if misused. The controls which apply to Schedule 2 also apply to drugs in this schedule, except:
(a) there is a difference in the classes of persons who may possess and supply them;
(b) the requirements for an authorised witness to attend during the destruction of date expired stock does not apply in retail pharmacy, (unless the pharmacist is a "producer" of Schedule 3 Controlled Drugs, ie, they manufacture or compound these items);
(c) records in the register of Controlled Drugs need not be kept in respect of these drugs, (unless the pharmacist is a "producer" of these items, as above);
(d) while safe custody requirements apply, currently most drugs in this Schedule are exempted. Currently, the four Schedule 3 Controlled Drugs that do require safe custody are temazepam, diethylpropion, buprenorphine and flunitrazepam. Neither phenobarbitone nor midazolam require safe custody. The requirement for safe custody of the four Schedule 3 drugs listed above, also applies to these drugs when they are returned by patients for disposal, until such time as they are denatured. Any drugs added to Schedule 3 require safe custody, unless specifically exempted. Invoices need to be retained by retail dealers.

Schedule 4 drugs (CD Benz POM or CD Anab POM)

Schedule 4 is split into two parts. Part I (CD Benz POM) contains most of the benzodiazepines. Part II (CD Anab POM) contains most of the anabolic and androgenic steroids,

together with clenbuterol (adrenoceptor stimulant) and growth hormones (5 polypeptide hormones). The restrictions applicable to Schedule 3 drugs apply to them with the following relaxations:

(a) if the substance from Part II (CD Anab POM) is in the form of a medicinal product and is for administration by a person to himself a Home Office import or export licence is not required for the importation and exportation of this substance (a Home Office import or export licence would still be required for the importation and exportation of substances in Part I [CD Benz POM] and Part II [CD Anab POM] of Schedule 4 not falling under the above exemption);
(b) there is no restriction on the possession of any Schedule 4 Part II (CD Anab POM) when contained in a medicinal product;
(c) the labelling requirements of the Misuse of Drugs Regulations 2001, as amended, do not apply. However, the labelling requirements falling under the controls of the Medicines Act 1968 would still apply;
(d) prescription requirements under the Misuse of Drugs Regulations 2001, as amended, do not apply, except for the validity of a prescription being limited to 28 days; prescription requirements falling under the controls of the Medicines Act 1968 continue to apply;
(e) Controlled Drug register entries need not be kept by retailers;
(f) the requirement for an authorised witness for the destruction of Schedule 4 CDs applies only to importers, exporters and manufacturers;
(g) there are no safe custody requirements.

Schedule 5 drugs (CD Inv. P or CD Inv. POM)

Schedule 5 contains preparations of certain Controlled Drugs, for example, codeine, pholcodine and morphine, which are exempt from full control when present in medicinal products of low strength. There is no restriction on the import, export, possession or administration of these preparations, and safe custody requirements do not apply. A practitioner or pharmacist acting in his capacity as such, or a person holding an appropriate licence, may manufacture or compound any of them.

No record in the register of Controlled Drugs need be made in respect of drugs obtained or supplied by a person lawfully conducting a retail pharmacy business unless that person is a "producer", ie, a manufacturer or compounder of such items. The invoices or copies of Schedule 5 Controlled Drugs obtained or supplied must be kept for two years. No authorised witness is required to witness the destruction of these drugs, and there are no special labelling requirements other than the labelling requirements of the Medicines Act 1968.

Possession and supply of Controlled Drugs

It is unlawful for any person to be in possession of Controlled Drugs in Schedules 2, 3 and 4 unless:
(a) that person holds an appropriate licence from the Home Office; or
(b) that person is a member of a class specified in the Regulations; or

(c) the Regulations provide that possession of that drug or group of drugs is not unlawful, for example there is no restriction on the possession of any Schedule 4 Part II (CD Anab POM) drug when contained in a medicinal product; or

(d) they have been lawfully prescribed for that person (or for that person's animal).

In any case, possession or supply is not lawful unless the person concerned is acting in his capacity as a member of his class, or in accordance with the terms of his licence or group authority.

Practitioners and pharmacists when acting in their capacity as such are amongst those who have a general authority to possess, supply and procure all Controlled Drugs except those in Schedule 1.

Certain other persons, including wholesalers, importers and exporters, must obtain licences from the Secretary of State. "Wholesale dealer" in this context means a person who carries on the business of selling drugs to persons who buy to sell again.

Any person who is lawfully in possession of a Controlled Drug may supply that drug to the person from whom he lawfully obtained it. Other legislation (such as waste legislation), however, may prevent Controlled Drugs being transferred back to a pharmacy from certain sources.

Secretary of State prohibitions

The Home Secretary also has the power, under the Misuse of Drugs Act 1971, to make a direction against a practitioner prohibiting him from having in his possession, prescribing, administering, manufacturing, compounding and supplying, and from authorising the administration and supply of those Controlled Drugs specified in the direction. In order to confirm whether or not a practitioner has had a direction made against him under the Misuse of Drugs Act 1971, prohibiting him from dealing with Controlled Drugs as indicated above, pharmacists are advised to contact the Home Office directly on 020 7035 4848.

Safe custody of Controlled Drugs

The regulations relating to safe custody apply to all Controlled Drugs included in Schedules 1, 2 (except quinalbarbitone [secobarbital]) and 3 (except any 5,5 disubstituted barbituric acid, cathine, ethchlorvynol, ethinamate, mazindol, meprobamate, methylphenobarbitone, methprylone, midazolam, pentazocine, phentermine or any stereoisomeric form of the above, or any salts of the above). Phenobarbitone (Phenobarbital) is a 5,5 disubstituted barbituric acid and therefore does not require safe custody.

Any liquid preparations designed for administration otherwise than by injection which contain any of the following substances and products are exempt from safe custody requirements:

(a) amphetamine
(b) benzphetamine
(c) chlorphentermine
(d) fenethylline
(e) mephentermine
(f) methaqualone
(g) methylamphetamine
(h) methylphenidate

(i) phendimetrazine
(j) phenmetrazine
(k) pipradrol
(l) any stereoisomeric form of a substance specified in (a) to (k) or any salt of a substance specified in (a) to (l).

However, pharmacists may wish to keep these drugs in the Controlled Drug cupboard.

Retail dealers and care homes must comply with the requirements for safe custody where they apply and must ensure that the relevant Controlled Drugs are kept in a locked safe, cabinet or room which is so constructed and maintained in accordance with the Misuse of Drugs (Safe Custody) Regulations 1973, as amended. This requirement does not apply in respect of any Controlled Drug which is for the time being constantly under the direct personal supervision of a pharmacist, for example, when dispensing a prescription.

The specifications with which safes, cabinets and rooms must comply are given in great detail in the Regulations (obtainable from The Stationery Office, *www.tso.co.uk*.) The owner of a pharmacy may, however, elect to apply, as an alternative, to the police for a certificate that his safes, cabinets or rooms provide an adequate degree of security. Applications must be made in writing. The certificate may specify conditions to be observed.

The requirement for safe custody for certain Controlled Drugs applies equally to patient returned and out-of-date Controlled Drugs, which until such time that they can be denatured and be rendered irretrievable, must be kept in the Controlled Drug cabinet. Patient returned Controlled Drugs must be kept segregated from stock Controlled Drugs, and clearly marked as such to minimise the risk of errors and inadvertent supply.

Requisitions for Schedules 1, 2 and 3 Controlled Drugs

A requisition in writing must be obtained by a supplier before he delivers any Schedule 2 or 3 Controlled Drug. The requisition does not have to be in the recipient's handwriting but must:

(a) be signed by the recipient;
(b) state the recipient's name;
(c) state the recipient's address;
(d) state the recipient's profession or occupation;
(e) specify the total quantity of the drug;
(f) specify the purpose for which it is required.

The supplier must be reasonably satisfied that the signature is that of the person purporting to sign the requisition and that he is engaged in the occupation stated.

The requisition must be obtained prior to supply to any of the following:

(a) a practitioner (a practitioner urgently requiring a drug and unable to supply a written requisition before delivery may be supplied on his giving an undertaking to furnish a requisition within the next 24 hours; failure to furnish the requisition within 24 hours is an offence on the part of the practitioner);

(b) the person or acting person in charge of a hospital or care home (a requisition from the person in charge of a hospital or care home must be signed by a doctor or dentist employed or engaged there);

(c) a person who is in charge of a laboratory the recognised activities of which consist in or include the conduct of scientific education or research and which is attached to a university, university college or such a hospital as aforesaid or to any other institution approved for such a purpose by the Secretary of State;

(d) the owner of a ship or the master of a ship which does not carry a doctor among the seamen employed on board;

(e) the installation manager of an offshore installation;

(f) the master of a foreign ship in a port in Great Britain (a requisition from the master of a foreign ship must contain a statement from the proper officer of the port health authority, or, in Scotland, the medical officer designated under section 14 of the National Health Service (Scotland) Act 1978 by the Health Board, within whose jurisdiction the ship is, that the quantity of drug is necessary for the equipment of the ship);

(g) a supplementary prescriber;

(h) a senior registered nurse or acting senior registered nurse for the time being in charge of any ward, theatre or other department of a hospital or care home who obtains a supply of a Controlled Drug from the person responsible for dispensing and supplying medicines at that hospital or care home must furnish a requisition in writing signed by the recipient which specifies the total quantity of the drug required. The recipient must retain a copy or note of the requisition. The person responsible for the dispensing and supply of the Controlled Drug must mark the requisition in such a manner as to show that it has been complied with and must retain the requisition in the dispensary;

(i) an operating department practitioner (ODP) can order Schedule 2, 3, 4 and 5 controlled drugs from a hospital pharmacy and the hospital pharmacy, in which the ODP is practising, can supply the ODP with these drugs.
Currently, when ordering Controlled Drugs from a hospital pharmacy, the ODP is under no legal obligation to provide a written requisition. However, pharmacists are advised as a matter of good practice and/or to comply with local standard operating procedures, supplies should be made on the receipt of a requisition signed by the ODP. The legislation is due to be changed to make the provision of a written requisition a legal requirement. (There is no provision to allow an ODP to obtain Controlled Drugs from a community pharmacy.)

Supply of Controlled Drugs stock from the community

Standardised requisition forms have been produced for use in England (FP10CDF), Scotland (CDRF) and Wales (WP10CDF). There is no legal requirement to use these standardised requisition forms, however, they should be used wherever possible as a matter of good practice. The standardised requisition forms can be obtained from the local Primary Care Organisation.

It is still lawful for a community pharmacist to supply against a requisition form written in a format other than on the newly introduced standardised forms as long as all the legal requirements for a requisition are complied with. When one community pharmacy supplies another community pharmacy, as a matter of good practice a written requisition should be obtained, and ideally this should be the standardised form.

In Scotland the arrangements for the requisition form used to obtain NHS stock remain unchanged. GP10A stock order forms should be used for NHS purposes. A duplicate GP10A will be required to be kept at the pharmacy. It should be noted that separate GP10A forms should be used for Schedule 1, 2 and 3 Controlled Drugs. Prescribers in Scotland who wish to obtain stocks of Schedule 1, 2 and 3 Controlled Drugs privately from a community pharmacy should use the standardised requisition form (CDRF). Those wishing to obtain a supply of CDRF forms must contact the local NHS Board to register as a private prescriber (if they are not already registered) and to order the forms.

On receipt of a requisition for a Schedule 1, 2 or 3 Controlled Drug by a pharmacist in a community setting (not a care home or a hospital), the pharmacist must:

(i) mark on the requisition (in ink or otherwise indelibly) the supplier's name and address. The Home Office has confirmed that a pharmacy stamp can be used to mark these details on the requisition if the address details appear in full and the information is clear and legible;

(ii) preserve and retain a copy of the requisition for two years from the date of supply;

(iii) send all original requisitions to the relevant National Health Service agency in accordance with arrangements specified by that agency.

The requirements to mark and send the requisition to the relevant NHS agency do not apply where the supplier is:

(a) a person responsible for the dispensing and supply of medicines at a hospital or care home. The original requisition must be kept for two years;

(c) a pharmaceutical manufacturer or pharmaceutical wholesaler;

(d) a person responsible for the supply of Controlled Drugs within a prison setting.

The requirements to mark and send the requisition to the relevant NHS agency do not apply to:

(a) midwives' supply orders. The arrangements for midwives' supply orders remain unchanged.

(b) veterinary requisitions. A "veterinary requisition" is a requisition which states that the recipient is a veterinary surgeon or veterinary practitioner. The requirements for a requisition, as described above, state that the requisition must specify "the recipient's profession or occupation". The original requisition must be kept for five years.

Where non-standardised Controlled Drug requisition forms have been used, these must also be marked on receipt, copied and sent to the relevant NHS agency, as above.

Collection by messenger

A messenger sent by a purchaser (recipient) to collect Controlled Drug stock in resppnse to a written requisition on the recipient's behalf may only be supplied with the Controlled Drug if he produces to the supplier a statement in writing given by the recipient to the effect that the messenger is empowered to receive the drugs on his behalf. The supplier must be reasonably satisfied that the document is genuine and must retain it for two years. The requirement for the written statement does not apply to a person carrying on a business as a carrier engaged by the supplier.

Controlled Drugs in hospitals

In hospitals additional requirements relating to administration and supply, prescriptions, requisitions and registers for Controlled Drugs include:

(a) A senior registered nurse or acting senior registered nurse, for the time being in charge of a ward, theatre, or other department, may not supply any drug otherwise than for administration to a patient in the ward, theatre or department in accordance with the directions of a doctor, dentist, supplementary prescriber acting under and in accordance with the terms of a clinical management plan, or of a nurse independent prescriber subject to the limited list of Controlled Drugs which they may prescribe which includes a specific purpose for which the drug may be prescribed (*see* p37)*.

(b) The senior registered nurse or acting senior registered nurse, for the time being in charge of a ward, theatre or other department is not required by the Misuse of Drugs Regulations 2001, as amended, to keep any register. However, Department of Health guidance and good practice should be followed, which may require such a register to be kept. It follows that ward stocks of Controlled Drugs may legally be destroyed without the attendance of an "authorised person." However, Department of Health guidance must again be taken into account.

(c) An operating department practitioner is authorised to order Schedule 2, 3, 4 and 5 Controlled Drugs from the hospital pharmacy, in which the ODP is practising. That hospital pharmacy would be able to supply an ODP with those drugs. ODPs are able to possess and supply Schedule 2–5 Controlled Drugs for the purposes of administration to a patient in a ward, theatre or other department, at the hospital in which they are practising, in accordance with the directions of a doctor, dentist, supplementary prescriber acting under and in accordance with the terms of a clinical management plan, or of a nurse independent prescriber. The directions given by a nurse prescriber relate only to the limited list of Controlled Drugs which they may prescribe, and are subject to restrictions on the purpose for which they may be prescribed.**

(d) The person in charge or acting person in charge of a hospital or care home having a pharmacist responsible for the dispensing and supply of medicines may not supply or offer to supply any drug.

(e) A prescription issued for the treatment of a patient in a hospital or care home may be written on the patient's bed-card or casesheet. Where a bed-card or casesheet is used as an authorisation to administer a Controlled Drug, it would not need to comply with the full prescription requirements for a Controlled Drug. However, where a bed-card or casesheet is used as an authorisation to supply a Controlled Drug to a patient it would need to fully comply with the prescription requirements of a Controlled Drug (*see* below).

---

* When legislation changes, it is anticipated that pharmacist independent prescribers and nurse independent prescribers will be able to prescribe any Controlled Drug for any condition

** When legislation changes, it is anticipated that this would also include supply in accordance with the directions of a pharmacist independent prescriber and the full range of Controlled Drugs by a nurse independent prescriber

(f) Private prescriptions for Schedule 2 or 3 Controlled Drugs that are to be supplied by a pharmacist in a hospital do not need to specify the prescriber identification number and do not need to be on a standardised form provided by the primary care organisation for the purposes of private prescribing.

(g) Requisitions for Schedule 2 or 3 Controlled Drugs that are to be supplied by a pharmacist in a hospital do not need to be sent to a National Health Service agency and do not need to be marked with the name and address of the supplying pharmacy.

Prescriptions for Controlled Drugs

No prescription is required under the Misuse of Drugs Regulations for the supply by a pharmacist of a Schedule 5 drug but, for preparations above certain strengths, a prescription is required under the Medicines Act 1968. Prescriptions are necessary for all other categories of Controlled Drugs which are always prescription-only medicines. The requirements of both the Misuse of Drugs Act 1971 and the Medicines Act 1968 must be satisfied. In the case of a prescription for an animal, *see* Section 1.8.1 (p91).

It is unlawful for a practitioner to issue a prescription containing a Schedule 2 or 3 Controlled Drug (except temazepam) or for a pharmacist to dispense it, unless it complies with the following requirements:

The prescription must:

(a) be signed by the person issuing it with his usual signature;

(b) be dated;

(c) be written so as to be indelible;

(d) except in the case of an NHS or local health authority prescription, specify the address of the person issuing it. NB: The Medicines Act requires that all prescriptions for prescription-only medicines contain the prescriber's address;

(e) in the case of a private prescription (including one for temazepam and midazolam) be on a standardised form, when dispensed in a community pharmacy or GP practice. The forms issued in England, Scotland or Wales, are called FP10PCD, PPCD(1) and WP10PCD respectively. NB: The requirement to use standardised prescription forms when prescribing Schedule 2 and 3 Controlled Drugs does not apply to veterinary prescriptions, but does apply to private prescriptions issued by doctors, dentists and non-medical prescribers (eg, nurse and pharmacist prescribers);

(f) in the case of a private prescription for human use (including temazepam and midazolam), contain the private prescriber's identification number on the prescription.

(g) specify the dose to be taken (NB: The Home Office has expressed the view that a dose of "as directed" or "when required" is not acceptable, but "one to be taken as directed/when required" is acceptable); and:

(i) in the case of preparations, the form and, where appropriate, the strength of the preparation;

(ii) and either the total quantity (in both words and figures) of the preparation, or the number (in both words and figures) of dosage units, as appropriate, to be supplied; in any other case, the total quantity (in both words and figures) of the Controlled Drug to be supplied (*see* Technical errors on Controlled Drug prescriptions, p34);

(h) have written on it, if issued by a dentist, the words "for dental treatment only";

(i) specify the name and address of the person for whose treatment it is issued;

(j) in the case of a prescription for a total quantity intended to be dispensed by instalments, contain a direction specifying the amount of the instalments which may be supplied and the intervals to be observed when supplying.

The Home Office has confirmed that an instalment prescription must have **both** a dose **and** an instalment amount on the prescription (ie, they both have to be specified separately.)

Prescriptions for Schedule 2 and 3 Controlled Drugs do not have to be written in the handwriting of the prescriber. Apart from the prescriber's signature, the entire prescription, including the date, may be computer generated.

The requirement for certain particulars to be on the prescription does not apply to prescriptions for temazepam (eg, total quantity in words and figures), or to prescriptions for Controlled Drugs in Schedule 4. For the purpose of prescription writing, temazepam can be written up as for any other prescription-only medicine (*see* Prescriptions for prescription-only medicines, p11)

A Schedule 2 or 3 Controlled Drug must not be supplied by any person on a prescription:

(a) unless the prescription complies with the provisions set out above (except temazepam);

(b) unless the prescriber's address on the prescription is within the United Kingdom;

(c) unless the supplier is either acquainted with the prescriber's signature and has no reason to suppose that it is not genuine, or has taken reasonably sufficient steps to satisfy himself that it is genuine;

(d) before the appropriate date on the prescription;

(e) in the case of an instalment prescription (FP10MDA or equivalent), unless the first instalment is dispensed within 28 days of the appropriate date. The remainder of the instalments can be dispensed in accordance with the instructions (even when this runs past the 28-day limit).

(f) later than 28 days after the appropriate date on the prescription. (This also applies to temazepam, midazolam and Schedule 4 Controlled Drugs.)

The "appropriate date" for the purposes of these Regulations is defined as "the later of the date on which it was signed by the person issuing it or the date indicated by him as being the date before which it shall not be supplied."

Where a prescriber wishes the 28-day period to start on a date other than the date of signing, he may specify a start date from which the period will begin. The start date specified can be more than 28 days from the date of signing / issue.

Owings of dispensed prescriptions for Schedule 2, 3 or 4 controlled drugs cannot be supplied more than 28 days after the appropriate date.

The date must be marked on the prescription at the time of supply of a Schedule 2 or 3 Controlled Drug.

Private Controlled Drug prescriptions

Private prescriptions for Schedule 2 and 3 Controlled Drugs (including temazepam) for human use that are to be dispensed in community, must:

(i) be on a standardised form (FP10PCD for England, PPCD(1) for Scotland and WP10PCD for Wales). Private Controlled Drug prescriptions which are not on the designated form must not be dispensed, and should not be accepted.

(ii) For Schedule 2 and 3 Controlled Drugs for human use, a private prescription that is to be dispensed in community must contain the private prescriber's identification number.

(iii) There is a requirement for pharmacists in England, Scotland and Wales to submit the original of Schedule 2 and 3 private prescription forms for human use to the relevant NHS agency. An identifying code, assigned to the pharmacy for this purpose, will be required to submit private Controlled Drug prescriptions to the PPD-NHSBSA (or equivalent).

No other items should be prescribed on a private standardised form (FP10PCD, PPCD(1) or WP10PCD) other than Controlled Drugs, as the prescription has to be sent away and pharmacists would therefore be unable to comply with the requirement to keep the private prescription of a POM for two years.

These requirements (i), (ii) and (iii) do not apply to certain prison arrangements in England and Wales. Where a service level agreement exists between a community pharmacy and a primary care organisation to supply items to a prison, the local primary care organisation should be consulted to determine whether it would not be necessary to use the standardised private prescription form for such supplies. Whether or not standardised private prescription forms are required, a robust audit trail must be maintained. Where it is determined that this is a private (not an NHS) arrangement, prescribers would need to use a standardised private prescription form for Schedule 2 or 3 Controlled Drugs to be supplied in a community setting. Where the private standardised form is required, the prescriber's identification number would also need to appear on the form.

These requirements (i), (ii) and (iii) do not apply to veterinary prescriptions for Controlled Drugs. Veterinary prescriptions do not need to be sent to any NHS agency but must be retained for at least five years (see pp91).

Sativex (a cannabis oro-mucosal spray) does not have to be prescribed on a standardised private prescription form when being dispensed in community.

Repeat prescriptions

Repeat prescriptions for Schedule 2 and 3 Controlled Drugs are not allowed. Instalment prescriptions allow Schedule 2 and 3 Controlled Drugs to be issued over a period of time.

With reference to Schedule 4 Controlled Drugs and repeats on prescriptions, after the first dispensing, legislation does not specify the time frame in which the repeat dispensing(s) of private prescriptions should be made. As long as the first dispensing of a repeat for a Schedule 4 Controlled Drug is within 28 days of the appropriate date, repeat dispensing of Schedule 4 Controlled Drugs can be made after 28 days. However, for the NHS repeat dispensing scheme in England and Wales, batch repeats are valid for a maximum of 12 months.

Prescribing for up to 30 days' clinical need

Although not a legal requirement, the Department of Health and the Scottish Executive have issued a strong recommendation that as good practice, the quantity of Schedule 2, 3 and 4 Controlled Drugs prescribed should not exceed 30 days' supply. Pharmacists may legally supply a quantity greater than 30 days' supply, if appropriate. Prescribers will need to be able to justify on the basis of clinical need, a supply of more than 30 days.

Technical errors on Controlled Drug prescriptions

Pharmacists may supply Schedule 2 or 3 Controlled Drugs (excluding temazepam) if the prescription contains a minor typographical error or spelling mistake. A supply can also be made if the total quantity of the preparation or the number of dosage units (as the case may be) is specified on the prescription in either words or figures, but not both. Pharmacists can make a supply against a prescription containing these technical errors provided that:

(a) having exercised all due diligence, the pharmacist is satisfied on reasonable grounds that the prescription is genuine;

(b) having exercised all due diligence, the pharmacist is satisfied on reasonable grounds that he or she is supplying the drug in accordance with the intention of the person issuing the prescription;

(c) the pharmacist amends the prescription in ink or otherwise indelibly to correct the minor typographical errors or spelling mistakes or so that the prescription complies with the requirement to contain the total quantity of the preparation or the number of dosage units in both words and figures; and

(d) the pharmacist marks the prescription so that the amendment he has made under (c) is attributable to him or her.

No other amendments, such as the date, the dose and the form can be made, or added if omitted, as minor typographical errors by the pharmacist.

Supply of Controlled Drugs to misusers

A person is regarded as being addicted to a drug if, and only if, he has as a result of repeated administration become so dependent on a drug that he has an overpowering desire for the administration of it to be continued.

No doctor may administer or authorise the supply of cocaine, diamorphine or dipipanone, or their salts, to an addicted person, except for the purpose of treating organic disease or injury, unless he is licensed to do so by the Secretary of State.

There is provision for misusers to receive daily supplies of cocaine or diamorphine on special prescriptions. This is an administrative arrangement under the National Health Service and does not form part of the Misuse of Drugs legislation.

Instalment prescriptions

In the case of instalment prescriptions for Schedule 2, 3 and 4 Controlled Drugs, the first instalment must be dispensed within 28 days of the appropriate date, with the remainder of instalments dispensed in accordance with the instructions.

The 28-day period of validity starts from the appropriate date on the prescription form. The appropriate date is the later of the date of signing or a date specified by the prescriber as being the date before which the Controlled Drug should not be supplied (start date) if the prescriber wishes the 28-day period to start on a date other than the date of signing.

The start date specified can be more than 28 days from the date of signing/issue.

Although there is no legal requirement for a starting date to be specified, where one is given in the prescription, it must be complied with and the instalment directions run from that date. In every other case the instalment direction will run from the date of first dispensing of the prescription. The prescription must be marked with the date of each dispensing.

It is a legal requirement that the instalment amount **and** the dose are specified separately on the prescription. Prescriptions which contain a direction that specified instalments of the total amount may be dispensed at stated intervals must not be dispensed otherwise than in accordance with the directions.

However, the Home Office has confirmed that if specified, approved wording is included in the prescription, it will enable those supplying Controlled Drugs to issue the remainder of an instalment prescription when the person fails to collect the instalment on the specified day. **If the prescription does not reflect such wording, the Regulations only permit the supply to be in accordance with the prescriber's instalment direction.** The direction must be clear and unambiguous.

The Home Office approved wording does not appear in the Misuse of Drugs Regulations 2001, as amended, and a strict interpretation of the legislation allows no scope for dispensing a prescription for a Schedule 2 or 3 Controlled Drug outside of a prescriber's directions, ie each supply against an instalment prescription must be dispensed on the date specified on the prescription. However, the Home Office has approved wording in the past that, in their opinion, would cover a pharmacist supplying when instalments have been missed or supplies for days on which the pharmacy is closed (see below).

The approved wording is not included in legislation but the fact that the wording (see below) has been approved by the Home Office gives the dispensing pharmacist a degree of protection against the consequences of supplying against a strictly unlawful prescription. An instalment prescription that contains wording different from that approved by the Home Office would not provide the dispensing pharmacist the security conferred by a prescription containing Home Office approved wording.

If a pharmacist decides to supply against an instalment prescription that utilises wording that is not approved by the Home Office the pharmacist must be aware that they do not have the protection afforded by Home Office approved wording. Therefore, in this situation a pharmacist would be advised to get the prescription amended to reflect the Home Office approved wording. It should be noted that the Home Office no longer approve any new versions of approved wording that vary from those that already exist.

Home Office approved wording is in addition to the usual Controlled Drug prescription requirements (ie all the other prescription requirements apply).

Where Home Office approved wording is included on the prescription, allowing a reduced amount of Controlled Drug to be supplied on a day other than that specified on the prescription, the pharmacist must still use his or her professional judgment in deciding whether making the supply, less the days missed, would be appropriate.

Two versions of Home Office approved wording for use when the day for an instalment to be collected is missed are as follows:

For supervised consumption: *"Supervised consumption of daily dose on specified days; the remainder of supply to take home. If an instalment prescription covers more than one day and is not collected on the specified day, the total amount prescribed less the amount prescribed for the day(s) missed may be supplied."*

For unsupervised consumption: *"Instalment prescriptions covering more than one day should be collected on the specified day; if this collection is missed the remainder of the instalment (i.e., the instalment less the amount prescribed for the day(s) missed) may be supplied."*

Other Home Office approved wording to be used when the pharmacy is closed is given here. This approved wording will enable those supplying Controlled Drugs to issue instalments on the day immediately prior to closure should the pharmacy be closed on days when instalments are due. The wording approved by the Home Office is: *"Instalments due on days when the pharmacy is closed should be dispensed on the day immediately prior to closure."*

Where a third party collects a Controlled Drug for a patient being treated for drug addiction, although not a legal requirement it is good practice that a letter of authorisation from the patient is obtained on every occasion that the representative collects the medicine, and that the letter should be retained in the pharmacy.

National Health prescriptions for the treatment of misusers

In England, prescription form FP10(MDA) is used for instalment prescribing by both drug treatment centres and GPs. A maximum of 14 days' supply of any Schedule 2 Controlled Drug, buprenorphine and diazepam can be prescribed for the treatment of addiction using this form.

In Scotland, forms HBP(A) and HBP are issued from drug misuse centres and hospitals respectively and can be used to prescribe, in instalments, any drug used in the treatment of addiction. General practitioners may prescribe by instalment for the treatment of addiction on a GP10 of GP10-SS form. The doctor may specify that the drug should be dispensed in instalments and the prescription must comply with the Misuse of Drugs Regulations 2001, as amended.

In Wales, two types of prescription form are used for the treatment of misusers by instalment: WP10(MDA), issued by general practitioners, and WP10(HP)Ad, used principally by drug treatment centres. Up to 14 days' supply of drugs listed in Schedules 2 to 5 of the Misuse of Drugs Regulations 2001, as amended, will be reimbursed.

Cocaine, diamorphine and dipipanone can only be prescribed for the treatment of addiction by specially authorised doctors who hold a Home Office licence.

Supplying drug paraphernalia

Legislation permits practitioners, pharmacists, persons employed or engaged in the lawful provision of drug treatment services and supplementary prescribers acting under and in accordance with the terms of a clinical management plan to supply specified drug paraphernalia to illicit drug users.

The items that a pharmacist can supply are:
- swabs;
- utensils for the preparation of Controlled Drugs;
- citric acid;
- ascorbic acid; and
- filters.

Pharmacists employed or engaged in the lawful provision of a drug treatment service can supply only in the course of those services:
- ampoules of sterile water for injection (on the condition that each ampoule does not contain more than 2ml).

A pharmacist who is not engaged or employed in such services, can only supply water for injection against a prescription or under a patient group direction.

Collection of Schedule 2 and 3 Controlled Drugs

Schedule 2 and 3 Controlled Drug prescriptions have a space on the reverse of the form for the person collecting to sign. There is no legal requirement for a signature on collection, but it is good practice to obtain one. The pharmacist must exercise their discretion as to whether or not to make a supply if the collector does not sign the back of the prescription.

Patients who collect their prescription in instalments via an FP10 (MDA) or equivalent are not required to sign for each instalment, nor will a third party collecting the CD on the patient's behalf. However, it would be good practice to have the back of the prescription signed on at least one occasion.

The patient may nominate a person to sign the back of the prescription on their behalf, who could be a delivery driver, or another representative. There should be a robust audit trail in place to show the successful delivery to the patient.

On collection of a Schedule 2 Controlled Drug, it is a legal requirement for the pharmacist asked to supply the drug on the prescription, to ascertain whether the person collecting is the patient, the patient's representative or a healthcare professional acting in their professional capacity on behalf of the patient.

Where a patient or their representative (other than a healthcare professional acting in their professional capacity) is collecting the Controlled Drug, the pharmacist may request evidence of that person's identity, and may refuse to make the supply if he is not satisfied as to the identity of that person.

Where a healthcare professional acting in their capacity as such is collecting the Controlled Drug on behalf of the patient, the pharmacist must obtain the healthcare professional's name and address, and unless acquainted with that professional, must request evidence of that professional's identity. The pharmacist may proceed with the supply even if he is not satisfied as to the healthcare professional's identity.

The Home Office has indicated that ID fields of the CDR should be completed in the case of supplies made against requisitions as well as against prescriptions.

Details regarding the person collecting Schedule 2 Controlled Drugs must be recorded in the Controlled Drug

Register (CDR). (*See* below and also table on p41 for further information.)

When a delivery driver is taking a dispensed Schedule 2 CD to a patient, either at their own home or in a care home, his/her details should be entered in the CD register. The delivery driver would be classed as the patient's representative. However, the pharmacy may wish to annotate the register to show that the person collecting was the delivery driver.

The requirements to check ID apply where Schedule 2 CDs are supplied. In a hospital, the porter should be asked for ID unless they are already known by the pharmacist, but legislation does not require the porter's name and address to be recorded.

Controlled Drug registers

Records must be kept by pharmacists of all Schedule 1 (except Sativex) and 2 Controlled Drugs received or supplied. The headings under which information must be recorded in the Controlled Drug register are as follows:

For Controlled Drugs obtained, the following must be recorded:
(a) date supply received;
(b) name and address from whom received;
(c) quantity received.

For Controlled Drugs supplied, the following must be recorded:
(a) date supplied;
(b) name/address of person or firm supplied;
(c) details of authority to possess – prescriber or licence holder's details;
(d) quantity supplied;
(e) person collecting Schedule 2 Controlled Drug (patient/patient's representative/healthcare professional), and if a healthcare professional collecting a Schedule 2 Controlled Drug, their name and address;
(f) was proof of identity requested of patient / patient's representative (Yes/No);
(g) was proof of identity of person collecting provided (Yes/No).

These particulars are the minimum fields of information that must be recorded in the Controlled Drug register. The regulations allow additional related information to be recorded. The proof of identity and evidence seen requirements apply to all CDRs that are required by legislation (ie, even to registered retail hospital pharmacy CDRs).

The following points must be complied with in relation to the keeping of Controlled Drug registers:
(a) Entries must be in chronological sequence.
(b) A separate register or separate part of the register must be used for each class of drugs. NB - Separate sections are required for amphetamines (which includes dexamphetamine) and methylamphetamine.
(c) In the separate register or separate part of the register used for each class of drug, a separate page shall be used for each strength and form of that drug.
(d) The class of the drug, its strength and form must be specified at the head of each page.
(e) Entries must be made on the day of the transaction or on the next day following.
(f) No cancellation, obliteration or alteration may be made; correction must be dated by marginal note or footnote.

(g) Entries must be in ink or otherwise indelible, or shall be in a computerised form.
(h) The computerised form must ensure every such entry is attributable and capable of being audited. Electronic Controlled Drug registers must comply with best practice guidance.
(i) The register must be kept at the premises to which it is related and a separate register must be kept for each premises of the business. Where the register is in computerised form, it must be accessible from those premises.
(j) With Home Office approval, separate registers may be kept for each department of a business.
(k) Particulars of stocks, receipts and supplies must be furnished to any authorised person on request (this includes inspectors of the Royal Pharmaceutical Society and Controlled Drug liaison officers). Other documents and stocks of drugs must also be produced if required.
(l) Registers must be kept for two years from the last date of entry.
(m) Records must be kept in their original form or copied and kept in an approved computerised form.
(n) A copy of the register, in its computerised or other specified form may be requested to be sent to persons authorised by the Secretary of State (eg, the Society's Inspectors).

Entries made in respect of drugs obtained and drugs supplied may be made on the same page or on separate pages in the register.

The following is good practice in relation to the keeping of Controlled Drug registers:

(a) It is good practice that all Controlled Drug registers contain a running balance.
(b) Where an entry has been made in the Controlled Drug register no entry need be made in the prescription-only register under the Medicines Act 1968, but it is good practice to make such entries.

Electronic Controlled Drugs registers

As an alternative to a bound book, pharmacists may elect to keep their Controlled Drug register electronically. They must be capable of printing or displaying the name, form and strength of the drug in such a way that the details appear at the top of each display or printout to comply with the new Regulations. Electronic Controlled Drug registers must also comply with best practice guidance. Current best practice guidance states that:
(a) Registers may only be kept in computerised form if safeguards are incorporated into the software to ensure all of the following:
    - the author of each entry is identifiable;
    - entries cannot be altered at a later date;
    - a log of all data entered is kept and can be recalled for audit purposes.
(b) Access control systems should be in place to minimise the risk of unauthorised or unnecessary access to the data in computerised registers.
(c) Adequate backups must be made of computerised registers.
(d) Arrangements should be made so that Inspectors can examine computerised registers during a visit with minimum disruption to the dispensing process.

The most up to date guidance can be found at the National Prescribing Centre website at (www.npc.co.uk) or on the Society's website at (www.rpsgb.org).

Controlled Drugs and supplementary prescribing

A supplementary prescriber is permitted, when acting under and in accordance with the terms of a clinical management plan (CMP) to administer and/or supply or direct any person to administer Controlled Drugs in Schedules 2, 3, 4 and 5.

In England, supplementary prescribers use FP10MDA-SS or FP10MDA-SP prescription forms for drug misusers, and FP10SP and FP10SS prescription forms for general practice patients. In Wales, WP10SP, WP10SP-SS and WP10HSP prescription forms are issued by supplementary prescribers for general practice patients and hospital outpatients. In Scotland, GP10(N), GP10(N)SS and HBPN prescription forms are issued by nurse supplementary prescribers for general practice patients and hospital outpatients. In Scotland, GP10P and HBPP prescription forms are issued by pharmacist supplementary prescribers for general practice patients and hospital outpatients.

Controlled Drugs and nurse independent prescribers

Currently, nurse independent prescribers are permitted to prescribe, supply, administer or direct any other person to administer the following Controlled Drugs, solely for the medical conditions indicated:

(a) Diamorphine hydrochloride (orally or parenterally), morphine hydrochloride (rectally), morphine sulphate (orally, parenterally or rectally), or oxycodone hydrochloride (orally or parenterally) for use in palliative care;
(b) Buprenorphine (by transdermal route) or fentanyl (by transdermal route) in palliative care;
(c) Diamorphine hydrochloride (orally or parenterally), or morphine hydrochloride (rectally), morphine sulphate (orally, parenterally or rectally) for pain relief in respect of suspected myocardial infarction or for relief of acute or severe pain after trauma, including in either case post-operative pain relief;
(d) Chlordiazepoxide hydrochloride (orally) and diazepam (orally, parenterally or rectally) for treatment of initial or acute alcohol withdrawal symptoms;
(e) Codeine phosphate (orally), dihydrocodeine tartrate (orally) and co-phenotrope (orally) (no restriction on medical conditions).
(f) Diazepam (orally, parenterally or rectally), lorazepam (orally or parenterally) or midazolam (parenterally or via buccal route) for use in palliative care or treatment of tonic-clonic seizures.

This situation is currently being changed. Further guidance will be issued following the amendments to legislation.

In England, independent nurse prescribers use FP10P prescription forms for general practice patients and FP10SS for hospital outpatients. In Wales, independent nurse prescribers use WP10PN prescription forms for general practice patients, WP10IP by hospital independent prescribers, WP10CN by community nurses and WP10HP for hospital outpatients. In Scotland, independent nurse prescribers use GP10(N) prescription forms for general practice patients and HBPN for hospital outpatients.

Controlled Drugs and pharmacist independent prescribers

Pharmacist independent prescribers are not currently permitted to prescribe, administer in their own right or direct the administration of Controlled Drugs. The restriction applies to all Controlled Drugs including Schedule 5 Controlled Drugs (these may appear in pharmacy only preparations that are available for over the counter sale).

This situation is currently being changed. Further guidance will be issued following the amendments to legislation.

Controlled Drugs and midwives

A registered midwife may possess diamorphine, morphine, pethidine and pentazocine in her own right so far as is necessary for the practice of her profession (see p18). Supplies of diamorphine, morphine, pethidine and pentazocine may only be made to her on the authority of a midwife's supply order signed by the "appropriate medical officer" who is a doctor authorised in writing by the local supervising authority for the region or area, or the person appointed by the local supervising authority to exercise supervision over midwives within their area. The order must be in writing and must contain the following particulars:

(a) the name of the midwife;
(b) the occupation of the midwife;
(c) the purpose for which the Controlled Drug is required:
(d) the total quantity to be obtained;
(e) the signature of the "appropriate medical officer"

A midwife is required to keep a record of supplies of diamorphine, morphine and pethidine received and administered in a book used solely for that purpose. She must not destroy surplus stock but may surrender it to the "appropriate medical officer."

The pharmacist should retain the midwives supply order for two years. As diamorphine, morphine and pethidine are Schedule 2 Controlled Drugs, an appropriate entry is required in the Controlled Drug register. Pentazocine is a Schedule 3 Controlled Drug and therefore no entry is required in the Controlled Drug register, although an entry should be made in the prescription-only register.

Controlled Drugs and operating department practitioners

An operating department practitioner (ODP) may, when acting in their capacity as such, supply Controlled Drugs for administration to a patient in a ward, theatre or other department in accordance with the directions of a doctor, dentist, supplementary prescriber acting under and in accordance with the terms of a clinical management plan, or of a nurse independent prescriber. The Controlled Drugs to which this relates are those which have been supplied to the ODP by a person responsible for the dispensing and supply of medicines at that hospital.

The directions given by a nurse independent prescriber relate only to the limited list of Controlled Drugs which they may prescribe and are subject to restrictions on the purpose for which the drug may be prescribed (see above)

An ODP can order Schedule 2, 3, 4 and 5 controlled drugs from a hospital pharmacy. The hospital pharmacy in which the ODP is practising, can supply the ODP with these drugs. ODPs are able to possess and supply Schedule 2–5 Controlled Drugs for the purposes of administration to a patient in a ward, theatre or other department, at the hospital in which they are practising, in accordance with the directions of an appropriate practitioner for that particular drug.

Currently, when ordering Controlled Drugs from a hospital pharmacy, the ODP is under no legal obligation to provide a written requisition. However, pharmacists are advised as a matter of good practice and/or to comply with local standard operating procedures, supplies should be made on the receipt of a requisition signed by the ODP. The legislation is due to be changed to make the provision of a written requisition a legal requirement. There is no provision to allow an ODP to obtain Controlled Drugs from a community pharmacy.

Controlled Drugs and patient group directions

There are currently only three circumstances in which certain Controlled Drugs may be administered or supplied under a patient group direction (PGD). These are outlined below:
(a) A registered nurse may, when acting in her capacity as such, supply or administer diamorphine under a PGD for the treatment of cardiac pain to a person admitted as a patient to a coronary care unit or accident and emergency department of a hospital.
(b) A registered nurse, pharmacist or any of the other named healthcare professionals listed in Schedule 8 of the Misuse of Drugs Regulations 2001, as amended, may, when acting in their capacity as such, supply or administer any Schedule 5 CD in accordance with a valid PGD.
(c) A registered nurse, pharmacist or any of the other named healthcare professionals listed in Schedule 8 of the Misuse of Drugs Regulations 2001, as amended, may, when acting in their capacity as such, supply or administer any Part 1 Schedule 4 CD or midazolam in accordance with a valid PGD provided that it is not a drug in parenteral form for the treatment of addiction.

Midazolam is the only Schedule 3 Controlled Drug that can be included in a PGD. Under no other circumstances can a Controlled Drug be considered for inclusion in a PGD.

The list of Controlled Drugs that can be included in a PGD and the circumstances in which they can be supplied or administered is currently being reviewed and may be extended. Further guidance will be issued when changes in legislation have been made.

Standard operating procedures for Controlled Drugs

In England, Scotland and Wales, all healthcare providers who hold a stock of Controlled Drugs on their premises, including community pharmacies, must have up to date standard operating procedures (SOPs) in place that cover the following matters:
(a) who has access to the Controlled Drugs;
(b where the Controlled Drugs are stored;
(c) security in relation to the storage and transportation of Controlled Drugs as required by misuse of drugs legislation;
(d) disposal and destruction of Controlled Drugs;

(e) who is to be alerted if complications arise (which may include details of when and how the relevant accountable officer (see p3) (within a primary care organisation, trust or independent hospital) should be made aware of incidents); and
(f) record keeping, including:
(i) maintaining relevant Controlled Drugs registers under misuse of drugs legislation, and
(ii) maintaining a record of the Controlled Drugs specified in Schedule 2 to the Misuse of Drugs Regulations 2001, as amended, that have been returned by patients.

The Department of Health (in England) has issued guidance giving more detailed advice on the areas that may need to be covered by the SOP. The guidance is entitled the "Safer management of Controlled Drugs: guidance on standard operating procedures for Controlled Drugs" and is available on the Department of Health website at *www.dh.gov.uk*. The Scottish Executive Health Department has also issued more detailed advice in the document "Safer management of Controlled Drugs: standard operating procedures", which is available on *www.sehd.scot.nhs.uk*. The Department for Health and Social Services in Wales will issue guidance on what should be covered by SOPs in Wales in the near future.

Although the recording of patient returned Controlled Drugs is not a current legal requirement in relation to the Misuse of Drugs Regulations 2001, as amended, the Controlled Drugs (Supervision of Management and Use) Regulations 2006 and Controlled Drugs (Supervision of Management and Use) (Wales) Regulations 2008 as described in (f)(ii), above, require SOPs to be in place for maintaining a record of Schedule 2 Controlled Drugs that have been returned by patients.

Pharmacists are therefore advised to keep a record of patient returned Schedule 2 Controlled Drugs, and their destruction, and to ensure that another member of staff, preferably a pharmacist or pharmacy technician if available, witnesses the destruction. The record of destruction should be made somewhere other than the Controlled Drug register, for example at the back of the private prescription register or in a separate book designated for that purpose.

It is recommended that the following details are recorded:
• the date of return of the Controlled Drugs;
• details of the Controlled Drugs:
(i) name of the Controlled Drug
(ii) quantity of the Controlled Drug;
(iii) strength of the Controlled Drug; and
(iv) form of the Controlled Drug;
• the role of the person who returned the Controlled Drugs (if known);
• the name and signature of the person who received the Controlled Drugs;
• the patient's name and address (if known);
• the names, positions and signatures of:
(i) the person destroying the Controlled Drugs; and
(ii) the person witnessing the destruction; and
• the date of destruction.

The recommendation is that these records be retained for a period of at least seven years.

Forms to record these details are available from the Society's website, *www.rpsgb.org*. Other bodies, organisations and suppliers may produce a record book specifically designed for this purpose.

Marking of containers for Controlled Drugs

A container in which a Controlled Drug other than a preparation is supplied must be plainly marked with the amount of drug contained in it.

If the drug is a preparation made up into tablets, capsules or other dosage units, the container must be marked with the amount of Controlled Drug(s) in each dosage unit and the number of dosage units in it. For any other kind of preparation, the container must be marked with the total amount of the preparation in it and the percentage of each of its components which are Controlled Drugs in the preparation.

These requirements do not apply to certain Schedule 3 Controlled Drugs, Schedule 4 and 5 Controlled Drugs, to poppy straw, to the supply of a Controlled Drug by or on the prescription of a practitioner or supplementary prescriber, to the supply of a Controlled Drug for administration in a clinical trial or a medicinal test on animals, or any exempt products.

Destruction of Controlled Drugs

Obsolete, expired and unwanted stock Controlled Drugs

Until they can be destroyed, obsolete, expired and unwanted stock CDs requiring safe custody, according to arrangements appropriate to their Schedule, must be kept segregated from other CDs in the CD cupboard. Stock CDs awaiting destruction must be clearly marked in order to minimise the risk of errors and inadvertent supply to patients.

Pharmacists (and persons conducting a retail pharmacy business) that produce (ie, manufacture or compound) Schedule 3 and Schedule 4 Controlled Drugs, or import or export Schedule 3 and Schedule 4 Controlled Drugs are required to keep records relating to this activity. Therefore, they must have the destruction of these drugs witnessed, as must those persons licensed by the Home Office to produce and supply these items.

The Home Office has advised that Schedule 2, 3 and 4 Part I Controlled Drugs must be denatured before being placed into waste containers.

The destruction of Schedule 5 Controlled Drugs (stock and patient returned medication) does not need to be witnessed by an authorised person, regardless of the activity.

Particulars of the drug name, form and strength, the date of destruction, and the quantity destroyed must be entered in the register of Controlled Drugs and signed by the authorised person in whose presence the drug is destroyed. The authorised person may take a sample of the drug which is to be destroyed.

The master of a ship or the installation manager of an offshore installation may not destroy any surplus drugs, but must make arrangements to dispose of these items by surrendering it to a constable or contacting the appropriate authority to arrange disposal.

There are conditions on the storage of waste in general that apply to all waste (including waste Controlled Drugs), that must be adhered to. The regulatory authority for waste legislation in England and Wales is the Environment Agency (08708 506506); in Scotland it is the Scottish Environment Protection Agency (01786 457700). They should be contacted for further advice on methods of destruction and for further guidance and information on waste storage conditions. The

Home Office should also be contacted for further advice on methods of destruction.

Authorised witness

Certain persons are required by the Regulations to keep records of certain Controlled Drugs obtained and supplied. Pharmacists are required to keep records of Schedule 1 and 2 drugs obtained and supplied. Therefore they may only destroy their stock of such drugs (including out of date stock) in the presence of a person authorised as a witness by the Secretary of State either personally or as a member of a class. The latter includes inspectors of the Royal Pharmaceutical Society and Controlled Drugs liaison officers (certain police officers). The following people are also among those authorised to witness the destruction of Controlled Drugs: chief executives of NHS trusts and medical directors of primary care trusts in England; Chief Dental Officer of the Department of Health or a senior dental officer to whom authority has been delegated; senior officers in an NHS trust who report directly to the trust Chief Executive and who have responsibility for health and safety, security or risk management matters in the trust; primary care trust Chief Pharmacist or pharmaceutical/prescribing adviser who reports directly to the Chief Executive or to a director of the primary care trust. A list of the groups of people authorised to witness the destruction of Controlled drugs can be found at *www.dh.gov.uk/assetRoot/04/13/97/03/04139703.pdf*

In addition to a Secretary of State, accountable officers (*see* p3) are able to authorise a person or class of persons to be an authorised witness. An accountable officer however must not be an authorised witness. Any person nominated to witness destruction should have appropriate training and be accountable for this activity directly to the accountable officer. Practitioners who are actively involved in the day-to-day management of CDs should not be asked to witness the destruction of CDs in that GP practice. A list of accountable officers in England can be found on the Care Quality Commission website, *www.cqc.org.uk*

In Scotland the classes of people currently authorised by the Secretary of State to witness the destruction of CDs is currently being updated. However accountable officers can authorise certain individuals to witness the destruction of CDs. A list of accountable officers in Scotland can be found at *www.sehd.scot.nhs.uk/mels/CEL2009_07.pdf*

In Wales, pharmacists should contact their local health board or NHS trust to determine who is authorised to witness the destruction of Controlled Drugs.

Patient-returned Controlled Drugs

Currently, a pharmacist (or a practitioner) may destroy Controlled Drugs returned to him by a patient or a patient's representative, from their own homes or from care homes providing residential care without the presence of an authorised person. Such Controlled Drugs must not be returned to stock.

Pharmacies in England and Wales are not able to accept waste medicines, including Controlled Drugs, from care homes that provide nursing care or CDs produced by a doctor, dentist, vet, midwife or nurse. However, in Scotland, pharmacies are able to accept a range of waste, including CDs, from individuals, households and "Care services" as defined by Section 2 of the Regulation of Care (Scotland) Act 2001. It

Table A: Summary of legal requirements for Controlled Drugs as they apply to pharmacists

	Schedule 2	Schedule 3	Schedule 4, Part I	Schedule 4, Part II	Schedule 5
Designation as shown in Alphabetical list of medicines for human use	CD POM	CD No Reg POM	CD Benz POM	CD Anab POM	CD Inv P or CD Inv POM
Prescription requirements (see Note A1)	Yes	Yes, except temazepam	No	No	No
Validity of prescription (see Note A2)	28 days	28 days	28 days	28 days	6 months (if POM)
Address of prescriber must be in the UK	Yes	Yes	No	No	No
Repeats allowed on prescription	No	No	Yes	Yes	Yes
Emergency supplies allowed	No	No, except phenobarbitone for epilepsy	Yes	Yes	Yes
Requisitions necessary (see Note A3)	Yes	Yes	No	No	No
Requisition to be marked by the supplier (see Note A4)	Yes	Yes	No	No	No
Requisition to be sent to relevant NHS agency (see Note A5)	Yes	Yes	No	No	No
Invoices to be retained for two years	No	Yes	No	No	Yes
Safe custody	Yes, except quinalbarbitone	Yes, but see exemptions under "Safe custody of Controlled Drugs" (p30)	No	No	No
Licences required for import and export	Yes	Yes	Yes	Yes, unless the substance is in the form of a medicine and for administration by a person to himself	No

Notes

A1. *Prescription requirements:* This refers to the particulars which must be present for a prescription to be valid as a prescription for a Controlled Drug, ie, it must include dose, form, strength (where appropriate) and a total quantity of the preparation in both words and figures (see also p32). These requirements do not apply to temazepam prescriptions, which need only comply with the usual prescription requirements for prescription-only medicines (see p11)

A2. *Validity of prescriptions:* Where a drug in Schedule 4 is prescribed on a repeatable prescription, the first supply must be made within 28 days of the date of issue, or the appropriate date specified by the prescriber as the valid period for that drug. An NHS repeatable prescription for a Schedule 4 Controlled Drug is valid for 12 months. Where a drug in Schedule 5 is prescribed on a repeatable prescription, the first supply must be made within six months of the date of issue of the prescription

A3. *Requisitions necessary:* ie, whether a requisition is necessary before supply may be made to practitioners, persons in charge of hospitals, masters of ships, etc (see also p30)

A4. *Requisitions to be marked by the supplier:* On receipt of a requisition for a Schedule 2 or 3 CD, it should be marked with the supplying pharmacy's name and address. The Home Office has confirmed that a pharmacy stamp can be used to mark these details on the requisition. This does not apply where the supplier is a pharmacist in a hospital or a care home, or where it is a veterinary requisition (see p31)

A5 *Requisitions to be sent to relevant NHS agency:* Requisitions for Schedule 2 or 3 CDs should be sent to the relevant NHS agency in accordance with arrangements specified by that agency. This does not apply where the supplier is a pharmacist in a hospital or a care home, or where it is a veterinary requisition (see p31)

should be noted however that the definition of "care services" may exclude certain NHS premises.

Although recording of patient-returned CDs is not a current legal requirement in relation to the Misuse of Drugs Regulations 2001, as amended, The Controlled Drugs (Supervision of Management and Use) Regulations 2006 and The Controlled Drugs (Supervision of Management and Use) (Wales) Regulations 2008 require standard operating procedures to be in place for maintaining a record of the CDs specified in Schedule 2 that have been returned by patients.

Pharmacists are therefore advised to record patient returned Schedule 2 CDs and their destruction, and to ensure another member of staff, preferably a pharmacist or pharmacy technician if available, witnesses the destruction.

The record of destruction should currently be made somewhere other than the CD register, for example, at the back of the private prescription register or in a separate book designated for that purpose (see "Standard operating procedures for Controlled Drugs", p38, for details of what should be recorded). The Society recommends that these records be retained

Table B: Additional requirements for private prescriptions for Controlled Drugs

	Schedule 2	Schedule 3	Schedule 4, Part I	Schedule 4, Part II	Schedule 5
Private prescriber identification number required on private prescription (*see* Note B1)	Yes	Yes	No	No	No
Private CD prescriptions to be written only on standardised form (*see* Note B2)	Yes	Yes	No	No	No
Private CD prescription forms to be sent to relevant NHS agency (*see* Note B3)	Yes	Yes	No	No	No

Notes

B1. *Private prescriber identification number:* This number is required on private prescriptions for human use intended to be dispensed in community. Private prescriptions for temazepam must also contain the prescriber's identification number

B2. *Private prescription standardised forms:* Private prescriptions for human use intended to be dispensed in community must be issued on the relevant standardised form. Private prescriptions for temazepam must also be on the standardised form

B3. *Submission of private CD prescriptions:* The original of a Schedule 2 or 3 private CD prescription for human use must be sent to the relevant NHS agency in accordance with their arrangements for collection and analysis purposes (*see* p31)

Table C: Requirements for record keeping of Controlled Drugs

	Schedule 2	Schedule 3	Schedule 4, Part I	Schedule 4, Part II	Schedule 5
Records to be kept in CD register	Yes	No	No	No	No
Pharmacist must ascertain the identity of the person collecting CD (*see* Note C1)	Yes	No	No	No	No
Pharmacist must record in the CD register whether the person collecting is the patient, the patient's representative or a healthcare professional	Yes	No	No	No	No
Pharmacist must record in the CD register, where the person collecting is a healthcare professional, their name and address (*see* Note C2)	Yes	No	No	No	No
Pharmacist must record in the CD register whether proof of identity was requested of the patient/ patient's representative	Yes	No	No	No	No
Pharmacist must record in the CD register whether proof of identity was provided by the person collecting)	Yes	No	No	No	No

Notes

C1. *Identity of person collecting:* The pharmacist must ascertain the role of anyone collecting a Schedule 2 Controlled Drug. It must be ascertained whether the person is the patient, the patient's representative or a healthcare professional acting within their professional capacity as such. If a healthcare professional is collecting, their name and address (which may be their professional/work address) must be obtained and if they are not known to the pharmacist, ID must be requested (*see* p35)

C2. *Healthcare professional collecting:* The name and address of the healthcare professional collecting a Schedule 2 CD must be recorded in the CD register. The Home Office has confirmed that this may be their professional/work address.

for a period of at least seven years. Forms to record these details are available from the Society's website at *www.rpsgb.org.uk/pdfs/restooldestrcd.pdf*

The requirement for safe custody for certain Controlled Drugs applies equally to patient returned Controlled Drugs, which until such time that they can be denatured and be ren-

dered irretrievable, must be kept in the Controlled Drug cabinet. Patient returned Controlled Drugs must be kept segregated from stock Controlled Drugs, and clearly marked as such to minimise the risk of errors and inadvertent supply.

As the quantity of Controlled Drugs being returned can often pose a storage problem as well as an increased security risk, pharmacists are encouraged to destroy patient returned Controlled Drugs as soon as possible, as they currently do not require an authorised witness.

England and Wales

The Hazardous Waste (England and Wales) Regulations 2005 only allow community pharmacists in England and Wales to accept patient returned medication which is classified as household waste. For further information *see* Section 1.2.13: Handling of waste medicines (p27-28).

Schedule 3 to the Waste Management Licensing Regulations 1994 has been revoked and replaced by Schedule 3 to the Environmental Permitting (England and Wales) Regulations 2007 which contains an updated list of the exemptions.

The Environment Agency has confirmed that the sorting of waste medicines and denaturing (destruction) of Controlled Drugs returned to a pharmacy from households and by individuals is a "low risk waste activity". The Agency has stated that it does not believe it is in the public interest to expect pharmacies to obtain an environmental permit for these activities. The Environment Agency, however, emphasises that it may amend or revoke its position at any time and will continue to consider enforcement in all circumstances where an activity has or is likely to cause pollution or harm to health.

Controlled Drug waste from a care home providing nursing care (previously this would have been designated as a nursing home) or produced by a doctor, dentist, vet, midwife or nurse would be classed as industrial waste and would require licences for the storage and treatment (destruction) of that waste from the Environment Agency. Therefore, a pharmacy which does not hold such licences, cannot accept this type of waste for destruction and disposal.

Scotland

In Scotland, pharmacies should register an exemption under paragraph 39 of Schedule 3 to the Waste Management Licensing Regulations 1994 (as amended) with the Scottish Environment Protection Agency (SEPA). The exemption covers the secure storage of CDs at a pharmacy prior to subsequent collection and disposal. SEPA has currently accepted that the denaturing of CDs forms part of the exempt activity of secure storage. However, SEPA may reconsider this position and pursue enforcement action if the denaturing activity causes, or is likely to cause, pollution of the environment or harm to human health.

Waste regulations in Scotland (the Waste Management Licensing Amendment (Scotland) Regulations 2006) allow pharmacies to accept a range of waste, including CDs, from individuals, households and "Care Services" as defined by section 2 of the Regulation of Care (Scotland) Act 2001, without the need for a waste management licence, subject to certain conditions. It should be noted however that the definition of "care services" may exclude certain NHS premises. For a list of "care services" from which pharmacies in Scotland may accept returned waste, *see* Section 1.2.13, p28

Methods and procedures

All medicines should be disposed of in a safe and appropriate manner. Medicines should be disposed of in relevant waste containers which are then sent for incineration and should not be disposed of in the sewerage system. All CDs in Schedule 2, 3 and 4 (Part I) must be rendered irretrievable (ie by denaturing) before being placed into waste containers. Wherever practicable, pharmacists are advised to use CD denaturing kits in order to denature CDs. CD denaturing kits can be obtained from some PCOs and waste contractors. Pharmacists should ensure that where alternative methods are used to denature Controlled Drugs, these should protect the environment and workers who might be affected by this activity.

Controlled Drugs should be deblistered and then denatured. In England and Wales, deblistering is only permitted by the Environment Agency for Controlled Drugs, in order to remove the solid dosage form from the loose blister strip or tablet bottle, in order to denature the drug and render it irretrievable.

Tablets and capsules should be removed from their outer packaging, removed from blister packaging and placed in a CD denaturing kit. Best practice would be to use a commercially produced CD denaturing kit to ensure that whole tablets or capsules are not readily recoverable. An alternative method of denaturing is to crush/grind the solid dose formulation and place it into a small amount of hot, soapy water ensuring that the drug has been dissolved or dispersed. The resultant mixture should then be placed in an appropriate waste disposal bin.

Controlled Drug liquids can be added to the normal CD denaturing kit where it will mix with the other waste materials, thus rendering it irretrievable. An alternative method of disposing of a large quantity of a liquid controlled drug is by adding and adsorbing it into an appropriate amount of cat litter, or similar product in accordance with Health and Safety regulations. The cat litter or similar product should be disposed of for incineration via the usual waste disposal methods for medicines.

Fentanyl and buprenorphine patches should have the backing removed and the patch folded over onto itself and placed in the waste disposal bin, or preferably a Controlled Drug denaturing kit.

Ampoules should be opened, the liquid poured into the Controlled Drug denaturing kit and the ampoule itself be put in the sharps bin. An ampoule that contains powder can have water added to it to dissolve the powder, and the resulting mixture can be poured into the Controlled Drug denaturing kit.

Aerosol formulations should be expelled into water (to prevent droplets of drug entering the air) and the resultant liquid disposed of as a liquid formulation.

For further information and advice on safe methods of destruction and precautions to be followed, see the guidance document "Guidance for Pharmacists on the safe destruction of Controlled Drugs, England, Scotland and Wales" on the Society's website *www.rpsgb.org*.

Summary of legal requirements for possession and supply of Controlled Drugs

The tables on pp40-41 summarise the legal requirements of the Regulations for Schedules 2 to 5 for the possession and supply of Controlled Drugs by pharmacists.

1.3: Alphabetical list of medicines for human use

This list of medicines for human use brings together medicines listed in the "Prescription Only Medicines" Order, the "General Sale List" Order and the Misuse of Drugs Regulations 2001. Generic medicines not specifically named in legislation are listed with the legal status granted under the marketing authorisation of the proprietary products in which they are contained.

However, changes to the reclassification procedure for medicines since 2003 mean that the legal status of a product now becomes part of its marketing authorisation rather than being determined by the active substance listed in secondary legislation.

Because a change of legal status will be conferred only on products that are the subject of an application for reclassification, users of this list should refer to the entry for the specific proprietary product and not rely on the entry for the active substance.

Since the POM Order remains in force, entries for active substances will remain in the list but will include cross references wherever proprietary products have been reclassified.

Further guidance or clarification on the status of individual products can be obtained from manufacturers or from the Medicines and Healthcare products Regulatory Agency (tel 020 7084 2000; e-mail info@mhra.gsi.gov.uk; website *www.mhra.gov.uk*).

The Royal Pharmaceutical Society's Legal and Ethical Advisory Service welcomes, in writing, details of any errors or omissions in this list.

KEY TO ANNOTATIONS

CD Lic: A substance controlled by the Misuse of Drugs Act 1971 to which the restrictions of the Regulations apply and, in addition, the production, possession and supply of which is limited in the public interest to purposes of research or other special purposes. A Home Office licence is required for such purposes. CD Lic substances are listed in Schedule 1 of the Misuse of Drugs Regulations 2001, as amended

CD POM: A substance controlled by the Misuse of Drugs Act 1971 to which the principal restrictions of the Misuse of Drugs Regulations 2001 apply. CD POM substances are listed in Schedule 2 of the Misuse of Drugs Regulations 2001, as amended

CD No Register POM: A substance controlled by the Misuse of Drugs Act 1971 to which the restrictions of the Regulations apply except that no entry in the Controlled Drugs Register is required and invoices must be retained for two years. CD No Register POM substances are listed in Schedule 3 of the Misuse of Drugs Regulations 2001, as amended

CD Benz POM: A substance controlled by the Misuse of Drugs Act 1971 to which the restrictions of the Regulations apply but with the following relaxation: prescription and labelling requirements do not apply (except those under the Medicines Act 1968), records in the CD register need not be kept by retailers, destruction requirements apply only to importers, exporters and manufacturers, there are no safe custody requirements. CD Benz POM substances are listed in Schedule 4, Part I of the Misuse of Drugs Regulations 2001, as amended

CD Anab POM: A substance controlled by the Misuse of Drugs Act 1971 to which the restrictions of the Regulations apply but with the following relaxation: prescription and labelling requirements do not apply (except those under the Medicines Act 1968), records in the CD register need not be kept by retailers, destruction requirements apply only to importers, exporters and manufacturers, there are no safe custody requirements. There is no restriction on possession when contained in a medicinal product. A Home Office import or export licence is required for the importation and exportation of these substances, unless they are imported or exported in the form of a medicinal product by a person for administration to himself. CD Anab POM substances are listed in Schedule 4, Part II of the Misuse of Drugs Regulations 2001, as amended

CD Inv. POM: A substance controlled by the Misuse of Drugs Act 1971 but which is exempt from all restrictions under the Regulations except that the invoice or a copy of it must be kept for two years. CD Inv. POM substances are listed in Schedule 5 of the Misuse of Drugs Regulations 2001, as amended

POM: A substance which, by virtue of an entry in the Prescription Only Medicines (Human Use) Order 1997, as amended, or by virtue of its marketing authorisation may be sold or supplied to the public only on a practitioner's prescription or in accordance with another legal authority, eg, patient group direction

P: A substance which is a pharmacy medicine by virtue of its marketing authorisation or a substance which is not subject to the prescription-only requirements of the Prescription Only Medicines (Human Use) Order 1997, as amended, and which is not included in the Medicines (Products Other Than Veterinary Drugs) (General Sale List) Order 1984, as amended

GSL: A substance which is licensed as a general sale list medicine or one which is described in the Medicines (Products Other Than Veterinary Drugs) (General Sale List) Order 1984, as amended, made under the Medicines Act 1968

PO: A substance which contains GSL ingredients but is licensed for sale through pharmacies only

md (maximum dose), ie, the maximum quantity of the substance contained in the amount of a medicinal product which is recommended to be taken or administered at any one time

mdd (maximum daily dose), ie, the maximum quantity of the substance that is contained in the amount of a medicinal product which is recommended to be taken or administered in any period of 24 hours

ms (maximum strength), ie, either or, if so specified, both of the following: (a) the maximum quantity of the substance by weight or volume that is contained in the dosage unit of a medicinal product; or (b) the maximum percentage of the substance contained in a medicinal product calculated in terms of w/w, w/v, v/w or v/v, as appropriate

External use means for application to the skin, teeth, mucosa of the mouth, throat, nose, eye, ear, vagina or anal canal when a local action only is necessary and extensive systemic absorption is unlikely to occur.
Note: The following are not regarded as for external use: throat sprays, throat pastilles, throat lozenges, throat tablets, nasal drops, nasal sprays, nasal inhalations or teething preparations

Parenteral administration means administration by breach of the skin or mucous membrane

A

A and P infant powders GSL
AAA mouth and throat spray P
Abacavir POM
Abciximab POM
Abelcet infusion POM
Abidec drops GSL
Abietis oil GSL
Abilify preparations POM
Abraxane POM
Abstral sublingual tablets CD POM
Abtrim P
AC Vax POM
Acamprosate tablets POM
Acarbose POM
Accolate tablets POM
Accupro tablets POM
Accuretic tablets POM
Accusite injectable gel POM
Acebutolol hydrochloride POM
Acea gel POM
Aceclofenac tablets POM
Acemetacin POM
Acenocoumarol/Nicoumalone POM
Acepril tablets POM
Acepromazine POM
Acepromazine maleate POM
Acerola GSL
Acetanilide POM
Acetarsol POM
Acetazolamide POM
Acetazolamide sodium POM
Acetic acid, if internal use maximum
    strength 7.5 per cent or external use
    maximum strength 15.0 per cent
    GSL
Acetohexamide POM
Acetone, external use only GSL
Acetorphine; its salts, esters and ethers
    CD POM
Acetylcholine chloride POM but if
    external use and maximum strength
    0.2 per cent, P
Acetylcysteine POM
Acetyldihydrocodeine CD POM
Acezide tablets POM
Achromycin ear/eye ointment POM
Achromycin preparations POM
Aci-Jel GSL
Aciclovir POM but if external for treat-
    ment of herpes simplex virus infec-
    tions of the lips and face (Herpes
    labialis) and maximum strength 5.0
    per cent, and container or package
    contains not more than 2g of medic-
    inal product, P or GSL. Please refer to
    proprietary names for the classifica-
    tion granted under the marketing
    authorisation (See Zovirax products)
Acid-eze tablets P
Acidex GSL
Acipimox POM
Acitak tablets P
Acitretin POM
Aclacin POM
Aclarubicin hydrochloride POM
Aclasta solution for infusion POM
Acnamino MR POM
Acnecide gel 10% P
Acnecide gel 5% P
Acnidazil cream P
Acnisal P
Acnocin tablets POM
Acoflam Retard tablets POM
Acoflam SR tablets POM
Acoflam tablets POM
Acomplia POM
Aconite POM but if external and maxi-
    mum strength 1.3 per cent, P
Acorvio P
Acorvio plus POM
Acriflex cream GSL
Acrivastine POM but if 24 mg (MDD)
    and container or package containing
    not more than 240mg of acrivastine,
    P; if for internal use for the sympto-
    matic relief of allergic rhinitis,

including hayfever, and chronic idio-
    pathic urticaria in adults and chil-
    dren 12-65 years with a maximum
    strength of 8mg, 8mg (MD) 24mg
    (MDD) in a pack containing no more
    than 21 doses (168mg acrivastine),
    GSL. Please refer to proprietary
    names for the classification granted
    under the marketing authorisation
    (see Benadryl Allergy Relief products)
Acrosoxacin POM
ACT-HIB POM
ACT-HIB DTP POM
Actal pastils PO
Actal tablets GSL
ACTH injection POM
Actidose Aqua Advance suspension P
Actidose Aqua suspension P
Actifed Chesty P
Actifed Linctus CD Inv P
Actifed syrup P
Actifed tablets P
Actilyse POM
Actinac POM
Actinomycin C POM
Actinomycin D POM
Actinomycin D inj POM
Actiq lozenges CD POM
Activated Attapulgite GSL
Activated dimeticone/dimethicone GSL
Actonel Combi preparations POM
Actonel Once a Week tablets POM
Actonel tablets POM
Actonorm gel P
Actonorm powder P
Actos tablets POM
Actrapid insulins POM
Acular ophthalmic solution POM
Acumed patch GSL
Acupan preparations POM
ACWY Vax vaccine POM
Adalat capsules POM
Adalat LA tablets POM
Adalat Retard tablets POM
Adalimumab POM
Adapalene gel POM
Adartrel tablets POM
Adcal chewable tablets P
Adcal D3 P
Adcortyl in Orabase POM
Adcortyl in Orabase for mouth ulcers
    (PL 0034/0321) P
Adcortyl preparations POM
Adcortyl with Graneodin preparations
    POM
Addamel POM
Addiphos solution POM
Additrace solution POM
Adefovir Dipivoxil POM
Adenocor injection POM
Adenoscan vials POM
Adenosine POM
Adgyn Combi tablets POM
Adgyn Estro tablets POM
Adgyn Medro tablets POM
Adios P
Adipine MR POM
Adipine XL tablets POM
Adizem SR preps POM
Adizem XL capsules POM
Adizem XL Plus capsules POM
Adrenaline POM but if (1) by inhaler,
    (2) external (except ophthalmic), P
Adrenaline acid tartrate POM but if (1)
    by inhaler, (2) external, P
Adrenaline hydrochloride POM but if
    (1) by inhaler, (2) external, P
Adrenocortical extract POM
Adsorbed diphtheria and tetanus vac-
    cine POM
Adsorbed diphtheria vaccine POM
Adsorbed diphtheria, tetanus and per-
    tussis vaccine POM
Adsorbed tetanus vaccine POM
Advate solution for injection POM
Advil cold and sinus tablets P
Advil extra strength 400mg pack sizes
    24s P

Advil tablets 200mg pack sizes 12s GSL
Advil tablets pack sizes 24s P
Aerobec Autohaler POM
Aerobec Forte Autohaler POM
Aerocrom inhaler POM
Aerocrom Syncrone POM
Aerodiol nasal spray POM
Aerolin Autohaler POM
Aerrane POM
Aezodent P
Afrazine nasal preparations GSL
After-bite GSL
Agalsidase alfa POM
Agalsidase Beta POM
Agarol P
Agenerase preparations POM
Aggrastat POM
Agnus castus (Chaste Tree) GSL
Agrimony GSL
Agrippal POM
Agropyron (triticum) GSL
Ailax Forte suspension POM
Ailax suspension POM
Air GSL
Airbron POM
Airomir autohaler POM
Airomir inhaler POM
Akineton preparations POM
Aklomide POM
Aknemin capsules POM
Aknemycin Plus POM
Albendazole POM
Albufilm GSL
Albumin Human (Immuno) POM
Albumin Human (Kabi) POM
Albumin Microspheres Human (3M)
    POM
Albuminar preps POM
Albutein preps POM
Alclofenac POM
Alclometasone dipropionate POM
Alcobon preparations POM
Alcoderm preparations P
Alcohol GSL
Alcon Isopto alkaline, eye drops P
Alcon Isopto atropine 1% eye drops
    POM
Alcon Isopto carbachol 3% eye drops
    POM
Alcon Isopto carpine 0.5%, 1%, 2%, 3%,
    4% POM
Alcon Isopto Frin, eye drops P
Alcon Isopto Plain, eye drops P
Alcon Maxidex eye drops POM
Alcon Maxitrol eye drops POM
Alcon Maxitrol oint POM
Alcon Mydriacyl 0.5% drops POM
Alcon Mydriacyl 1% drops POM
Alcon tears naturale eye drops P
Alcowipes GSL
Alcuronium chloride POM
Aldactide tablets POM
Aldactone tablets POM
Aldara cream POM
Aldesleukin POM
Aldioxa (aluminium dihydroxyallan-
    toinate), external use only GSL
Aldomet preparations POM
Aldosterone POM
Aldurazyme POM
ALEC vials POM
Alemtuzumab POM
Alendronic acid tablets POM
Alexitol sodium GSL
Alfa D capsules POM
Alfacalcidol POM
Alfentanil CD POM
Alfuzosin hydrochloride POM
Algesal cream P
Algicon tabs and suspension P
Alginic acid GSL
Algitec Chewtab POM
Algitec suspension POM
Algitec tablets POM
Alglucerase vials POM
Alimemazine/Trimeprazine POM
Alimemazine/Trimeprazine tartrate POM
Alimta POM

Alka Rapid crystals GSL
Alka-Seltzer GSL
Alka-Seltzer XS tablets GSL
Alkaline eye drops BPC P
Alkanna, external use only GSL
Alkeran preparations POM
n-Alkyl isoquinolinium bromide, exter-
    nal use only GSL
Allantoin, external use only GSL
Allegron preparations POM
Allens chesty cough GSL
Allens dry tickly cough GSL
Allens pine & honey balsam GSL
Aller-eze Plus preparations P
Aller-eze tablets P
Allergen Extracts POM
Allergy therapeutics POM
Allerief P
Allertek GSL
Allevyn Adhesive 17cm x 17cm GSL
Allevyn Lite GSL
Alli 60mg capsules P
Alloferin injection POM
Allopurinol POM
Allyloestrenol POM
Allylprodine CD POM
Almodan capsules POM
Almodan syrup POM
Almogran tablets POM
Almond oil GSL
Almotriptan POM
Aloes, Barbados, up to 50mg (MD) GSL
Aloes, Cape, up to 100mg (MD) GSL
Aloin, up to 20mg (MD) GSL
Alomide Allergy ophthalmic solution P
Alomide ophthalmic POM
Alophen pills P
Aloxiprin POM but if non-effervescent
    tablets or capsules with ms 620mg
    supplied in a container not exceed-
    ing 32 (unless the number of tablets,
    capsules or a combination of both
    supplied to a person at any one time
    exceeds 100) P; or if powders or gran-
    ules maximum strength 800mg, or
    non-effervescent tablets or capsules
    with ms 400mg supplied in a con-
    tainer not exceeding 16 (unless the
    number of tablets, capsules or a com-
    bination of both supplied to a person
    at any one time exceeds 100), GSL
    (when combined with aspirin, the
    aspirin limits apply to the combina-
    tion of aspirin and aspirin equiva-
    lent)
Alpha Keri bath oil P
Alpha tocopheryl acid succinate GSL
Alpha-pinene, external use only GSL
Alphacetylmethadol; its salts CD POM
Alphaderm cream POM
Alphadolone acetate POM
Alphagan eye drops POM
Alphaglobin POM
Alphameprodine; its salts CD POM
Alphamethadol; its salts esters and
    ethers CD POM
Alphaparin POM
Alphaprodine; its salts CD POM
Alphavase tablets POM
Alphaxalone POM
Alphosyl 2 in 1 shampoo GSL
Alphosyl cream P
Alphosyl HC cream POM
Alphosyl lotion P
Alprazolam CD Benz POM
Alprenolol POM
Alprenolol hydrochloride POM
Alprostadil POM
Alseroxylon POM
Altacite Plus suspension 500ml P
Altacite Plus suspension 100ml GSL
Altacite suspension P
Altargo POM
Alteplase inj POM
Altretamine capsules POM
Alu-Cap P
Aludrox liquid GSL

Aspirin legal status

Product	Container size	Legal status	Where it can be sold	Maximum that can be sold to a person at any one time (*see* Note 2)
Aspirin tablets (non-effervescent) and capsules up to 325mg (including 75mg preparations)	Up to 16	GSL	Pharmacies and non-pharmacy retail outlets	Not more than 100 tablets or capsules
Aspirin tablets (non-effervescent) and capsules up to 325mg (including 75mg preparations)	Between 17 and 32	P (*see* Note 3)	Pharmacies only	Not more than 100 tablets or capsules
Aspirin enteric-coated tablets up to 75mg	Up to 28	GSL	Pharmacies and non-pharmacy retail outlets	Not more than 100 tablets or capsules
Aspirin tablets (non-effervescent) and capsules up to 75mg	Between 17 and 100	P (*see* Note 3)	Pharmacies only	Not more than 100 tablets or capsules
Aspirin tablets (non-effervescent) and capsules above 325mg and up to 500mg	Up to 32	P	Pharmacies only	Not more than 100 tablets or capsules
Aspirin tablets (non-effervescent) and capsules above 325mg and up to 500mg	Greater than 32	POM	Pharmacies only	To be sold or supplied only in accordance with a prescription
Aspirin tablets (effervescent) up to 325mg (*see* Note 1)	Up to 30	GSL	Pharmacies and non-pharmacy retail outlets	No legal limit
Aspirin tablets (effervescent) up to 325mg (*see* Note 1)	Greater than 30	P (*see* Note 3)	Pharmacies only	No legal limit
Aspirin tablets (effervescent) above 325mg and up to 500mg (*see* Note 1)	Up to 20	GSL	Pharmacies and non-pharmacy retail outlets	No legal limit
Aspirin tablets (effervescent) above 325mg and up to 500mg (*see* Note 1)	Greater than 20	P (*see* Note 3)	Pharmacies only	No legal limit
Aspirin powders up to 650mg	Up to 10	GSL	Pharmacies and non-pharmacy retail outlets	No legal limit
Aspirin powders up to 650mg	Greater than 10	P (*see* Note 3)	Pharmacies only	No legal limit

Note 1: Effervescent preparations in relation to a tablet, means containing not less than 75 per cent, by weight of the tablet, of ingredients included wholly or mainly for the purpose of releasing carbon dioxide when the tablets is dissolved or dispersed in water

Note 2: While several products have no legal limit for the amount that may be sold or supplied, pharmacists are expected to exercise professional control to limit the amount of aspirin which may be stored in a patient's home

Note 3: Strictly speaking, aspirin is a POM or GSL product, but limited to sale through pharmacies under certain conditions and exemptions. Products would be pharmacy medicines unless specifically licensed otherwise

Note 4: When aspirin is in combination with a pharmacy medicine (eg, low-strength codeine) or a prescription-only medicine (eg, dextropropoxyphene), the more stringent legal category applies

Alum BP, external use only GSL
Aluminium carbonate (Basic) GSL
Aluminium glycinate GSL
Aluminium hydroxide GSL
Aluminium oxide GSL
Aluminium sulphate, external use only GSL
Alupent aerosol inhalation POM
Alupent syrup POM
Alupent tablets POM
Alvedon suppositories P
Alvercol granules P
Alverine P
Alvesco POM
Amantadine hydrochloride POM

Amaranth GSL
Amaryl tablets POM
Ambenonium chloride POM
Amber oil, external use only GSL
Ambisome injection POM
Ambutonium bromide POM
Amcinonide POM
Ametazole hydrochloride POM
Amethocaine see Tetracaine
Ametop gel P
Amfetamine/Amphetamine; its salts CD POM
Amfipen preparations POM
Amias tablets POM
Amidone see Methadone

Amidopyrine POM
Amidox tablets POM
Amifostine infusion POM
Amikacin sulphate POM
Amikin injections POM
Amil-Co tablets POM
Amilamont solution POM
Amilmaxco 5/50 tablets POM
Amiloride hydrochloride POM
Amilospare tablets POM
Aminacrine see Aminoacridine
Aminoacetic acid (Glycine) GSL

Aminoacridine/aminacrine hydrochloride, external use only GSL

Aminobenzoic acid, if internal 30mg (MD) or external GSL
Aminocaproic acid POM
Aminoglutethimide POM
Aminogran food supplement P
Aminogran mineral mixture P
Aminophylline injection BP POM
Aminoplex preparations POM
Aminopterin sodium POM
Aminorex CD Benz POM
Amiodarone hydrochloride POM
Amiphenazole hydrochloride POM
Amisulpride tablets POM
Amitriptyline POM
Amitriptyline embonate POM

Amitriptyline hydrochloride POM
Amix preps POM
Amlodipine besylate POM
Amlodipine maleate POM
Amlostin POM
Ammonaps POM
Ammonia, solutions of, up to maximum strength 5.0 per cent of NH3 (ammonia) in all preparations except smelling salts or 15.0 per cent of NH3 (ammonia) in smelling salts GSL
Ammonium acetate solution strong GSL
Ammonium bicarbonate GSL
Ammonium bromide POM
Ammonium carbonate GSL
Ammonium chloride GSL
Amnivent 225-SR tablets P
Amobarbital sodium/Amylobarbitone sodium CD No Register POM
Amobarbital/Amylobarbitone CD No Register POM
Amodiaquine hydrochloride POM
Amoram preps POM
Amorolfine hydrochloride POM; but in the form of a nail lacquer for the treatment of mild cases of distal and lateral subungual onychomycoses caused by dermatophytes, yeasts and moulds; treatment is limited to 2 nails, max strength 5% amorolfine (as the base), max pack 3ml of product, P
Amoxapine POM
Amoxicillin/Amoxycillin POM
Amoxicillin/Amoxycillin sodium POM
Amoxicillin/Amoxycillin trihydrate POM
Amoxil preparations POM
Amoxycillin see Amoxicillin
Amphetamine see Amfetamine
Amphocil infusion POM
Amphomycin calcium POM
Amphotericin POM
Ampicillin POM
Ampicillin sodium POM
Ampicillin trihydrate POM
Ampitrin preps POM
Amprenavir POM
Amsacrine POM
Amsidine preparations POM
Amyben POM
Amygdalin POM
Amyl nitrite POM but if sold or supplied by pharmacists to persons to whom cyanide salts may be sold by virtue of Section 3 (regulation of poisons) or Section 4 (exclusion of sales by wholesale and certain other sales) of the Poisons Act 1972 or by virtue of article 5 and the sale or supply shall only be so far as is necessary to enable an antidote to be available to persons at risk of cyanide poisoning P
Amylmetacresol, if internal 0.6mg (MD), or external except mouthwash maximum strength 0.5 per cent, or mouthwash maximum strength 0.001 per cent final concentration GSL

Amylobarbitone see Amobarbital
Amylobarbitone sodium see Amobarbital sodium
Amylocaine hydrochloride POM but if non-ophthalmic use P
Amyloglycosidase Concentrate GSL
Amytal tablets CD No Register POM
Ana-Kit POM
Anabact gel POM
Anacal preparations P
Anadin capsules, Maximum Strength P
Anadin Cold Control preparations GSL
Anadin Extra soluble tablets pack sizes 8s, 16s GSL
Anadin Extra tablets pack sizes 8s, 12s, 16s GSL; 32s P

Anadin Ibuprofen tablets pack sizes 16s GSL
Anadin Paracetamol tablets pack sizes 8s, 16s GSL; 32s P
Anadin tablets pack sizes 6s, 12s, 16s GSL; 32s P
Anadin Ultra capsules pack sizes 8s, 16s GSL; 32s P
Anadin Ultra Double Strength P
Anaflex cream P
Anafranil preparations POM
Anafranil SR tablets POM
Anagrelide POM
Anaguard POM
Anakinra POM
Anapen POM
Anapen Junior POM
Anastrazole tablets POM
Anbesol Adult Strength gel GSL
Anbesol liquid P
Anbesol teething gel P
Ancotil POM
Ancrod POM
Andrews Antacid tablets GSL
Andrews Liver Salts GSL
Andrews Plus GSL
Androcur tablets POM
Andropatch CD Anab POM
4-Androstene-3,17-dione CD Anab POM
5-Androstene-3,17-diol CD Anab POM
Androsterone POM
Anectine injection POM
Anethaine cream P
Anethole GSL
Anexate injection POM
Angelica GSL
Angeliq tablets POM
Angettes tablets P
Angettes-75 tablets P
Angeze SR capsules POM
Angeze tablets P
Angilol tablets POM
Angiopine 40 LA tablets POM
Angiopine capsules POM
Angiopine LA tablets POM
Angiopine MR tablets POM
Angiotensin amide POM
Angiox POM
Angiozem CR tablets POM
Angiozem tablets POM
Angitak spray P
Angitil SR capsules POM
Angitil XL capsules POM
Anhydrol Forte P
Anileridine; its salts CD POM
Animalintex GSL
Anise Oil GSL
Aniseed (Anise) GSL
Anistreplase POM
Anodesyn preparations GSL
Anquil tablets POM
Antabuse tablets POM
Antepsin suspension POM
Antepsin tablets POM
Anterior Pituitary Extract POM
Anthisan Bite & Sting cream GSL
Anthisan cream P
Anthisan Plus spray GSL
Anthrax vaccine (Bacillus Anthracis) POM
Anti-D (Rh:) Immuno globulin inj POM
Antihepatitis B Immunoglobulin inj POM
Antimony barium tartrate POM
Antimony dimercaptosuccinate POM
Antimony lithium thiomalate POM
Antimony pentasulphide POM
Antimony potassium tartrate POM
Antimony sodium tartrate POM
Antimony sodium thioglycollate POM
Antimony sulphate POM
Antimony trichloride POM
Antimony trioxide POM
Antimony trisulphide POM
Antipeol GSL
Antipressan tablets POM
Antirabies Immunoglobulin inj POM
Antirobe capsules POM

Antistreplase inj POM
Antitetanus Immunoglobulin inj POM
Antivaricella-zoster Immunoglobulin inj POM
Anturan tablets POM
Anugesic-HC preparations POM
Anusol Plus HC ointment (0018/0223) P
Anusol Plus HC suppositories (0018/0224) P
Anusol preparations GSL
Anusol-HC preparations POM
Anzemet preparations POM
Apidra preparations POM
Apiol POM
APO-go pen injector POM
Apomorphine POM
Apomorphine hydrochloride POM
APP stomach powder and tablets POM
Apraclonidine ophthalmic solution 0.5%; 1% POM
Apramycin POM
Aprepitant POM
Apresoline preparations POM
Aprinox tablets POM
Aprotinin POM
Aprovel tablets POM
Apsin preparations POM
Apsolol tablets POM
Apstil tablets POM
Aptivus capsules POM
APV Acellular Pertussis Vaccine POM
Aquaban tablets GSL
Aquaban Herbal GSL
Aquadrate cream P
Aquaform GSL
Aqualette tablets GSL
Aquasept skin cleanser GSL
Aquasol sachets P
Aqueous cream BP GSL
Arachis oil GSL
Aramine injection POM
Aranesp injection POM
Arava tablets POM
Arbralene tablets POM
Arcoxia tablets POM
Arecoline hydrobromide POM
Aredia Dry Powder inj POM
Aredia vials POM
Arelix capsules POM
Argipressin POM
Aricept tablets POM
Aricept Evess POM
Aridil tablets POM
Arilvax yellow fever vaccine POM
Arimidex tablets POM
Aripiprazole POM
Aristolochia POM
Aristolochia Clematitis POM
Aristolochia Contorta POM
Aristolochia Debelis POM
Aristolochia Fang-chi POM
Aristolochia Manshuriensis POM
Aristolochia Serpentaria POM
Arixtra injection POM
Arlevert POM
Arnica, external use only GSL
Aromasin tablets POM
Arpicolin syrup POM
Arpimycin suspension POM
Arret capsules P
Arrowroot GSL
Arsenic POM
Arsenic triiodide POM
Arsenic trioxide POM
Arsphenamine POM
Artelac eye-drops P
Artesunate POM
Arthrocin tablets POM
Arthrofen tablets POM
Arthrotec 50 tablets POM
Arthrotec 75 tablets POM
Arthroxen tablets POM
Artichoke GSL
Artilan tablets POM
Arythmol tablets POM
Asacol foam enema POM
Asacol suppositories POM
Asacol MR tablets POM

Asafetida GSL
Asasantin Retard POM
Ascabiol P
Ascorbic acid GSL
Asendis tablets POM
Aserbine cream P
Aserbine solution P
Ashbourne emollient GSL
Ashton and Parsons infants powders GSL
Asilone Heartburn GSL
Asilone liquid GSL
Asilone suspension GSL
Asilone tablets GSL
Asilone Windcheaters GSL
Askit preparations GSL
Asmabec Clickhaler POM
Asmabec Spacehaler POM
Asmal tablets POM
Asmanex Twisthaler POM
Asmasal Clickhaler POM
Asmasal Spacehaler POM
Asmaven Inhaler POM
Asmaven tablets POM
Aspav tablets CD Inv POM
Aspergum P
Aspirin (see table p45) POM but if (1) non-effervescent tablets and capsules above 325mg up to maximum strength 500mg, and the quantity sold or supplied in one container or package does not exceed 32, and the quantity sold or supplied to a person at any one time does not exceed 100 P; or (2) non effervescent tablets and capsules maximum strength 75mg, and the quantity sold or supplied in one container or package does not exceed 100, and the quantity sold or supplied to a person at any one time does not exceed 100 GSL (Note there is a pack size limit in non- pharmacy premises); (3) in the case of non-effervescent tablets where they are enteric coated, maximum strength 75mg and not more than 28 tablets, GSL; (4) non-effervescent tablets and capsules maximum strength 325mg (and the quantity sold or supplied at any one time does not exceed 100), powder or granules maximum strength 650mg or effervescent tablets maximum strength 500mg GSL (Note there is a pack size limit in non-pharmacy premises)
Aspirin (dispersible) and papaveretum tablets (Cox) CD Inv POM
Aspro Clear maximum strength GSL
Aspro Clear pack sizes 18s, 30s GSL
Astemizole POM
AT 10 P
Atamestane CD Anab POM
Atazanavir POM
Atarax preparations POM
Atenix tablets POM
AtenixCo 100 POM
AtenixCo 50 POM
Atenolol POM
Athranol 2.0% POM
Atimos Modulite inhaler POM
Ativan preparations CD Benz POM
Atomoxetine POM
Atorvastatin tablets POM
Atosiban POM
Atovaquone suspension POM
Atracurium POM
Atracurium besylate POM
Atriance POM
Atro arnica pain relief gel GSL
Atromid-S capsules POM

Atropine POM but if (1) in inhalers P; or (2) in preparations for internal use (other than inhalers) with md 300mcg and mdd 1mg P; or (3) in preparations for external use (except preparations for local ophthalmic use POM) P

Atropine methobromide POM but if (1) in inhalers P; or (2) in preparations for internal use (other than inhalers) with md 400mcg and mdd 1.3mg P; or (3) in preparations for external use (except preparations for local ophthalmic use POM) P

Atropine methonitrate POM but if (1) internal by inhaler P; or (2) in preparations for internal use (other than inhalers) with md 400mcg and mdd 1.3mg P

Atropine oxide hydrochloride POM but if (1) in inhalers P; (2) in preparations for internal use (other than inhalers) with md 360mcg and mdd 1.2mg P; or (3) in preparations for external use (except preparations for local ophthalmic use POM) P

Atropine sulphate POM but if (1) in inhalers P; (2) in preparations for internal use (other than inhalers) with md 360mcg and mdd 1.2mg P; or (3) in preparations for external use (except preparations for local ophthalmic use POM) P

Atrovent Aerocaps POM
Atrovent Autohalers POM
Atrovent CFC-free inhaler POM
Atrovent Forte inhaler POM
Atrovent inhaler POM
Atrovent Nebuliser solution POM
Audax ear drops P
Audicort ear drops POM
Augmentin Duo suspension POM
Augmentin preparations POM
Auralgan ear drops P
Auranofin POM
Aureocort preparations POM
Aureomycin eye ointment POM
Aureomycin preparations POM
Aurothiomalate sodium inj POM
Avamys spray POM
Avandamet tablets POM
Avandia tablets POM
Avastin concentrate for solution for infusion POM
Avaxim vaccine POM
Avelox tablets POM
Avena (oats) GSL
Aviral cream P
Avloclor tablets POM but for prophylaxis of malaria P
AVOCA P
Avodart capsules POM
Avomine tablets P
Avonex injection POM
Axid capsules POM
Axid injection POM
Axsain cream POM
Ayrton preparations GSL
Azactam injection POM
Azamune tablets POM
Azapropazone POM
Azatadine preps P
Azathioprine POM
Azathioprine sodium POM
Azelaic Acid POM
Azelastine hydrochloride POM but if for nasal administration, for the treatment of seasonal allergic rhinitis or perennial allergic rhinitis for use in adults and children not less than five years, as a non-aerosol, aqueous form 140mcg per nostril (MD), 280mcg per nostril (MDD) and container or package contains not more than 5,040mcg of azelastine hydrochloride, P
Azidocillin potassium POM
Azidothymidine POM
Azilect tablets POM
Azithromycin POM but if for the treatment of confirmed aysmptomatic Chlamydia trachomatis genital infection in individuals aged 16 years and over, and for the epidemiological treatment of their sexual partners, 1g

(MD), 1g (MDD) in a maximum pack size of 1g, P
Azlocillin sodium POM
Azopt eye-drops POM
Aztreonam POM

B

Baby Meltus cough syrup GSL
Babyhaler GSL
Bacampicillin hydrochloride POM
Bach flower remedies GSL
Bach rescue cream GSL
Bach rescue remedy GSL
Bach spray GSL
Bacillus Calmette-Guerin vaccine POM
Bacillus Calmette-Guerin Vaccine, Isoniazid-Resistant POM
Bacillus Calmette-Guerin Vaccine, Percutaneous POM
Bacitracin POM
Bacitracin methylene disalicylate POM
Bacitracin zinc POM
Baclofen POM
Baclospas tablets POM
Bacticlor MR POM
Bactigras P
Bactroban cream POM
Bactroban nasal POM
Bactroban ointment POM
Balanced Salt Solution POM
Balgifen tablets POM
Balm GSL
Balm of Gilead GSL
Balmosa cream GSL
Balneum preparations GSL
Balneum Plus preparations GSL
Balsalazide capsules POM
Balto foot balm GSL
Bambec tablets POM
Bambuterol hydrochloride POM
Bansor mouth antiseptic GSL
Baraclude POM
Baratol tablets POM
Barberry Bark GSL
Barbitone CD No Register POM
Barbitone sodium CD No Register POM
Baritop 100 P
Baritop Plus powder P
Barium carbonate POM
Barium chloride POM
Barium sulphide POM
Basiliximab injection (powder for reconstitution) POM
Baxan preparations POM
Bay oil, external use only GSL
Bayberry GSL
Baycaron tablets POM
Bazetham MR capsules POM
Bazuka gel P
Becaplermin POM
Beclamide POM
Beclazone Easi-Breathe POM
Beclazone inhaler POM
Beclo-Aqua nasal spray POM
Becloforte Diskhaler POM
Becloforte Easi-Breathe POM
Becloforte inhaler POM
Becloforte Integra Inhaler POM
Beclometasone/Beclomethasone POM
Beclometasone/Beclomethasone dipropionate POM but if for nasal administration (non-aerosol), for the prevention and treatment of allergic rhinitis in persons aged 18 years and over, 100mcg per nostril (MD) 200mcg per nostril (MDD) for a maximum period of 3 months and container or package contains not more than 20,000mcg of beclometasone dipropionate, please refer to proprietary names for classification granted under the marketing authorisation (see Beconase products)
Beclomethasone see Beclometasone
Beclomist nasal spray P
Becodisks POM
Beconase Allergy nasal spray P

Beconase Hayfever nasal spray GSL
Beconase nasal spray (aqueous) POM
Becotide 50, 100, 200 inhaler POM
Becotide Easi-Breathe POM
Becotide Rotacaps POM
Bedol tablets POM
Bedranol SR capsules POM
Beechams All-in-One GSL
Beechams cold & flu GSL
Beechams decongestant plus with paracetamol capsules GSL
Beechams Flu Plus caplets pack sizes 16s GSL; 24s P
Beechams Flu-Plus sachets GSL
Beechams for Natural Defence zinc and vitamin C tablets GSL
Beechams hydrocortisone ointment (PL 0079/0203) P
Beechams powders capsules GSL
Beechams powders pack sizes 10s GSL; 20s P
Beechams sore throat relief max strength lozenges GSL
Beechams Tablets lemon GSL
Beechams Throat-Plus lozenges GSL
Beeswax GSL
Begrivac vaccine POM
Belladonna herb POM but if internal and 1 mg of the alkaloids (MDD), or external, P
Belladonna root POM but if internal and 1 mg of the alkaloids (MDD), or external, P
Bemegride POM
Bemegride sodium POM
Bemiparin POM
Benactyzine hydrochloride POM
Benadryl Allergy Relief capsules 12s P; 12s GSL; 24s P
Benadryl allergy relief solution 70ml GSL; 100ml P
Benadryl for Children Allergy Solution GSL
Benadryl cream and lotion P
Benadryl One A Day tablets GSL
Benadryl Plus capsules P
Benadryl Skin Allergy Relief preparations P
Benapryzine hydrochloride POM
Bencard skin testing solutions POM
Bendrofluazide see Bendroflumethiazide
Bendroflumethiazide/Bendrofluazide POM
Benefix recombinant factor IX POM
Benemid tablets POM
Benerva tablets GSL
Benethamine Penicillin POM
Benoral granules P
Benoral suspension P
Benoral tablets P
Benoxaprofen POM
Benoxyl 10 lotion P
Benoxyl 5 cream P
Benoxyl 5 lotion P
Benperidol POM
Benquil POM
Benserazide hydrochloride POM
Bentiromide POM
Benuryl POM
Benylin 4-Flu liquid and tablets P
Benylin Active Response oral solution GSL
Benylin Day and Night cold treatment P
Benylin chesty cough (drowsy) P
Benylin for Chesty Coughs (non-drowsy formulation) 125ml, 300ml GSL
Benylin childrens chesty cough GSL
Benylin childrens chesty cough sachets GSL
Benylin for Children's Coughs and Colds P
Benylin childrens dry cough P
Benylin for Children's Night Coughs P
Benylin childrens tickly cough GSL
Benylin cold & flu max strength capsules GSL
Benylin cold & flu max strength hot drink sachets GSL

Benylin cough and congestion P
Benylin dry cough (drowsy and non-drowsy) P
Benylin Fortified linctus P
Benylin Mentholated linctus P
Benylin Paediatric P
Benylin sachets GSL
Benylin Sore Throat lozenges GSL
Benylin tickly cough (non-drowsy) GSL
Benylin with codeine CD Inv P
Benzalkonium chloride, if external use, or internal (pastilles, lozenges, throat tablets) max strength 600mcg GSL
Benzamycin gel POM
Benzathine penicillin POM
Benzatropine/Benztropine mesylate POM
Benzbromarone POM
Benzethidine; its salts CD POM
Benzethonium chloride, external use only GSL
Benzfetamine/Benzphetamine; its salts CD No Register POM
Benzhexol see Trihexyphenidyl
Benzilonium bromide POM
Benzocaine POM but any use except ophthalmic use P, except preparations with maximum strength 3% for use in adults and in children aged 12 years and over GSL; in spray form for use in adults and children aged 2 years and over with maximum strength 1% and maximum pack size 22g of product GSL; as a dental gel for the temporary relief of toothache pain associated with open carious lesions and for use in adults and children aged 12 years and over with a maximum strength of 10% and maximum pack size 5.3g of product GSL; benzocaine throat spray delivering 1mg per spray for the symptomatic relief of sore throat pain in adults and children aged 6 years and over, maximum dose 3mg, maximum daily dose 24mg, maximum pack size 106.5mg of benzocaine GSL; in combination with mepyramine maleate, for the treatment of insect bites and stings, nettle stings and jellyfish stings in adults and children aged 2 years and over, maximum pack size 22g of the product GSL, please refer to proprietary names for the classification granted under the marketing authorisation (See Waspeze preparations and Orajel Dental Gel)
Benzocaine 10% mouth gel for temporary relief from the pain and tenderness associated with mouth ulcers and from wearing dentures GSL
Benzoctamine hydrochloride POM
Benzoic acid, if internal maximum strength 0.2 per cent or external maximum strength 5.0 per cent GSL
Benzoin Tincture, Compound BP, if external use or internal (pastilles maximum strength 0.8 per cent or vapour inhalations) GSL
Benzoyl peroxide POM but if external maximum strength 10.0 per cent P; or for the treatment of spots or pimples on the face maximum strength 2.5 per cent GSL
N-Benzoyl sulphanilamide POM
Benzphetamine see Benzfetamine
Benzquinamide POM
Benzquinamide hydrochloride POM
Benzthiazide POM
Benztropine see Benzatropine
Benzydamine P
Benzyl alcohol, if external use or internal (pastilles, lozenges, throat tablets maximum strength 4mg) GSL
Benzyl benzoate, external use only GSL
Benzyl cinnamate, external use only GSL

Benzyl nicotinate, external use only GSL
Benzylmorphine (3-benzylmorphine) CD POM
Benzylpenicillin calcium POM
Benzylpenicillin potassium POM
Benzylpenicillin sodium POM
Bepro Cough syrup CD Inv P
Beractant POM
Beractant suspension POM
Berberis P but if equivalent to 500mcg berberine (MD) (Bitter, Stomachic), GSL
Berkatens tablets POM
Berkmycen preparations POM
Berkolol tablets POM
Berkozide tablets POM
Berocca Vit B effervescent tablets GSL
Berotec inhaler POM
Beta-Adalat capsules POM
Beta-aminoisopropylbenzene see Amfetamine
Beta-Cardone preparations POM
Beta-Prograne capsules POM
Betacap scalp application POM
Betacarotene, up to 6mg (MD) GSL
Betacetylmethadol; its salts CD POM
Betadine alcoholic solution P
Betadine antiseptic paint GSL
Betadine cream P
Betadine dry powder spray GSL
Betadine gargle and mouthwash P
Betadine ointment GSL
Betadine scalp and skin cleanser GSL
Betadine shampoo GSL
Betadine skin cleanser GSL
Betadine spare parts pump dispenser GSL
Betadine Standardised antiseptic Solution P
Betadine surgical scrub P
Betadine vaginal gel P
Betadine vaginal pessaries P
Betadine VC Kit P
Betaferon injection POM
Betagan POM
Betahistine hydrochloride POM
Betaine Hcl P
Betaloc injection POM
Betaloc SA tablets POM
Betaloc tablets POM
Betameprodine; its salts CD POM
Betamethadol; its salts, esters and ethers CD POM
Betamethasone POM
Betamethasone adamantoate POM
Betamethasone benzoate POM
Betamethasone dipropionate POM
Betamethasone sodium phosphate POM
Betamethasone valerate POM
Betaprodine CD POM
Betaxolol hydrochloride POM
Bethanechol chloride POM
Bethanidine sulphate POM
Betim tablets POM
Betinex tablets POM
Betnelan tablets POM
Betnesol preparations POM
Betnesol-N eye, ear and nose drops POM
Betnovate preparations POM
Betnovate RD preparations POM
Betnovate-C preparations POM
Betnovate-N preparations POM
Betoptic eye drops POM

Bettamousse POM
Bevacizumab POM
Bexarotene POM
Bextra tablets POM
Bezafibrate POM
Bezalip tablets POM
Bezalip-Mono tablets POM
Bezitramide; its salts CD POM
Bicalutamide tablets POM
Bi-Carzem SR POM
Bi-Carzem XL POM
Bicillin injection POM
BiCNU injection POM

Bifonazole P but if for external use for the treatment of athlete's foot, in a cream with a maximum strength of 1 per cent and a maximum pack size of 30g of product, GSL
Bimatoprost POM
Binocrit prefilled syringes POM
Binovum tablets POM
Biolax tablets pack sizes 10s GSL; 30s P
Biolon syringe P
Bioplex granules for mouthwash POM
Bioral gel P
Biorphen oral solution POM
Biostrath elixir GSL
Bio-strath natural herb remedies GSL
Biotene dry mouth sensitive toothpaste GSL
Biotene oralbalance dry mouth moisturising liquid GSL
Biotin GSL
Biovital liquid P
Biovital tablets P
Biperiden hydrochloride POM
Biperiden lactate POM
Bipranix POM
Bisacodyl, if internal tablets (other than for use by children under 10 years of age) with a maximum strength of 5mg, 10mg (MD), not more than 40 tablets GSL
Bismuth aluminate, up to 6mg (MD), calculated as bismuth oxide GSL
Bismuth carbonate GSL
Bismuth citrate GSL
Bismuth glycollylarsanilate POM
Bismuth oxide GSL
Bismuth subgallate, external use only GSL
Bismuth subnitrate GSL
Bisodol Extra GSL
Bisodol Heartburn GSL
Bisodol tablets and powders GSL
Bisodol tablets extra strong mint GSL
Bisodol tablets flip top GSL
Bisodol wind relief tablets GSL
Bisoprolol fumarate POM
Bitrex GSL
Bivalirudin POM
Black Bryony, external use only GSL
Black Catechu GSL
Black Currant GSL
Black Haw GSL
Black Root GSL
Blackberry GSL
Bladderwrack (Fucus) GSL
Blemix tablets POM
Bleo-Kyowa POM
Bleomycin POM
Bleomycin sulphate POM
Blistex relief cream GSL
Blisteze cream GSL
Blocadren tablets POM
Blue Cohosh (Caulophyllum), up to 265mg (MD) GSL
Blue Flag, up to 600mg (MD) GSL
Bocasan P
Bolandiol CD Anab POM
Bolasterone CD Anab POM
Bolazine CD Anab POM
Boldenone CD Anab POM
Boldo, up to 1.5g (MD) GSL
Bolenol CD Anab POM
Bolmantalate CD Anab POM
Bondronat preparations POM
Bonefos preparations POM
Boneset (Eupatorium perfoliatum) GSL
Bonjela gel GSL
Bonviva solution for injection POM
Bonviva tablets POM
Borax (sodium borate), if maximum strength 5.0% in all preparations except ophthalmic lotions; or maximum strength 0.7% in ophthalmic lotions (external use only) GSL
Boric acid, maximum strength 2.5% (external use only) GSL
Bornyl acetate, external use only GSL
Bortezomib POM

Bosentan POM
Botox injection POM
Botulinium A toxin-Haemagglutinin complex injection POM
Botulinum B toxin POM
Botulism antitoxin POM
Bradosol lozenges GSL
Bradosol Plus lozenges P
Braggs Charcoal tablets GSL
Bran GSL
Brasivol 1 Fine GSL
Brasivol 2 Medium GSL
Bretylate injection POM
Bretylium tosylate POM
Brevibloc POM
Brevinor tablets POM
Brevoxyl cream P
Brexidol tablets POM
Bricanyl preparations POM
Bricanyl SA tablets POM
Bridion POM
Brietal sodium injections POM
Brimonidine tartrate POM
Brinzolamide POM
Britaject pens POM
Britaject preparations POM
BritLofex POM
Brochlor P
Broflex syrup POM
Brolene eye drops P
Brolene eye ointment P
Bromazepam CD Benz POM
Bromhexine hydrochloride POM
Bromocriptine mesylate POM
4-Bromo-2,5-dimethoxy-a-methylphenethylamine CD Lic
Bromperidol POM
Bromvaletone POM
Bronalin Decongestant P
Bronalin Dry Cough P
Bronalin Expectorant P
Bronalin Junior P
Bronchodil POM
Brotizolam CD Benz POM
Brovon asthma inhalant POM
Brufen preparations POM
Brufen Retard POM
Bruiseze GSL
Brulidine cream GSL
Buccastem M tablets P
Buccastem tablets POM
Buchu GSL
Buckthorn GSL
Budenofalk capsules POM
Budesonide POM but for nasal administration, for the prevention or treatment of seasonal allergic rhinitis in persons aged 18 years and over as a non-aerosol, aqueous form, 200mcg per nostril (MD) 200mcg per nostril (MDD), for a maximum period of 3 months and container or package contains not more than 10mg of budesonide, P
Budeneside Easyhaler POM
Bufexamac POM
Bufotenine; its salts, esters and ethers CD Lic
Bugleweed GSL
Bumetanide POM
Buphenine hydrochloride POM but if 6mg (MD) 18mg (MDD), P
Bupivacaine POM but any use except ophthalmic use P
Bupivacaine hydrochloride POM but any use except ophthalmic use, P
Buprenorphine CD No Register POM
Bupropion POM
Burgundy Pitch, external use only GSL
Burinex A tablets POM
Burinex K tablets POM
Burinex preparations POM
Burneze P
Buscopan ampoules POM
Buscopan IBS Relief GSL
Buscopan tablets, pack sizes 56s POM
Buserelin acetate POM
Buserelin nasal spray POM

Busilvex concentrate for solution for infusion POM
Buspar tablets POM
Buspirone hydrochloride POM
Busulfan/busulphan POM
Busulphan see Busulfan
Butacaine sulphate POM but any use except ophthalmic use, P
Butacote tablets POM
Butalbital CD No Register POM
Butobarbital/Butobarbitone CD No Register POM
Butobarbital/Butobarbitone sodium CD No Register POM
Butobarbitone see Butobarbital
Butorphanol tartrate POM
BuTrans CD No Reg POM
Butriptyline hydrochloride POM
Buttercup infant cough syrup GSL
Buttercup medicated sweets GSL
Buttercup syrup GSL
Butternut (White Walnut) GSL
Byetta POM

C

C-View GSL
Cabaser tablets POM
Cabdrivers Adult cough linctus P
Cabergoline POM
Cacit D3 granules P
Cacit tablets P
Cade oil, external use only GSL
Caelyx for infusion POM
Cafergot suppositories POM
Cafergot tablets POM
Caffeine GSL
Caffeine citrate GSL
Caffeine injection POM
Cajuput oil GSL
Calaband GSL
Calabren tablets POM
Caladryl cream P
Caladryl lotion P
Calamine, external use only GSL
Calamus (Sweet Flag) GSL
Calanif capsules POM
Calazem tablets POM
Calceos tablets P
Calchan MR POM
Calcicard CR tablets POM
Calcichew Forte tablets P
Calcichew tablets P
Calcichew-D3 Forte tablets P
Calcichew-D3 tablets P
Calcidrink sachets P
Calciferol injection POM
Calciferol tablets P
Calcijex injection POM
Calcimax syrup P
Calciparine injection POM
Calcipotriol POM
Calcisorb P
Calcitare POM
Calcitonin POM
Calcitonin (salmon)/Salcatonin POM
Calcitonin (salmon)/Salcatonin acetate POM
Calcitriol POM
Calcium alginate, external use only GSL
Calcium amphomycin POM
Calcium ascorbate GSL
Calcium benzamidosalicylate POM
Calcium bromide POM
Calcium bromidolactobionate POM
Calcium carbimide POM
Calcium carbonate GSL
Calcium chloride GSL
Calcium chloride injection POM
Calcium folinate POM
Calcium gluconate GSL
Calcium gluconate injection POM
Calcium glycerophosphate GSL
Calcium heptagluconate GSL
Calcium hydrogen phosphate GSL
Calcium lactate GSL
Calcium leucovorin preparations POM
Calcium metrizoate POM

Calcium pantothenate GSL
Calcium phosphate GSL
Calcium resonium P
Calcium sulphaloxate POM
Calcium undecylenate, external use only GSL
Calcium with vitamin D tablets BPC P
Calcium-Sandoz syrup P
Calcort tablets POM
Calendula (Marigold), external use only GSL
Calfovit D3 POM
Calgel GSL
Califig GSL
Califig, Junior GSL
Calimal P
Callanish Nutritional preparations GSL
Calmurid cream P
Calmurid HC cream POM
Calpol Fast melts 6+ tablets 12 P; 12 GSL; 24 P
Calpol infant sachets sugar-free GSL
Calpol Infant suspension 70ml P; 100ml GSL; 140ml P; 200ml P
Calpol infant suspension sugar-free 100ml GSL; 140ml P; 200ml P
Calpol Paediatric suspension P
Calpol sachets GSL
Calpol 6+ sugar-free sachets GSL
Calpol Six Plus suspension P
Calprofen paediatric suspension POM
Calprofen sachets GSL
Calprofen suspension 100ml P; 100ml GSL
Calsalettes P
Calsynar POM
Caltrate tablets GSL
Calumba GSL
Calusterone CD Anab POM
CAM P
Camazepam CD Benz POM
Camcolit tablets POM
Camphor oil, external use only GSL
Camphor up to 20mg (MD), 30mg (MDD) GSL
Camphorated opium tincture BP CD Inv POM
Campral EC tablets POM
Campto infusion POM
Cancidas POM
Candesartan cilexitil POM
Candicidin POM
Candida Yeast Extract GSL
Candiden preparations P
Canesten 1 vaginal Tablet P
Canesten 10% VC POM
Canesten 2% vaginal cream POM
Canesten AF GSL
Canesten AF Once Daily P
Canesten Cream Combi GSL
Canesten Combi GSL and POM
Canesten Complete P
Canesten cream P
Canesten dermatological spray P
Canesten Duo P
Canesten Duopack POM
Canesten HC cream 30g POM
Canesten hydrocortisone 15g P
Canesten Internal P
Canesten Oasis GSL
Canesten Once P
Canesten Oral P
Canesten pessary 500mg P and POM
Canesten powder P
Canesten solution P
Canesten thrush cream P
Canesten vaginal cream P
Canesten vaginal tablets P
Cannabinol CD Lic
Cannabinol derivatives not being dronabinol or its stereoisomers CD Lic
Cannabis and cannabis resin CD Lic
Canrenoic Acid POM
Cantharidin POM but if external maximum strength 0.01 per cent, P
Canusal injection POM
Capasal P
Capastat injection POM

Capecitabine POM
Caplenal tablets POM
Capoten tablets POM
Capozide LS tablets POM
Capozide tablets POM
Capreomycin sulphate POM
Caprin 75mg tablets P
Caprin 300mg tablets POM
Capsaicin POM
Capsicum GSL
Capsicum oleoresin (water soluble), external use only GSL
Capsicum oleoresin BPC 1923 GSL
Capsicum oleoresin BPC 1973, if internal 1.2mg (MD) and 1.8mg (MDD) or external maximum strength 2.5 GSL
Capsicum oleoresin, external use only GSL
Capsuvac capsules POM
Capto-co POM
Captopril POM
Carace 10 Plus tablets POM
Carace 20 Plus tablets POM
Carace tablets POM
Caralpha tablets POM
Caramet CR POM
Caraway GSL
Caraway oil GSL
Carbachol POM
Carbadox POM
Carbagen CR tablets POM
Carbaglu POM
Carbalax suppositories GSL
Carbamazepine POM
Carbaryl POM
Carbasalate calcium POM
Carbellon tablets P
Carbenicillin sodium POM
Carbenoxolone sodium POM but if (1) Pellet 5mg (MD) 25mg (MDD); (2) Gel maximum strength 2.0 per cent; (3) Granules for mouthwash in adults and children not less than 12 years, 20mg (MD) 80mg (MDD) and maximum strength 1.0 percent and container or package containing not more than 560mg of carbenoxolone sodium, P
Carbetocin POM
Carbex P
Carbidopa POM
Carbidopa monohydrate POM
Carbimazole POM
Carbo-Cort cream POM
Carbo-Dome cream GSL
Carbocisteine POM
Carbomix P
Carbon Black GSL
Carbon tetrachloride POM
Carboplatin POM
Carboprost Trometamol POM
Carbromal POM
Carbuterol hydrochloride POM
Cardamom GSL
Cardamom Oil GSL
Cardene capsules POM
Cardene SR capsules POM
Cardicor tablets POM
Cardilate MR tablets POM
Cardinol tablets POM
Cardioplen XL tablets POM
Cardura tablets POM
Cardura XL tablets POM
Care ammonia & ipecacuanha mixture GSL
Care antiseptic first aid cream GSL
Care antiseptic mouthwash GSL
Care aqueous cream GSL
Care arnica tincture GSL
Care aspirin dispersible 75mg P
Care calamine aqueous cream GSL
Care calamine lotion GSL
Care castor oil GSL
Care Cetirizine Hayfever Relief tablets P
Care chlorhexidine antiseptic mouthwash GSL
Care clotrimazole cream P

Care clove oil GSL
Care codeine oral solution CD Inv P
Care codeine linctus CD Inv P
Care Cystitis Relief Sachets GSL
Care ephedrine nasal drops P
Care epsom salts GSL
Care eucalyptus oil GSL
Care flu-strength liquid all-in-one P
Care fluconazole capsules P
Care friars balsam GSL
Care fullers earth cream GSL
Care gees linctus CD Inv P
Care glycerin GSL
Care glycerin suppositories GSL
Care glycerin, lemon & honey GSL
Care glycerin, lemon, honey & ipecacuanha GSL
Care haemorrhoid relief ointment GSL
Care hay fever relief nasal spray P
Care Heartburn & Indigestion liquid PO
Care Heartburn Relief tablets P
Care hydrogen peroxide GSL
Care ibuprofen gel 5% GSL
Care ibuprofen gel 10% P
Care ibuprofen suspension P
Care ibuprofen tablets P
Care indian brandee GSL
Care iodine tincture GSL
Care ipecacuanha & morphine mixture CD Inv P
Care kaolin & morphine mixture CD Inv P
Care kaolin mixture GSL
Care kaolin paediatric mixture GSL
Care loperamide capsules GSL
Care magnesium sulphate paste GSL
Care magnesium trisilicate mixture GSL
Care menthol & eucalyptus inhalation GSL
Care paracetamol junior suspension P
Care paraffin liquid P
Care pholcodine oral solution sugar-free CD Inv P
Care pholcodine linctus CD Inv P
Care potassium citrate mixture P
Care senna tablets GSL
Care simple linctus GSL
Care simple paediatric linctus GSL
Care sleep aid tablets P
Care sodium bicarbonate GSL
Care surgical spirit GSL
Care terpin with codeine linctus CD Inv P
Care white embrocation GSL
Care witch hazel GSL
Care zinc & castor oil cream GSL
Careline products GSL
Carfecillin sodium POM
Carfentanil; its stereoisomers, salts, esters and ethers CD POM
Carglumic acid POM
Carindacillin sodium POM
Carisoma tablets POM
Carisoprodol POM
Carmellose sodium GSL
Carmil XL P
Carmustine POM
Carnation Callous caps GSL
Carnation Corn caps GSL
Carnation Verruca treatment GSL
Carnitine POM
Carnitor preparations POM
Carperidine POM
Carrot GSL
Carteolol hydrochloride POM
Carvedilol POM
Carylderm lotion POM
Carylderm shampoo POM

Cascara GSL
Cascor POM
Casodex tablets POM
Caspofungin infusion POM
Cassia Oil GSL
Castor Oil GSL
Catapres preparations POM
Catarrh-Eeze tablets GSL
Catechu GSL

Cathine its salts, stereoisomers (other than phenylpropanolamine), their salts CD No Register POM
Cathinone; its salts, stereoisomers, esters and ethers CD Lic
Caverject injection POM
CCNU POM
Ceanel concentrate P
Cedar wood oil, external use only GSL
Cedax capsules POM
Cedax suspension POM
Cedocard Retard tablets POM
Cefaclor POM
Cefaclor MR tablets POM
Cefadroxil POM
Cefalexin/Cephalexin POM
Cefalexin/Cephalexin sodium POM
Cefamandole nafate/Cephamandole nafate POM
Cefazedone sodium POM
Cefazolin/Cephazolin sodium POM
Cefdinir POM
Cefixime POM
Cefizox injection POM
Cefodizime sodium POM
Cefotaxime sodium POM
Cefoxitin sodium POM
Cefpirome POM
Cefpodoxime proxetil POM
Cefprozil POM
Cefradine/Cephradine POM
Cefrom vials POM
Cefsulodin sodium POM
Ceftazidime POM
Ceftizoxime sodium POM
Ceftriaxone sodium POM
Cefuroxime axetil POM
Cefuroxime sodium POM
Cefzil preparations POM
Celance tablets POM
Celebrex capsules POM
Celecoxib POM
Celectol tablets POM
Celery oil GSL
Celery seed GSL
Celevac tablets GSL
Celiprolol hydrochloride POM
Cellcept capsules POM
Cellcept powder for infusion POM
Cellcept powder for oral suspension POM
Cellcept tablets POM
Cellulose GSL
Celluvisc P
Centaury GSL
Centella, external use only GSL
Centrapryl tablets POM
Centyl K tablets POM
Cephalexin see Cefalexin
Cephaloridine POM
Cephalothin sodium POM
Cephamandole nafate see Cefamandole nafate
Cephazolin see Cefazolin
Cephradine see Cefradine
Ceplac GSL
Ceporex preparations POM
Ceprotin injection POM
Cepton Medicated cleansing lotion GSL
Cepton Medicated skinwash GSL
Cerazette POM
Cerebrovase tablets POM
Ceredase Concentrate POM
Cerezyme powder for reconstitution POM
Cerium oxalate POM
Cerivastatin POM
Cerivastatin sodium POM
Cernevit POM
Cerubidin powder for reconstitution POM
Ceruletide diethylamine POM
Cerumol ear drops P
Cetalkonium chloride, if external use or internal (teething gel maximum strength 0.01 per cent) GSL
Cetanorm cream GSL
Cetavlex cream GSL

Cetec GSL

Cetirizine hydrochloride POM but if 10mg (MDD) P; or if maximum strength 10mg, in tablet form for the symptomatic relief of perennial rhinitis, seasonal allergic rhinitis and idiopathic chronic urticaria in adults and children aged 6 years and over, 10mg (MDD), in an individual container or package containing not more than 14 tablets, GSL. If liquid preparations with a maximum strength of 1mg/ml for the symptomatic relief of perennial rhinitis, seasonal allergic rhinitis and idiopathic chronic urticaria in adults and children aged 6 years and over with a maximum pack size of no more than 70ml, GSL. Please refer to the proprietary names for classification granted under the marketing authorisation (see Galpharm Hayfever and Allergy Relief syrup)

Cetomacrogol, external use only GSL

Cetostearyl alcohol, external use only GSL

Cetraben Emollient bath additive GSL

Cetraben Emollient cream GSL

Cetrimide, external use only GSL

Cetrorelix POM

Cetrotide injection POM

Cetuximab POM

Cetylpyridinium chloride, all preparations other than liquid preparations for oral administration 3mg (MD) and liquid preparations for oral administration 5mg (MD) GSL

Chalk GSL

Chamomile GSL

Chamomile oil, external use only GSL

Champix POM

Charas see Cannabis

Charcoal tabs GSL

Charcoal, medicinal GSL

Charcodote suspension P

Check-Mate pregnancy testing strips GSL

Chemotrim preparations POM

Chemydur 60XL tablets POM

Chenodeoxycholic acid POM

Chickenpox vaccine POM

Chickweed GSL

Chimax tablets POM

Chirocaine POM

Chloractil tablets POM

Chloral betaine see Cloral betaine

Chloral hydrate POM but if external, P

Chlorambucil POM

Chloramphenicol POM

Chloramphenicol cinnamate POM

Chloramphenicol ear drops POM

Chloramphenical eye drops POM, but containing 0.5% chloramphenicol, for the treatment of acute bacterial conjunctivitis in adults and children aged 2 years and over, maximum length of treatment 5 days, and pack size 10ml; Please refer to proprietary names for the classification granted under the marketing authorisation

Chloramphenicol eye/ear ointment POM

Chloramphenicol 1% eye ointment POM, but containing 1% chloramphenicol, for the treatment of acute bacterial conjunctivitis in adults and children aged 2 years and over, maximum length of treatment 5 days, and pack size 4g; please refer to proprietary names for the classification granted under the marketing authorisation

Chloramphenicol palmitate POM

Chloramphenicol sodium succinate POM

Chlorbutol see Chlorobutanol

Chlordiazepoxide CD Benz POM

Chlorhexadol POM

Chlorhexidine acetate, external use only GSL

Chlorhexidine gluconate, external use only GSL

Chlorhexidine hydrochloride, if external use or internal (pastilles, lozenges, throat tablets maximum strength 5mg) GSL

Chlormadinone acetate POM

Chlormerodrin POM

Chlormethiazole see Clomethiazole

Chlormethine/Mustine hydrochloride POM

Chlormezanone POM

Chlorobutanol/chlorbutol, if internal (solid preparations 150mg (MD) or liquid preparations maximum strength 0.5 per cent), or external (except toothache gel) maximum strength 2.5 per cent, or external (toothache gel) maximum strength 7.0 per cent GSL

Chlorocresol, if maximum strength 0.2 per cent (external use only) GSL

Chlorodyne BPC CD Inv POM

Chloroform POM but if (1) internal maximum strength 5.0 per cent, P; (2) internal maximum strength 0.5 per cent, GSL, (3) external GSL

4-Chloromethandienone CD Anab POM

Chloromycetin preparations POM

Chlorophene, if maximum strength 1.25 per cent (external use only) GSL

Chlorophenols, if internal maximum strength 1mg or external maximum strength 0.6 per cent GSL

Chloroquine phosphate POM but for prophylaxis of malaria, P

Chloroquine sulphate POM but for prophylaxis of malaria, P

Chlorothiazide POM

Chlorotrianisene POM

Chloroxylenol, if internal maximum strength 0.5 per cent or external maximum strength 5.0 per cent GSL

Chlorphenamine/Chlorpheniramine P

Chlorphenesin, external use only GSL

Chlorpheniramine see Chlorphenamine

Chlorphenoxamine hydrochloride POM

Chlorphentermine; its salts CD No Register POM

Chlorpromazine POM

Chlorpromazine embonate POM

Chlorpromazine hydrochloride POM

Chlorpropamide POM

Chlorprothixene POM

Chlorprothixene hydrochloride POM

Chlortalidone/Chlorthalidone POM

Chlortetracycline POM

Chlortetracycline calcium POM

Chlortetracycline hydrochloride POM

Chlorthalidone see Chlortalidone

Chlorzoxazone POM

Cholera vaccine POM

Cholestyramine see Colestyramine

Choline salicylate, if external use or internal (teething gel maximum strength 9.0 per cent) GSL

Chondrus GSL

Choragon injection CD Anab POM

Chorionic Gonadotrophin (HCG) CD Anab POM

Christy caplets P

Chymol emollient balm GSL

Cialis tablets POM

Cialis Once-A-Day tablets POM

Cibral tablets POM

Cibral XL tablets POM

Cicafem POM

Cicatrin preparations POM

Ciclacillin POM

Ciclesonide POM

Ciclobendazole POM

Ciclosporin/Cyclosporin POM

Cidofovir POM

Cidomycin preparations POM

Cilastatin sodium POM

Cilazapril POM

Cilest POM

Cilostazol POM

Ciloxan eye drops POM

Cimetidine POM but if (1) For the short-term symptomatic relief of heartburn, dyspepsia, indigestion, acid indigestion and hyperacidity and for the prophylaxis of meal-induced heartburn 200mg (MD) 800mg (MDD) for a maximum period of 14 days; or (2) For the prophylactic management of nocturnal heartburn by a single dose taken at night 100mg (MD) to be taken as a single dose at night, for a maximum period of 14 days, P

Cimetidine hydrochloride POM

Cimicifuga (Black Cohosh), up to 200mg (MD) GSL

Cinacalcet POM

Cinaziere 15 tablets P

Cinchocaine POM but if non-ophthalmic use maximum strength 3.0 per cent, P

Cinchocaine hydrochloride POM but if non-ophthalmic use maximum strength equivalent of 3.0 per cent of cinchocaine, P

Cinchophen POM

Cinnamic acid, if external use or internal (pastilles, lozenges, throat tablets maximum strength 500 GSL

Cinnamon GSL

Cinnamon oil GSL

Cinnarizine P

Cinobac capsules POM

Cinoxacin POM

Cipralex oral drops POM

Cipralex tablets POM

Cipramil preparations POM

Ciprofibrate POM

Ciprofloxacin POM

Ciprofloxacin hydrochloride POM

Ciproxin preparations POM

Circadin prolonged-release tablets POM

Cisatracurium besylate POM

Cisapride POM

Cisplatin POM

Citalopram POM

Citanest preparations POM

Citramag P

Citric acid GSL

Citronella oil, external use only GSL

Cladribine POM

Claforan injection POM

Clairette 2000/35 POM

Clarelux cutaneous foam POM

Clariteyes eye drops P

Clarithromycin POM

Clarityn preparations P; except Clarityn Allergy tablets pack size 7s GSL

Clarosip POM

Clarosip granules for suspension POM

Clavulanic acid POM

Clear complexion tablets GSL

Clear Ear GSL

Clearasil Max 10 P

Clearsore cream P

Clemastine P

Clenbuterol CD Anab POM

Clenil Modulite POM

Clexane injection POM

Clidinium bromide POM

Climagest POM

Climanor tablets POM

Climaval tablets POM

Climesse tablets POM

Clindamycin POM

Clindamycin hydrochloride POM

Clindamycin palmitate hydrochloride POM

Clindamycin phosphate POM

Clinitar preparations P

Clinorette tablets POM

Clinoril tablets POM

Clioquinol POM but if (1) external (other than treatment of mouth ulcers); (2) treatment of mouth ulcers

350mg (MDD) and maximum strength 35mg, P

Clivarine injection POM

Clivers GSL

Clobazam CD Benz POM

Clobetasol propionate POM

Clobetasone butyrate POM but if cream for external use for the short term symptomatic treatment and control of patches of eczema and dermatitis (excluding seborrhoeic dermatitis) in adults and children 12 years and over, maximum strength 0.05 per cent, in a container or packaging containing not more than 15g of medicinal product P

Cloburate eye drops POM

Clofarabine POM

Clofazimine POM

Clofibrate POM

Clomethiazole/Chlormethiazole POM

Clomethiazole/Chlormethiazole edisylate POM

Clomid tablets POM

Clomifene/Clomiphene citrate POM

Clomiphene see Clomifene

Clomipramine POM

Clomipramine hydrochloride POM

Clomocycline POM

Clomocycline sodium POM

Clonazepam CD Benz POM

Clonidine POM

Clonidine hydrochloride POM

Clonitazene; its salts CD POM

Clopamide POM

Clopenthixol decanoate POM

Clopenthixol hydrochloride POM

Clopidogrel hydrogen sulphate POM

Clopixol Acuphase injection POM

Clopixol injection POM

Clopixol tablets POM

Cloprostenol sodium POM

Cloral betaine/Chloral betaine POM

Clorazepic acid CD Benz POM

Clorexolone POM

Clostebol CD Anab POM

Clostet vaccine POM

Clotam Rapid tablets POM

Clotiazepam CD Benz POM

Clotrimazole POM but if external and in the case of vaginal use only external use for the treatment of vaginal candidiasis, P; if in a combination pack containing a maximum of one 500mg pessary (for the treatment of candidal vaginitis) and 2% cream with a maximum of 200mg of clotrimazole per pack (for the treatment of candidal vulvitis and as an adjunct to treatment of candidal vaginitis), GSL; please refer to proprietary names for classification granted under the marketing authorisation (see Canesten Combi); if maximum strength 1.0% for the external treatment of tinea pedis (athlete's foot) only, powders for the prevention of, or as an adjunct to the treatment of tinea pedis, and all preparations other than powders, for the treatment of tinea pedis and tinea cruris, in a pack containing no more than 500mg of clotrimazole with a maximum strength 1%, GSL

Clove GSL

Clove Oil GSL

Clover (Red Clover) GSL

Cloxacillin benzathine POM

Cloxacillin sodium POM

Cloxazolam CD Benz POM

Clozapine POM

Clozaril tablets POM

Co-amilofruse POM

Co-amilozide POM

Co-amoxiclav POM

Co-Aprovel tablets POM

Co-beneldopa POM

Co-Betaloc SA tablets POM

Co-Betaloc tablets POM
Co-careldopa POM
Co-codamol 30/500 preparations
  CD Inv POM
Co-codamol 8/500 effervescent
  CD Inv P
Co-codamol 8/500 pack sizes 32s CD
  Inv P; greater than 32s CD Inv POM
Co-codaprin eff CD Inv P
Co-codaprin pack sizes 32s CD Inv P;
  sizes greater than 32s CD Inv POM
Co-cyprindiol tablets POM
Co-danthramer POM
Co-danthrusate POM
Co-dergocrine mesylate POM
Co-diovan tablets POM
Co-dydramol CD Inv POM
Co-fluampicil POM
Co-flumactone POM
Co-phenotrope CD Inv POM
Co-prenozide POM
Co-proxamol CD Inv POM
Co-tenidone POM
Co-tetroxazine POM
Co-triamterzide POM
Co-trimoxazole POM
Co-zidacapt POM
Coal tar, external use only GSL
Cobadex cream POM
Cobalin-H injection POM
Cobalt sulphate, if MDD equivalent to
  0.25mg elemental cobalt GSL
Coca alkaloids see Cocaine
Coca leaf CD Lic
Cocaine; its salts CD POM
Cocculus Indicus POM
Cocillana GSL
Cocois scalp application GSL
Cod liver oil as for Vitamin A and
  Vitamin D GSL
Codafen Continus tablets CD Inv POM
Codalax Forte suspension POM
Codalax suspension POM
Codeine; its salts CD POM but if for
  non-parenteral use and (a) in undi-
  vided preparations with ms 2.5%
  (calculated as base) CD Inv POM; or
  (b) in single dose preparations with
  ms per dosage unit 100mg (calculat-
  ed as base) CD Inv POM; or (c) in
  unit preparations diluted to at least
  one part in a million (6X) in
  response to a specific request, CD Inv
  P; or (d) in unit preparations diluted
  to at least one part in a million mil-
  lion (6C), CD Inv P
Codipar Caplets CD Inv POM
Codis 500 soluble tablets CD Inv P
Cogentin preparations POM
Colaspase POM
Colazide capsules POM
Colchicine POM
Colestid preparations POM
Colestipol hydrochloride POM
Colestyramine/Cholestyramine POM
Colfosceril palmitate POM
Colgate Chlorohex 1200 oral rinse GSL
Colgate Chlorohex 2000 oral rinse P
Colgate dental cream tartar control
  50ml GSL
Colgate dental cream ultra cavity pro-
  tection 25ml GSL
Colgate dental cream ultra cavity pro-
  tection 50ml GSL
Colgate Fluorigard alcohol-free daily
  rinse GSL
Colgate Fluorigard daily drops P
Colgate Fluorigard daily rinse GSL
Colgate Fluorigard Gelkam gel P
Colgate Fluorigard tablets P
Colgate sensitive products GSL
Colgate Total products GSL
Colgate Total + whitening GSL
Colgate Total fresh stripe GSL
Colgate triple cool stripe gel GSL
Colgate ultra cavity protection GSL
Colifoam aerosol POM
Colistimethate sodium/Colistin

sulphomethate sodium POM
Colistin sulphate POM
Colistin sulphomethate POM
Colistin sulphomethate sodium see
  Colistimethate sodium
Collins elixir P
Collis Browne's mixture, J. CD Inv P
Collis Browne's tablets, J. CD Inv P
Colloidal sulphur, external use only GSL
Colofac 100 tablets P
Colofac IBS tablets P
Colofac liquid POM
Colofac MR capsules POM
Colofac tablets POM
Colomycin preparations POM
Colophony, external use only GSL
Colpermin capsules GSL
Colsor cream GSL
Colsor lotion GSL
Combivent aerosol POM
Combigan eye-drops POM
Combivent UDV POM
Combivir tablets POM
Comfrey root, external use only GSL
Comixco Suspension POM
Competact POM
Compound W P
Comtess tablets POM
Concavit preparations P
Concentrate of poppy-straw CD Lic
Concerta XL tablets CD POM
Concordin tablets POM
Condrotec POM
Condyline liquid POM
Congescor POM
Coniine POM
Conium leaf POM but if external maxi-
  mum strength 7.0 per cent, P
Conotrane cream GSL
Conray POM
Contac capsules P
Contiflo XL POM
Contigen POM
Contimin tablets POM
Contraflam capsules POM
Contraflam tablets POM
Convulex capsules POM
Copaxone injection POM
Copegus tablets POM
Copper carbonate, if MDD equivalent to
  1mg elemental copper GSL
Copper sulphate, if internal equivalent
  to 4mg elemental copper (MDD) or
  external maximum strength 1.0 per
  cent GSL
Coracten SR capsules POM
Coracten XL capsules POM
Cordarone X preparations POM
Cordilox preparations POM
Corgard tablets POM
Corgaretic tablets POM
Coriander GSL
Coriander oil GSL
Corlan Pellets (PL 0039/0397) P
Coro-Nitro spray P
Coroday MR POM
Corsodyl dental gel P
Corsodyl mouthwash GSL
Corsodyl spray P
Corticotrophin see Corticotropin
Corticotropin/Corticotrophin POM
Cortisone POM
Cortisone acetate POM
Cortisyl tablets POM
Corwin tablets POM
Cosalgesic tablets CD Inv POM
Cosmegen, Lyovac POM
Cosmofer POM
Cosopt eye-drops POM
Cosuric tablets POM
Cough Nurse Night Time liquid P
Coversyl Plus tablets POM
Coversyl tablets POM
Covonia Bronchial balsam original P
Covonia catarrh relief formula GSL
Covonia cold & flu formula P
Covonia menthol cough mixture expec-
  torant GSL

Covonia night time formula P
Covonia throat spray P
Covonia vapour drops GSL
Cozaar tablets POM
Cozaar-Comp tablets POM
Crampex tablets P
Cranesbill (Geranium) GSL
Cranesbill tabs GSL
Cremalgin GSL

Creon 10,000 P
Creon 25,000 capsules POM
Creon 40,000 POM
Creon granules P
Creon Micro granules P
Creosote, if internal 0.125ml (MD) or
  external maximum strength 0.5 per
  cent GSL
Crestor tablets POM
Crinone gel POM
Crisantaspase POM
Crixivan capsules POM
Cromogen preps POM
Cromolux eye drops POM
Cromolux hayfever P
Cropropamide POM
Crotamiton, external use only GSL
Crotethamide POM
Croton oil POM
Croton seed POM
Crystacide cream P
Crystapen injections POM
Cubicin injection POM
Cuplex gel P
Cuprofen preparations P
Curanail nail lacquer P
Curare POM
Curatoderm ointment POM
Curosurf POM
Cutipen POM
Cutivate cream POM
Cutivate ointment POM
Cuxson Gerrard belladonna plasters
  BPC white cloth P
CX powder P
Cyanocobalamin, up to 10mcg (MDD)
  GSL
4-Cyano-2-dimethylamino-4,4-
  diphenylbutane CD POM
4-Cyano-1-methyl-4-phenylpiperidine
  CD POM
Cyclimorph injections CD POM
Cyclizine hydrochloride tablets P
Cyclizine hydrochloride injection POM
Cyclo-Progynova tablets POM
Cyclobarbitone CD No Register POM
Cyclobarbitone calcium CD No Register
  POM
Cyclodox Caps POM
Cyclofenil POM
Cyclogest suppositories POM
Cyclomin tabs POM
Cyclopenthiazide POM
Cyclopentolate hydrochloride POM
Cyclophosphamide POM
Cycloserine POM
Cyclosporin see Ciclosporin
Cyclothiazide POM
Cyklokapron preparations POM
Cymalon GSL
Cymbalta capsules POM
Cymevene capsules POM
Cymevene vials POM
Cymex GSL
Cymex Ultra cream GSL
Cypripedium GSL
Cyproheptadine P
Cyprostat tablets POM
Cyproterone acetate POM
Cystagon caps POM
Cystemme cystitis sachets 6 PO
Cystocalm sachets GSL
Cystofem sachets PO
Cystopurin granules GSL
Cystrin tablets POM
Cytacon liquid P
Cytacon tablets P
Cytamen injection POM

Cytarabine POM
Cytarabine hydrochloride POM
Cytosar injection POM
Cytotec tablets POM

D

Dacarbazine POM
Dactinomycin POM
Daclizumab POM
Daktacort cream POM
Daktacort HC cream P
Daktacort ointment POM
Daktarin (Janssen-Cilag) cream 2% P
Daktarin (Janssen-Cilag) oral gel POM
Daktarin cream 2% 15g P
Daktarin dual action cream 2% 15g
  GSL; 30g GSL
Daktarin dual action powder 2% 20g
  GSL
Daktarin spray powder 2% 100g GSL
Daktarin oral gel 15g P
Daktarin powder 2% P
Daktarin Aktiv cream, powder and spray
  powder GSL
Daktarin Gold P
Dalacin C preparations POM
Dalacin cream 2% POM
Dalacin T preps POM
Dalfopristin POM
Dalivit drops GSL
Dalmane caps CD Benz POM
Dalteparin sodium POM
Damiana GSL
Danaparoid sodium POM
Danazol POM
Dandelion GSL
Dandrazol Antidandruff shampoo P
Dandrazol Dandruff Shampoo GSL
Dandrazol shampoo POM
Danlax syrup POM
Danol capsules POM
Danthron see Dantron
Dantrium preparations POM
Dantrolene sodium POM
Dantron/Danthron POM
Daonil tablets POM
Dapsone POM
Dapsone ethane ortho sulphonate POM
Daptomycin POM
Daraprim tablets POM
Darbopoetin alfa POM
Darifenacin POM
Dasatinib POM
Daunorubicin hydrochloride POM
Daunoxome injection POM
Davenol linctus CD Inv P
Day and Night Nurse capsules P
Day Nurse preparations CD Inv P
Dayleve cream P
DDAVP Melt POM
DDAVP preps POM
DDD preps GSL
De Witts analgesic pills pack sizes 16s
  GSL; 32s P
De Witts antacid powder GSL
De Witts antacid tablets GSL
De Witts antibiotic throat lozenges P
De Witts Kidney and Bladder pills GSL
De Witts Placidex syrup P
De Witts Secron catarrh syrup for chil-
  dren P
De Witts Secron susp P
De Witts worm syrup P
De-capeptyl SR vial POM
De-Nol P
De-Noltab tablets P
Deanol bitartrate POM but if 26mg
  (MDD) P
Debrisan P
Debrisoquine sulphate POM
Deca-Durabolin injection CD Anab
  POM
Decadron preparations POM
Decan POM
Decapeptyl SR injection POM
Decubal cream GSL
Deep Freeze cold gel GSL

Deep Freeze pain relief spray GSL
Deep Heat Liniment, rub, spray GSL
Deep Relief pack sizes 15g GSL; 30g GSL; 50g GSL; 100g P
Defanac POM
Defanac Retard POM
Deferasirox POM
Deferiprone POM
Deflazacort POM
Delfen foam GSL
Delorazepam CD Benz POM
Delta-9-tetrahydrocannabinol see Dronabinol
Deltacortril Enteric tablets POM
Deltaprim tabs POM
Deltastab injection POM
Delvas tablets POM
Demecarium bromide POM
Demeclocycline POM
Demeclocycline calcium POM
Demeclocycline hydrochloride POM
Demix caps POM
Demser capsules POM
Dencyl capsules P
Denes medicine products GSL
Denorex shampoo 125ml PO
Denorex shampoo with conditioner 125ml PO
Dentinox Infant Colic drops GSL
Dentinox shampoo GSL
Dentinox teething gel GSL
Dentogen gel GSL
Dentogen liquid GSL
Dentomycin gel POM
Denzapine tablets POM
Deoxycoformycin POM
Deoxycortone acetate POM
Deoxycortone pivalate POM
Depakote tablets POM
Depixol preparations POM
DepoCyte POM
Depodur suspension for injection CD POM
Depo-Medrone injection POM
Depo-Medrone with lidocaine POM
Depo-Provera injections POM
Deponit 10 P
Deponit 5 P
Depostat injection POM
Deptropine citrate POM
Dequa Spray P
Dequacaine lozenges P
Dequadin lozenges P
Dequalinium chloride POM but if (1) internal: throat lozenges or throat pastilles maximum strength 0.25mg, P; (2) external: paint maximum strength 1.0 percent, P; minor infections of the mouth and throat 0.25mg (MD) 2mg (MDD), GSL
Derbac M P
Dermabond GSL
Dermacort hydrocortisone cream (PL 8265/0002) P
Dermalo bath emollient GSL
Dermamist spray P
Dermax shampoo P
Dermestril transdermal patches POM
Dermestril-Septem transdermal patches POM
Dermidex P
Dermol P
Dermol 200 P
Dermol 500 lotion P
Dermol 600 bath emollient P
Dermovate preparations POM
Dermovate-NN skin preparations POM
Deseril tablets POM
Deserpidine POM
Desferal injection POM
Desferrioxamine mesylate POM
Desflurane POM
Desipramine hydrochloride POM
Deslanoside POM
Desloratadine POM
DesmoMelt POM
Desmopressin POM
Desmopressin acetate POM

Desmospray intranasal spray POM
Desmotabs POM
Desogestrel POM
Desomorphine; its salts, esters and ethers CD POM
Desonide POM
Desoximetasone/Desoxymethasone POM
Desoxymethasone see Desoximetasone
Destolit tablets POM
Detoclo preparations POM
Detrunorm POM
Detrunorm XL POM
Detrusitol tablets POM
Detrusitol XL capsules POM
Dettol anti-bacterial cleanser GSL
Dettol antiseptic cream GSL
Dettol antiseptic pain relief spray P
Dettol antiseptic wash GSL
Dettol disinfectant spray GSL
Dettol liquid GSL
Dexa-Rhinaspray Duo POM
Dexamethasone POM
Dexamethasone acetate POM
Dexamethasone isonicotinate POM
Dexamethasone phenylpropionate POM
Dexamethasone pivalate POM
Dexamethasone sodium metasulphobenzoate POM
Dexamethasone sodium phosphate POM
Dexamethasone troxundate POM
Dexamfetamine CD POM
Dexedrine preparations CD POM
Dexemel POM
Dexfenfluramine hydrochloride POM
Dexibuprofen POM
Dexketoprofen POM
Dexomon SR POM
Dexpanthenol GSL
Dexpanthenol (Panthenol, Pantothenol) GSL
Dexrazoxane POM
Dexsol POM
Dextran POM
Dextrodiphenopyrine see Dextromoramide
Dextromethorphan hydrobromide POM but if internal (1) In the case of a prolonged release preparation: equivalent of 30mg of dextromethorphan (MD) equivalent of 75mg of dextromethorphan (MDD), P; (2) in any other case: equivalent of 15mg of dextromethorphan (MD) equivalent of 75mg of dextromethorphan (MDD), P
Dextromoramide; its salts CD POM
Dextropropoxyphene; its salts, esters and ethers CD POM but if in a preparation for oral use containing not more than 135mg of dextropropoxyphene (calculated as base) per dosage unit or with a total concentration of not more than 2.5% (calculated as base) CD Inv POM
Dextrose GSL
Dextrose injection POM
Dextrose monohydrate GSL
Dextrothyroxine sodium POM
DF 118 forte tabs CD Inv POM
DHC Continus tablets CD Inv POM
Diabact UBT POM
Diabetamide tabs POM
Diacetylmorphine see Diamorphine
Diagesil inj CD POM
Diaglyk tabs POM
Diah-Limit capsules GSL
Dialar POM
Diamicron MR tablets POM
Diamicron tablets POM
Diamorphine; its salts CD POM
Diamox preps POM
Diampromide; its salts CD POM
Dianette tablets POM
Diaquitte P
Diarrest liquid CD Inv POM
Diasorb capsules P

Diazemuls injection CD Benz POM
Diazepam CD Benz POM
Diazoxide POM
Dibenyline preparations POM
Dibenzepin hydrochloride POM
Dibromopropamidine see Dibrompropamidine
Dibrompropamidine/Dibrompropamidine isethionate, external use only GSL
Dichloralphenazone POM
Dichlorobenzyl alcohol, if external use or internal (pastilles, lozenges, throat tablets maximum strength 2mg) GSL
Dichlorodifluoromethane (Propellant 12), external use only GSL
Dichlorodifluoromethane (Propellant 21), external use only GSL
Dichlorophen, if maximum strength 1.0 per cent (external use only) GSL
Dichlorotetrafluroethane, external use only GSL
Dichloroxylenol, if internal maximum strength 0.5 per cent or external maximum strength 5.0 per cent GSL
Dichlorphenamide POM
Diclofenac diethylammonium POM but if external for local symptomatic relief of pain and inflammation in trauma of the tendons, ligaments, muscles and joints, eg, due to sprains, strains and bruises; localised forms of soft tissue rheumatism, for use in adults and children aged 12 years and over, for a maximum period of 7 days, maximum strength 1.16 per cent and container or package containing not more than 50g of medicinal product, GSL. Please refer to proprietary names for the classification granted under the marketing authorisation (See Voltarol Pain-Eze Emulgel)
Diclofenac potassium POM but if for the short term relief of headache, dental pain, period pain, rheumatic and muscular pain, backache and the symptoms of colds and flu, including fever, in adults and children aged 14 years and over, maximum strength 12.5mg, 25mg (MD), 75mg (MDD), for a maximum duration of 3 days' treatment and in a maximum pack size of 18 tablets, P
Diclofenac sodium POM; but for the local symptomatic relief of mild to moderate pain and inflammation following acute blunt trauma of small and medium-sized joints and periarticular structures, such as trauma of the tendons, ligaments, muscles and joints eg due to sprains and strains, maximum length of treatment without medical advice 7 days, maximum dose 40mg, maximum daily dose 120mg, maximum strength 4%, maximum pack size 25g of product, P, please refer to proprietary names for the classification granted under the marketing authorisation
Diclofex 75mg SR tablets POM
Dicloflex Retard tablets POM
Dicloflex tablets POM
Diclomax Retard capsules POM
Diclomax SR capsules POM
Diclotard tablets POM
Diclovol tablets POM
Diclovol Retard POM
Diclozip tabs POM
Dicobalt edetate POM
Diconal tablets CD POM
Dicyclomine see Dicycloverine
Dicycloverine/Dicyclomine hydrochloride POM but if 10mg (MD) 60mg (MDD), P
Dicynene preparations POM
Didanosine POM
Didronel preps POM

Dienestrol/Dienoestrol POM
Dienoestrol see Dienestrol
Diethanolamine fusidate POM
Diethyl phthalate, external use only GSL
Diethylamine salicylate, external use only GSL
Diethylpropion; its salts CD No Register POM
Diethylstilbestrol/Stilboestrol POM
Diethylstilbestrol/Stilboestrol dipropionate POM
Diethylthiambutene; its salts CD POM
N,N-Diethyltryptamine; its salts CD Lic
Difenoxin CD POM but if in preparations containing per dosage unit, not more than 0.5mg of difenoxin and a quantity of atropine sulphate equivalent to at least 5% of the dose of difenoxin CD Inv POM
Differin gel POM
Difflam cream P
Difflam oral rinse P
Difflam spray P
Diffundox MR POM
Diflucan capsules POM
Diflucan infusion POM
Diflucan One capsule P
Diflucan Oral suspension POM
Diflucortolone valerate POM
Diflunisal POM
Diftavax vaccine POM
Digenac XL tabs POM
Digibind POM
Digitalin POM
Digitaline Nativelle preparations POM
Digitalis leaf POM
Digitalis prepared POM
Digitoxin POM
Digoxin POM
Dihydralazine sulphate POM
Dihydrocodeine; its salts CD POM but if for non-parenteral use and (a) in undivided preparations with ms 2.5% (calculated as base) CD Inv POM; or (b) in single dose preparations with ms per dosage unit 100mg (calculated as base) CD Inv POM; or (c) in unit preparations diluted to at least one part in a million (6X) in response to a specific request, CD Inv P; or (d) in unit preparations diluted to at least one part in a million million (6C), CD Inv P
Dihydrocodeineone O-carboxymethyloxime; its salts esters and ethers CD POM
Dihydroergotamine mesylate POM
Dihydroetorphine CD POM
Dihydrohydroxycodeinone see Oxycodone
Dihydrohydroxymorphinone see Oxymorphone
Dihydromorphine; its salts, esters and ethers CD POM
Dihydromorphinone see Hydromorphone
Dihydrone see Oxycodone
Dihydrostreptomycin POM
Dihydrostreptomycin sulphate POM
Dihydroxyaluminium sodium carbonate GSL
Dilcardia SR capsules POM
Dilcardia XL capsules POM
Dill Oil GSL
Diloxanide furoate POM
Diltiazem hydrochloride POM
Dilzem SR capsules POM
Dilzem XL capsules POM
Dimenhydrinate P
Dimenoxadole; its salts CD POM
Dimepheptanol; its salts, esters and ethers CD POM
Dimercaprol POM
Dimethicone see Dimeticone
Dimethisoquin hydrochloride POM but if non-ophthalmic use, P
Dimethisterone POM

Dimethothiazine mesylate POM
2,5-Dimethoxy-a,4-dimethylphenethy-
lamine; its salts CD Lic
Dimethyl sulfoxide/Dimethyl sulphox-
ide POM
Dimethyl sulphoxide see Dimethyl sul-
foxide
Dimethylthiambutene; its salts CD POM
N,N-Dimethyltryptamine; its salts CD
Lic
Dimethyltubocurarine bromide POM
Dimethyltubocurarine chloride POM
Dimethyltubocurarine iodide POM
Dimeticone/Dimethicone GSL
Dimetriose capsules POM
Dimorphone see Hydrocodone
Dimotane elixir P
Dimotane expectorant P
Dimotane LA tabs P
Dimotane Plus elixir P
Dimotane Plus Paediatric elixir P
Dimotane tablets P
Dimotane with Codeine CD Inv P
Dimotane with Codeine Paediatric CD
Inv P
Dimotapp elixir P
Dimotapp elixir Paediatric P
Dimotapp LA tablets P
Dindevan tablets POM
Dinnefords Teejel GSL
Dinoprost POM
Dinoprost Trometamol POM
Dinoprostone POM
Diocalm tablets CD Inv P
Diocalm Complete GSL
Diocalm Ultra pack sizes 6s GSL; 12s P
Diocaps POM
Dioctyl capsules P
Dioderm cream POM
Dioralyte pack sizes 6s GSL; 20s P
Dioralyte Relief pack sizes 6s GSL; 20s P
Diovan caps POM
Dioxaphetyl butyrate; its salts CD POM
Dipentum capsules POM
Dipeptiven POM
Diperodon hydrochloride, external use
only GSL
Diphenhydramine hydrochloride POM
but all preparations except liquid-
filled capsules, P
Diphenoxylate hydrochloride POM but
if maximum strength 2.5mg, in combination with atropine sulphate for
short term use as an adjunctive therapy to appropriate rehydration in
acute diarrhoea, for use in persons
aged 16 years and over, in tablet
form, with MDD 25mg, in a container or package containing not more
than 20 tablets, P
Diphenoxylate; its salts CD POM but if
in preparations with ms per dosage
unit 2.5mg of diphenoxylate (calculated as base), and a quantity of
atropine sulphate equivalent to at
least 1% of the dose of diphenoxylate CD Inv POM

Diphtheria and tetanus vaccine POM
Diphtheria vaccine POM
Diphtheria, tetanus and pertussis vac-
cine POM
Diphtheria, tetanus and poliomyelitis
vaccine POM
Diphtheria, tetanus, pertussis and
poliomyelitis vaccine POM
Dipipanone; its salts CD POM
Dipivefrine POM
Dipotassium clorazepate/Potassium clo-
razepate CD Benz POM
Diprivan injection POM
Diprobase cream and ointment GSL
Diprobath P
Diprosalic ointment and scalp applica-
tion POM
Diprosone preparations POM
Dipyridamole POM
Dirythmin SA tablets POM

Disipal POM
Disney multivitamins & minerals GSL
Disney vitamin C GSL
Disodium edetate, external use only
GSL
Disodium etidronate POM
Disodium pamidronate POM
Disogram SR POM
Disopyramide POM
Disopyramide phosphate POM
Dispello GSL
Disprin CV P
Disprin Direct tablets pack sizes 16s GSL
Disprin Extra tablets pack sizes 16s GSL
Disprin tablets pack sizes 8s, 16s GSL;
32s P
Disprol suspension sugar-free 100ml P
and GSL
Disprol soluble tablets pack sizes 16s
GSL
Disprol susp sachets pack sizes 12s GSL
Distaclor MR tablets POM
Distaclor preparations POM
Distalgesic tablets CD Inv POM
Distamine tablets POM
Distigmine bromide POM
Disulfiram POM
Ditemic Spansule P
Dithranol POM but if maximum
strength 1.0 per cent, P
Dithrocream 0.1%, 0.25%, 1% P
Dithrocream 2% POM
Dithrocream forte 0.5% P
Ditropan preparations POM
Diumide-K Continus tablets POM
Diurexan tablets POM
Diva tablets POM
Dixarit tablets POM
DMT see N,N-Dimethyltryptamine
Do-Do tablets P
Doans backache pills GSL
Dobutamine hydrochloride POM
Dobutrex ampoules POM
Docetaxel POM
Docosahexaenoic acid (DHA) GSL
Docusate sodium GSL
Docusol liquid P
Dolasetron mesilate POM
Dolmatil tablets POM
Dolobid tablets POM
Doloxene capsules CD Inv POM
Dolvan tablets P
Domical tablets POM
Dominion Pharma hayfever eye-drops P
Domiphen bromide GSL
Domperamol tabs POM
Domperidone POM but if for the relief
of post-prandial symptoms of exces-
sive fullness, nausea, epigastric bloat-
ing and belching, occasionally
accompanied by epigastric discom-
fort and heartburn, 10mg of domperidone (MD), 40mg of domperi-
done(MDD) in a container or package containing not more than
200mg of domperidone P
Domperidone maleate POM but if for
the relief of post-prandial symptoms
of excessive fullness, nausea, epigastric bloating and belching, occasionally accompanied by epigastric dis-
comfort and heartburn, 10mg of
domperidone as domperidone
maleate (MD), 40mg of domperidone
as domperidone maleate (MDD) in a
container or package containing not
more than 200mg of domperidone as
domperidone maleate P
Donepezil HCl POM
Dopacard injection POM
Dopamine hydrochloride POM
Dopexamine hydrochloride POM
Dopram injection POM
Doralese tiltabs tablets POM
Doribax POM
Dormonoct tabs CD Benz POM
Dornase alfa POM
Dorzolamide POM

Dostinex tablets POM
Dosulepin/Dothiepin POM
Dosulepin/Dothiepin hydrochloride
POM
Dothapax preps POM
Dothiepin see Dosulepin
Doublebase gel P
Dovobet ointment POM
Dovonex preps POM
Doxadura POM
Doxadura XL POM
Doxapram hydrochloride POM
Doxazosin mesylate POM
Doxepin hydrochloride POM
Doxorubicin POM
Doxorubicin hydrochloride POM
Doxycycline POM
Doxycycline calcium chelate POM
Doxycycline hyclate/Doxycycline
hydrochloride POM
Doxycycline hydrochloride see
Doxycycline hyclate
Doxylar capsules POM
Dozic liquid POM
Dozol liquid P
Dr. Greenfingers bumps & bruises oint-
ment GSL
Dr. Greenfingers cough soother GSL
Dr. Greenfingers cuts and grazes oint-
ment GSL
Dramamine tablets P
Drapolene cream GSL
Dreemon P
Driclor roll-on P
Dried smallpox vaccine POM
Dristan decongestant tablets P
Drogenil tablets POM
Droleptan preparations POM
Dromadol POM
Dronabinol CD POM
Droperidol POM
Drostanolone; its salts CD Anab POM
Drotebanol; its salts, esters and ethers
CD POM
Dryptal tablets POM
DTIC- Dome vial POM
DTP vaccine (pre-filled) POM
Duac Once Daily Gel POM
Dubam spray relief/cream GSL
Dukoral oral vaccine POM
Dulbalm P
Dulcoease GSL
Dulco-Lax children's suppositories P
Dulco-Lax liquid P
Dulco-Lax Perles pack sizes 20s GSL; 50s
P
Dulco-Lax suppositories P
Dulco-lax tablets pack sizes 10s GSL; 20s
GSL; 40s GSL; 60s P; 100s P
Duloxetine POM
Dumicoat denture lacquer POM
Duodopa intestinal gel POM
Duofilm P
DuoTrav eye drops POM
Duovent preparations POM
Duphalac Dry P
Duphalac syrup P
Duphaston HRT POM
Duphaston tablets POM
Duragel gel GSL
Duraphat 5000 toothpaste POM
Duraphat weekly rinse P
Duraphat 2800 POM
Durogesic patches CD POM
Durogesic DTrans patches CD POM
Duromine capsules CD No Register
POM
Dutasteride POM
Dutonin tablets POM
Dyazide tablets POM
Dydrogesterone POM
Dyflos POM
Dymotil tablets P
Dynamin tabs P
Dynastat injection POM
Dysman preps POM
Dyspamet POM
Dysport inj POM

Dytac capsules POM
Dytide capsules POM

E

E45 cream GSL
E45 Itch Relief GSL
Earcalm P
Earex ear drops GSL
Earex Plus P
Earex protector plugs GSL
Easyhaler preparations POM
Ebixa tablets and oral drops POM
Ebufac tablets POM
Eccoxolac capsules POM
Ecgonine; and any derivative of ecgo-
nine which is convertible to ecgo-
nine or to cocaine CD POM
Echinacea GSL
Echinacea tabs GSL
Econac preparations POM
Econacort cream POM
Econazole POM but if external, and in
the case of vaginal use only external
use for the treatment of vaginal can-
didiasis P
Econazole nitrate POM but if external,
and in the case of vaginal use only
external use for the treatment of
vaginal candidiasis P
Ecopace tabs POM
Ecostatin cream P
Ecostatin pessaries POM
Ecostatin Twinpack POM
Ecostatin-1 pessaries POM
Ecothiopate iodide POM
Edecrin preparations POM
Edetic acid, external use only GSL
Edible Bone Flour (bonemeal) GSL
Ednyt POM
Edronax tablets POM
Edrophonium chloride POM
Efalex caps GSL
Efalith ointment POM
Efalizumab POM
Efamast capsules POM
Efavirenz POM
Efcortelan cream, ointment POM
Efcortesol inj POM
Efexor capsules POM
Efexor XL tablets POM
Effentora buccal tablets CD POM
Effercitrate sachets GSL
Effercitrate tablets GSL
Effico GSL
Efient tablets POM
Eflornithine hydrochloride POM
Eformoterol see Formoterol
Efudix cream POM
Eicosapentaenoic acid (EPA) GSL
Elantan 10 tablets P
Elantan 20 tablets P
Elantan 40 tablets P
Elantan LA 25 capsules P
Elantan LA 50 capsules P
Elaprase POM
Elavil tablets POM
Eldepryl syrup POM
Eldepryl tablets POM
Elder GSL
Eldisine vials POM
Elecampane GSL
Electrolade sachets GSL
Eletriptan POM
Elidel cream POM
Elleste Duet POM
Elleste Duet Conti tablets POM
Elleste Solo MX40 patches POM
Elleste Solo MX80 patches POM
Elleste Solo tablets POM
Elliman's embrocation GSL
Elocon preparations POM
Elohaes IV inf POM
Eloxatin infusion POM
Elset rayon/elastic bandages GSL
Eltor vaccine POM
Eltroxin tablets POM
Eludril mouthwash GSL

Eludril spray P
Elyzol gel POM
Emadine eye drops POM
Emblon tabs POM
Embrel injection POM
Embutramide POM
Emcor LS tablets POM
Emcor tablets POM
Emedastine POM
Emend capsules POM
Emepronium bromide POM
Emeside preparations POM
Emetine POM but if maximum strength
    1.0 per cent, P
Emetine bismuth iodide POM
Emetine hydrochloride POM but if
    maximum strength equivalent of 1.0
    per cent of emetine, P
Emfib caps POM
Emflex capsules POM
Eminase injection POM
Emla cream P
Emmolate bath oil P
Emselex POM
Emtricitabine POM
Emtriva preparations POM
Emulsiderm P
Emulsifying ointment BP GSL
Emulsifying wax, external use only GSL
En-de-kay Fluodrops P
En-De-Kay Fluoride mouthrinse daily
    GSL
En-de-kay Fluorinse POM
En-de-kay Fluotabs 3-6 years tablets P
En-de-kay Fluotabs 6+ years tablets P
Enalapril maleate POM
Enbrel injection POM
Encephalitis Virus, Tick-borne, Cent Eur
    POM
Endoxana preparations POM
Enestebol CD Anab POM
Enfamil AR GSL
Enfuvirtide POM
Engerix B Paediatric vaccine POM
Engerix B vaccine POM
Enos powder GSL
Enoxacin POM
Enoxaparin sodium POM
Enoximone POM
Enprin tabs 28 P
Entecapone POM
Entecavir POM
Enterosan tablets CD Inv P
Entocort CR capsules POM
Entocort enemas POM
Entonox P
Entrocalm preparations GSL
Entrolax constipation relief tablets P
Entrolax laxative tablets GSL
Enzed tablets POM
Enzira POM
Epaderm emollient GSL
Epanutin preparations POM
Epaxal POM
Ephedrine POM but if (1) internal
    (other than nasal sprays or nasal
    drops) 30mg (MD) 60mg (MDD); (2)
    nasal sprays or nasal drops maxi-
    mum strength 2.0 per cent; (3) exter-
    nal, P
Ephedrine hydrochloride POM but if (1)
    internal (other than nasal sprays or
    nasal drops) equivalent of 30mg of
    ephedrine (MD) equivalent of 60mg
    of ephedrine (MDD); (2) nasal sprays
    or nasal drops maximum strength
    equivalent of 2.0 per cent of
    ephedrine; (3) external, P
Ephedrine sulphate POM but if (1)
    internal (other than nasal sprays or
    nasal drops) equivalent of 30mg of
    ephedrine (MD) equivalent of 60mg
    of ephedrine (MDD); (2) nasal sprays
    or nasal drops maximum strength
    equivalent of 2.0 per cent of
    ephedrine; (3) external, P
Ephynal tablets GSL
Epicillin POM

Epilim preparations POM
Epimaz tablets POM
Epinastine POM
Epinephrine see Adrenaline
Epipen pens POM
Epirubicin POM
Epirubicin hydrochloride POM
Episenta POM
Epithiazide POM
Epitiostanol CD Anab POM
Epivir solution POM
Epivir tablets POM
Eplerenone POM
Epoetin Alfa POM
Epoetin Beta POM
Epogam capsules POM
Epoprostenol sodium POM
Eposin POM
Eppy POM
Eprex injection POM
Eprosartan POM
Epsom salts BP GSL
Eptifibatide POM
Equagesic tablets CD No Register POM
Equanil tablets CD No Register POM
Equasym tablets CD POM
Equasym XL capsules CD POM
Equilon herbal caps GSL
Equilon tabs P
Equisetum GSL
Erbitux POM
Erdosteine POM
Erdotin POM
Erecnos injection POM
Ergometrine maleate POM
Ergometrine tartrate POM
Ergot, Prepared POM
Ergotamine tartrate POM
Erlotinib POM
Ertapenem POM
Ervevax vial POM
Erwinase inj POM
Eryacne gel POM
Erycen tabs POM
Erymax capsules POM
Erymin suspension POM
Erythrocin preparations POM
Erythromycin POM
Erythromycin estolate POM
Erythromycin ethyl succinate POM
Erythromycin ethylcarbonate POM
Erythromycin lactobionate POM
Erythromycin phosphate POM
Erythromycin stearate POM
Erythromycin thiocyanate POM
Erythroped A tablets POM
Erythroped preparations POM
Erythropoietin POM
Erythrosine E127 GSL
Escitalopram POM
Eskamel cream P
Eskazole tablets POM
Eskornade Spansule capsules P
Esmeron ampoules POM
Esmolol hydrochloride POM
Esomeprazole POM
Estazolam CD Benz POM
Estracombi POM
Estracyt capsules POM
Estraderm MX patches POM
Estraderm TTS POM
Estradiol implant POM
Estradiol/Oestradiol POM
Estradiol/Oestradiol benzoate POM
Estradiol/Oestradiol cypionate POM
Estradiol/Oestradiol dipropionate POM
Estradiol/Oestradiol diundecanoate
    POM
Estradiol/Oestradiol enanthate POM
Estradiol/Oestradiol phenylpropionate
    POM
Estradiol/Oestradiol undecanoate POM
Estradiol/Oestradiol valerate POM
Estradot POM
Estragest TTS POM
Estramustine phosphate POM
Estramustine sodium phosphate POM
Estrapak 50 POM

Estring POM
Estriol/Oestriol POM
Estriol/Oestriol succinate POM
Estrone/Oestrone POM
Estropipate POM
Etacrynic acid/Ethacrynic acid POM
Etafedrine hydrochloride POM
Etamsylate/Ethamsylate POM
Etanercept POM
Ethacrynic acid see Etacrynic acid
Ethambutol hydrochloride POM
Ethamivan POM
Ethamsylate see Etamsylate
Ethanolamine oleate POM
Ethchlorvynol CD No Register POM
Ether, up to 0.25ml (MD) GSL
Ethiazide POM
Ethimil tabs POM
Ethinamate CD No Register POM
Ethinyl androstenediol POM
Ethinylestradiol/Ethinyloestradiol POM
Ethinyloestradiol see Ethinylestradiol
Ethionamide POM
Ethisterone POM
Ethmozine tablets POM
Ethoglucid POM
Ethoheptazine citrate POM
Ethopropazine hydrochloride POM
Ethosuximide POM
Ethotoin POM
Ethyl biscoumacetate POM
Ethyl loflazepate CD Benz POM
Ethyl nicotinate, external use only GSL
Ethyl salicylate, external use only GSL
N-Ethylamfetamine; its salts; its
    stereoisomers; their salts CD Benz
    POM
Ethyleostrenol CD Anab POM
Ethylmethylthiambutene; its salts CD
    POM
Ethylmorphine (3-ethylmorphine); its
    salts CD POM but if for non-par-
    enteral use and (a) in undivided
    preparations with ms 2.5% (calculat-
    ed as base) CD Inv POM; or (b) in
    single dose preparations with ms per
    dosage unit 100mg (calculated as
    base) CD Inv POM; or (c) in unit
    preparations diluted to at least one
    part in a million (6X) in response to
    a specific request, CD Inv P; or (d) in
    unit preparations diluted to at least
    one part in a million million (6C),
    CD Inv P
Ethylmorphine hydrochloride see
    Ethylmorphine
Ethynodiol see Etynodiol
Ethyol infusion POM
Eticyclidine CD Lic
Etodolac POM
Etomidate POM
Etomidate hydrochloride POM
Etonitazene; its salts CD POM
Etonogestrel POM
Etopan XL POM
Etopophos injection POM
Etoposide POM
Etoposide for injection concentrate
    POM
Etoricoxib POM
Etorphine; its salts, esters and ethers CD
    POM
Etoxeridine; its salts, esters and ethers
    CD POM
Etretinate POM
Etryptamine CD Lic
Etynodiol/Ethynodiol diacetate POM
Eucalyptol GSL
Eucalyptus oil GSL
Eucardic tablets POM
Eucerin extremely dry skin cream GSL
Eucerin extremely dry skin lotion GSL
Eucreas tablets POM
Eudemine preparations POM
Euflexxa POM
Eugenol, external use only GSL
Euglucon tablets POM
Eugynon 30 tablets POM

Eumovate eczema and dermatitis cream
    P
Eumovate preparations POM
Euphorbia hirta (Euphorbia pilulifera,
    Pill-Bearing Spurge) GSL
Eurax cream GSL
Eurax HC cream (PL 0001/5010R) P
Eurax Hydrocortisone POM
Eurax lotion GSL
European Birch, external use only GSL
Evista tablets POM
Evoltra POM
Evorel Conti patches POM
Evorel Pak POM
Evorel patches POM
Evorel Sequi patches POM
Evotrox POM
Evra transdermal patches POM
Ex-Lax laxative chocolate GSL
Exelderm cream P
Exelon capsules POM
Exelon oral solution POM
Exemestane POM
Exforge POM
Exjade POM
Exocin eye drops POM
Exorex lotion GSL
Exosurf Neonatal POM
Expulin children's cough linctus P
Expulin decongestant linctus for babies
    and children P
Expulin Dry Cough CD Inv P
Expulin For Chesty Coughs GSL
Expulin Paediatric linctus CD Inv P
Extavia 250mcg/ml powder and solvent
    for solution for injection POM
Exterol ear drops P
Exubera tablets POM
Eye Dew eye drops P
Ezetimibe POM
Ezetrol tablets POM

F

Fabrazyme POM
Factor VIIA, VIII, IX POM
Factor XIII concentrate POM
Fam-Lax tablets POM
Famciclovir POM
Famel Original CD Inv P
Famotidine POM but if for the short-
    term symptomatic relief of heart-
    burn, dyspepsia, indigestion, acid
    indigestion and hyperacidity, and
    prevention of these symptoms when
    associated with food and drink,
    including nocturnal symptoms,
    10mg (MD) 20mg (MDD) for maxi-
    mum period of 14 days, P; in the
    case of a tablet, maximum strength
    10mg, for the short term sympto-
    matic relief of hearburn, indigestion,
    acid indigestion and hyperacidity,
    10mg (MD), 20mg (MDD) and not
    more than 12 tablets GSL
Famvir tablets POM
Fansidar tablets POM
Fareston tablets POM
Farlutal preparations POM
Fasigyn preparations POM
Faslodex injection POM
Fast Green FCF GSL
Fasturtec infusion POM
Faverin tablets POM
Fazadinium bromide POM
Fectrim preparations POM
Fedril preps P
Fefol Spansule capsules P
Fefol Z Spansule capsules P
Fefol-Vit Spansule capsules P
Fefol-Vit Z Spansule capsules P
Feiba Immuno POM
Felbinac POM but if external for the
    relief of rheumatic pain, pain of non-
    serious arthritic conditions and soft
    tissue injuries such as sprains, strains
    and contusions for use in adults and
    children not less than 12 years, for

maximum period of 7 days maximum strength 3.17 per cent and container or package containing not more than 30g of medicinal product, P

Feldene P gel P
Feldene capsules POM
Feldene Dispersible tablets POM
Feldene gel POM
Feldene IM POM
Feldene Melt POM
Feldene suppositories POM
Felendil XL POM
Felicium capsules POM
Felodipine POM
Felogen XL POM
Felotens XL POM
Felypressin POM
Femapak 40 HRT POM
Femapak 80 HRT POM
Femara tablets POM
Fematrix patches POM
Femeron cream P
Femeron pessaries P
Femfresh powder GSL
Femigraine P
Feminax tablets CD Inv P
Feminax Ultra tablets P
Feminine Balance GSL
Femodene preps POM
Femodette tablets POM
Femoston tablets POM
Femoston-conti tablets POM
FemSeven Conti patches POM
FemSeven patches POM
FemSeven Sequi patches POM
FemTab POM
FemTab Continuous POM
FemTab Sequi POM
Femulen tablets POM
Fenactol POM
Fenactol Retard POM
Fenbid Forte gel pack size 100g POM
Fenbid Forte gel pack size 30g P
Fenbid gel pack sizes 30g, 50g GSL; 100g P
Fenbid spansules POM
Fenbufen POM
Fenbuzip preps POM
Fencamfamin; its salts, stereoisomers CD Benz POM
Fenclofenac POM
Fendrix hepatitis B (rDNA) vaccine POM
Fenethylline; its salts and stereoisomers CD POM
Fenfluramine hydrochloride POM
Fenistil P
Fennel GSL
Fennel Oil GSL
Fennings Children's Cooling powder pack sizes 10s GSL; 20s P
Fennings Little Healers GSL
Fenofibrate POM
Fenogal capsules POM
Fenoket 200mg caps POM
Fenoprofen POM
Fenoprofen calcium POM
Fenopron tablets POM
Fenoterol hydrobromide POM
Fenox nasal drops P
Fenox nasal spray P
Fenpaed oral suspension P
Fenpaed sachets GSL
Fenproporex; its salts and stereoisomers CD Benz POM
Fentamox tabs POM
Fentanyl; its salts CD POM
Fentazin preparations POM
Fenticonazole nitrate POM but external use (but in the case of vaginal use, only for the treatment of vaginal candidiasis) P
Fenugreek GSL
Feospan Spansule capsules P
Feprapax POM
Feprazone POM
Ferfolic SV tablets POM
Feroglobin B12 caps GSL

Ferric ammonium citrate, if MD equivalent to 24 mg elemental iron GSL
Ferric chloride, if MD equivalent to 24mg elemental iron GSL
Ferriprox oral solution POM
Ferriprox tablets POM
Ferrograd C tablets P
Ferrograd Folic tablets P
Ferrograd tabs P
Ferrous arsenate POM
Ferrous carbonate, if MD equivalent to 24 mg elemental iron GSL
Ferrous fumarate, if MD equivalent to 24 mg elemental iron GSL
Ferrous gluconate, if MD equivalent to 24 mg elemental iron GSL
Ferrous sulphate, if internal (except for use as cyanide antidote) equivalent to 24 mg elemental iron (MD) or internal (for use as cyanide antidote only) maximum strength 15.8 per cent (FeSO4 7H2O) GSL
Fersaday tablets P
Fersamal syrup P
Fersamal tablets P
Fertiral injection POM
Fesovit Z Spansule capsules P
Feverfen P
Fexofenadine POM
Fibre, Vegetable GSL
Fibro-vein POM
Fiery Jack preparations GSL
Fig GSL
Filair preparations POM
Filgrastim POM
Filnarine SR tablets CD POM
Finacea POM
Finasteride POM
Fir Oil, Siberian GSL
Firazir POM
Firmagon powder and solvent for injection POM
Flagyl Compak POM
Flagyl injection POM
Flagyl suppositories POM
Flagyl tablets POM
Flagyl-S suspension POM
Flamatak preps POM
Flamatrol caps POM
Flamazine cream POM
Flamrase preps POM
Flavoxate hydrochloride POM
Flaxedil injection POM
Flecainide acetate POM
Fleet preps P
Fletchers' arachis oil retention enema P
Fletchers' enemette P
Fletchers' phosphate enema P
Fletchers' prednisolone retention enema (Predenema) POM
Flexin Continus tablets POM
Flexotard MR POM
Flexotard tablets POM
Flixonase Allergy nasal spray P
Flixonase aqueous spray POM
Flixonase nasules POM
Flixotide preps POM
Flolan POM
Flomax MR capsules POM
Flomaxtra XL tablets POM
Florinef tablets POM
Flosequinan POM
Floxapen preparations POM
Flu-amp caps POM
Fluanisone POM
Fluanxol tablets POM
Fluarix vaccine POM
Flubendazole POM
Fluclomix caps POM
Fluclorolone acetonide POM
Flucloxacillin magnesium POM
Flucloxacillin sodium POM
Flucloxin preps POM
Fluconazole POM but if for oral administration for the treatment of vaginal candidiasis or associated candidal balanitis in persons aged not less than 16 but less than 60 years,

150mg (MD) and container or package containing not more than 150mg of fluconazole, P
Flucytosine POM
Fludara POM
Fludara oral tablets POM
Fludarabine POM
Fludiazepam CD Benz POM
Fludrocortisone acetate POM
Fludroxycortide/Flurandrenolone POM
Flufenamic acid POM
Flumazenil POM
Flumetasone/Flumethasone POM
Flumetasone/Flumethasone pivalate POM
Flumethasone see Flumetasone
Flunisolide POM but if for the prevention and treatment of seasonal allergic rhinitis, including hay fever, in persons aged 18 years and over in the form of a non-pressurised nasal spray 50mcg per nostril (MD) 100mcg per nostril (MDD) for a maximum period of 3 months, maximum strength 0.025 per cent and container or package containing not more than 6,000mcg of flunisolide, P
Flunitrazepam CD No Register POM
Fluocinolone acetonide POM
Fluocinonide POM
Fluocortin butyl POM
Fluocortolone POM
Fluocortolone hexanoate POM
Fluocortolone pivalate POM
Fluor-A-Day tablets P
Fluorescein dilaurate POM
Fluorets P
Fluorigard Daily drops P
Fluorigard Daily rinse GSL
Fluorigard Gelkam gel P
Fluorigard tablets P
Fluorigard Weekly rinse P
Fluorometholone POM
Fluorouracil POM
Fluorouracil trometamol POM
Fluoxetine hydrochloride POM
Fluoxymesterone CD Anab POM
Flupenthixol see Flupentixol
Flupentixol/Flupenthixol decanoate POM
Flupentixol/Flupenthixol hydrochloride POM
Fluperolone acetate POM
Fluphenazine decanoate POM
Fluphenazine enanthate POM
Fluphenazine hydrochloride POM
Fluprednidene acetate POM
Fluprednisolone POM
Fluprostenol sodium POM
Flurandrenolone see Fludroxycortide
Flurazepam; its salts CD Benz POM
Flurbiprofen POM but if maximum strength 8.75mg, in the form of a throat lozenge, with a MDD 43.75mg and in a container or package containing not more than 140mg of flurbiprofen, P
Flurbiprofen sodium POM
Fluspirilene POM
Flutamide POM
Fluticasone propionate POM
Flutrimazole POM
Fluvastatin sodium POM
Fluvirin vaccine POM
Fluvoxamine maleate POM
Fluzone POM
FML Liquifilm ophthalmic suspension POM
FML-Neo eye drops POM
Folex-350 tablets P
Folic acid POM but if 500mcg (MDD), GSL
Folicare oral solution GSL
Follicle stimulating hormone POM
Follitropin alpha POM
Follitropin beta POM
Fomac tabs POM
Fondaparinux sodium POM

Foradil capsules (for inhalation) POM
Forceval capsules P
Forceval Junior P
Forceval-Protein P
Formaldehyde solution, if maximum strength 0.47% in a dentifrice or maximum strength 0.75% for external use other than as a dentifrice, GSL

Formebolone CD Anab POM
Formestane POM
Formocortal POM
Formoterol/Eformoterol fumarate POM
Forsteo POM
Fortagesic tablets CD No Register POM
Fortespan P
Fortipine LA 40 POM
Fortovase capsules POM
Fortum injection POM
Fosamax Once Weekly tablets POM
Fosamax tablets POM
Fosamprenavir POM
Fosavance tablets POM
Foscan POM
Foscarnet sodium POM
Foscavir infusion POM
Fosfestrol sodium POM
Fosfomycin trometamol POM
Fosinopril sodium POM
Fosphenytoin POM
Fosrenol POM
Fostimon POM
Frador GSL
Fragmin injection POM
Framycetin sulphate POM
Framyspray aerosol POM
Frangula GSL
Frangula bark GSL
Frangulin GSL
Franol Plus tablets P
Franol tablets P
Freederm gel P
Freezone P
Friars' balsam BP GSL
Fringe tree GSL
Frisium tabs CD Benz POM
Froben SR capsules POM
Froben suppositories POM
Froben tablets POM
Froop preps POM
Frovatriptan POM
Fru-Co tablets POM
Fructose injection POM
Frumil Forte tablets POM
Frumil LS tablets POM
Frumil tablets POM
Frusemide see Furosemide
Frusene tablets POM
Frusid tablets POM
Frusol oral solution POM
FSC waterfall caps GSL
FSME-Immun POM
Fucibet cream POM
Fucidin H preparations POM
Fucidin preparations POM
Fucithalmic drops POM
Fulcin preparations POM
Full Marks preps P
Fullers earth, external use only GSL
Fulvestrant POM
Fumitory, up to 160mg (MD) GSL
Fungederm cream P
Fungilin preparations POM
Fungizone injection POM
Furadantin preparations POM
Furamide tablets POM
Furazabol CD Anab POM
Furazolidone POM
Furethidine; its salts CD POM
Furosemide/Frusemide POM
Fusafungine POM
Fusidic acid POM
Fuzeon injection POM
Fybogel Mebeverine sachets pack sizes 10s P, 60s POM
Fybogel sachets pack sizes 10s, 30s PO
Fybozest Orange granules P

G

Gabapentin POM
Gabitril tablets POM
Gadoteridol POM
Galake tabs POM
Galantamine POM
Galcodine Linctus CD Inv P
Galcodine Linctus Paediatric CD Inv P
Galenamet tabs POM
Galenamox caps POM
Galenphol Linctus CD Inv P
Galenphol Linctus Paediatric CD Inv P
Galenphol Linctus Strong CD Inv P
Galenphol Original CD Inv P
Galfer preps P
Galfloxin capsules POM
Gallamine triethiodide POM
Galloway's Cough syrup GSL
Galpamol sachets GSL
Galpharm 3-in-1 antacid tablets GSL
Galpharm allergy eye drops P
Galpharm cold sore cream GSL
Galpharm dual action diarrhoea relief GSL
Galpharm extra power pain reliever tablets GSL
Galpharm Flu relief caps GSL
Galpharm flu strength all-in-one liquid P
Galpharm Hayfever and Allergy Relief Syrup GSL
Galpharm Hayfever and Allergy Relief Tablets pack sizes 7s GSL; 30s P
Galpharm Hayfever and Allergy Relief tablets non drowsy pack sizes 7s GSL; 30s P
Galpharm hot lemon powders flu strength GSL
Galpharm ibuprofen caplets 16s GSL; 24, 48, 96 P
Galpharm ibuprofen gel GSL
Galpharm ibuprofen 200mg tablets pack sizes 16s GSL
Galpharm ibuprofen 400mg tablets pack sizes 16s GSL; 96s P
Galpharm ibuprofen tablets max strength P
Galpharm migraine relief GSL
Galpharm Medical antiseptic cream GSL
Galpharm mouth ulcer treatment GSL
Galpharm nasal decongestant spray GSL
Galpharm paediatric suspension pack sizes 100ml P; 10 x 5ml GSL
Galpharm paracetamol caplets and tablets GSL
Galpharm senncalax GSL
Galpharm thrush preparations P
Galprofen cold & flu tablets GSL
Galprofen long lasting capsules 200mg GSL
Galprofen long lasting capsules 300mg P
Galpseud preps P
Galpseud Plus P
Galsud decongestant nasal spray GSL
Galsud linctus and tablets P
Galvus tablets POM
Gamanil tablets POM
Gamma Globulin (Kabi) ampoules POM
Gammabulin injection POM
Gammaderm cream GSL
Gammagard S/D POM
Gammahydroxy-butyrate (GHB) CD Benz POM
Ganciclovir POM
Ganciclovir sodium POM
Ganda eye drops POM
Ganfort eye drops POM
Ganirelix POM
Garamycin preparations POM
Gardasil POM
Gardenal sodium preparations CD No Register POM Note: emergency supply at request of patient not permitted except for use in the treatment of epilepsy
Garlic GSL

Garlic Oil GSL
Gastrobid Continus tablets POM
Gastrocote liquid P
Gastrocote tablets GSL
Gastroflux tabs POM
Gastromax capsules POM
Gastromiro POM
Gavilast pack sizes 6s GSL; 12s GSL; 48s P
Gavilast-P P
Gaviscon 250 tablets GSL
Gaviscon Advance PO
Gaviscon Cool preparations GSL
Gaviscon Double Action GSL
Gaviscon Extra Strength PO
Gaviscon infant sachets PO
Gaviscon liquid GSL
Gee's linctus BPC CD Inv P
Gelcosal P
Gelofusine POM
Gelsemine POM but if maximum strength 0.1 per cent, P
Gelsemium POM but if 25mg (MD) 75mg (MDD), P
Geltears P
Gemcitabine POM
Gemeprost POM
Gemfibrozil POM
Gemzar injection POM
Genalat retard tabs POM
Gencardia POM
Genotropin preps CD Anab POM
Gentamicin POM
Gentamicin Redibags POM
Gentamicin sulphate POM
Gentian GSL
Genticin preparations POM
Gentisone HC ear drops POM
Gentran IV inf POM
George's American Liniment GSL
Geranium oil, external use only GSL
Gerard House catarrh-eeze tablets GSL
Gerard House echinacea and garlic tablets GSL
Gerard House ginkgo tablets GSL
Gerard House hayfever aid tablets GSL
Gerard House herbulax tablets GSL
Gerard House reumalex tablets GSL
Gerard House serenity tablets GSL
Gerard House skin tablets GSL
Gerard House somnus tablets GSL
Gerard House water relief tablets GSL
Geref 50 POM
Germolene preparations GSL
Germoloids preparations GSL
Gestodene POM
Gestone injections POM
Gestonorone/Gestronol POM
Gestonorone/Gestronol hexanoate POM
Gestrinone POM
Gestronol see Gestonorone
Ginger GSL
Ginger tabs GSL
Ginseng GSL
Givitol capsules P
Glamin sol POM
Glatiramer acetate POM
Glau-opt eye drops POM
Glaucol eye drops POM
Gliadel POM
Glibenclamide POM
Glibenese tablets POM
Glibornuride POM
Gliclazide POM
Gliken tabs POM
Glimepiride POM
Glipizide POM
Gliquidone POM
Glisoxepide POM
Glivec preparations POM
Glucagen inj POM
Glucagon POM
Glucamet tabs POM
Glucobay tablets POM
Glucophage powder for oral solution in sachets POM
Glucophage SR POM
Glucophage tablets POM

Glucoplex preparations POM
Glucose, liquid GSL
Glurenorm tablets POM
Glutamic acid hydrochloride GSL
Glutaraldehyde P
Glutarol P
Glutethimide; its salts; its stereoisomers; their salts CD POM
Glycerin BP GSL
Glycerin suppositories BP GSL
Glycerin thymol compound BP GSL
Glycerol GSL
Glycerol and saline injection POM
Glycerophosphoric acid GSL
Glycol salicylate, external use only GSL
Glyconon tablets POM
Glycophos POM
Glycopyrronium bromide POM but if 1mg (MD) 2mg (MDD), P
Glykola tonic GSL
Glymese tablets POM
Glymidine POM
Glypressin injection POM
Glytrin spray P
Goddard's Embrocation GSL
Golden eye drops P
Golden eye ointment P
Golden Seal GSL
Gonadorelin POM
Gonal F preparations POM
Gonapeptyl Depot POM
Gopten capsules POM
Goserelin acetate POM
Gramicidin POM but if external maximum strength 0.2 per cent, P
Graneodin preparations POM
Granisetron hydrochloride POM
Granocyte injection POM
Gravel Root (Eupatorium purpureum) GSL
Grazax POM
Gregoderm ointment POM
Grepafloxacin POM
Grindelia GSL
Griseofulvin POM
Grisol AF P
Grisovin tablets POM
Ground Ivy GSL
Growth Hormone CD Anab POM
GTN 300mcg tablets P
Guaiacol, external use only GSL
Guaiacum resin, up to 200mg (MD) GSL
Guaifenesin/Guaiphenesin, up to 200mg (MD) GSL
Guaiphenesin see Guaifenesin
Guanethidine monosulphate POM
Guanfacine hydrochloride POM
Guanoclor sulphate POM
Guanor preparations P
Guanoxan sulphate POM
Guarem granules P
Guaza see Cannabis
Gum Ammoniacum GSL
Gutta Percha, external use only GSL
Gygel GSL
Gyne T 380 POM
Gyno-Daktarin preparations POM
Gyno-pevaryl preparations POM
Gynol II GSL
Gynomin P

H

Hactos cough mixture GSL
Haelan preparations POM
Haelan tape POM
Haemaccel infusion solution POM
Haes-steril IV inf POM
Halazepam CD Benz POM
Halciderm Topical POM
Halcinonide POM
Haldol decanoate injection POM
Haldol preparations POM
Half Beta-Prograne POM
Half Sinemet CR POM
Half-Inderal LA capsules POM
Half-Securon SR POM
Halfan tablets POM

Halibut liver oil as for Vitamin A and Vitamin D GSL
Halibut-Liver oil capsules BP GSL
Halita GSL
Halls childrens cough pastilles GSL
Halls max strength sore throat relief lozenges GSL
Halls Mentho-Lyptus GSL
Halls Soothers GSL
Halofantrine hydrochloride POM
Halogenated phenols, up to maximum strength 1.0 per cent GSL
Haloperidol POM
Haloperidol decanoate POM
Haloxazolam CD Benz POM
Halquinol, if maximum strength 0.6 per cent (external use only) GSL
Hamamelis GSL
Happinose GSL
Harmogen tablets POM
Hartmann's solution POM
Hashish see Cannabis
Havrix Junior vaccine POM
Havrix vaccine POM
Haycrom Aqueous eye drops POM
Haycrom Hayfever eye drops P
Hayleve P
Haymine tablets P
HBvaxPRO vaccine POM
HC45 hydrocortisone cream (PL 0327/0039) P
4head GSL
Healonid POM
Healthcheck No1, No 2 P
Healthy feet GSL
Heartsease GSL
Hedex Extra pack sizes 16s GSL; purse pack 12s GSL
Hedex tablets pack sizes 16s GSL; 32s P; purse pack 12s GSL
Hedex ibuprofen GSL
Hedrin P
Heliclear POM
Helicobacter Test HP Plus POM
Helicobacter Test Infai POM
HeliMet triple pack POM
Hemabate I/M solution POM
Heminevrin preparations POM
Hemlock Spruce (Pine Canadian) P but if 400mg (MD), GSL
Hemocane GSL
Hemohes POM
Hep-flush sol POM
Heparin POM but if external use only GSL
Heparin calcium POM but if external GSL
Heparin sodium POM
Heparinoid, if for external use, maximum strength 1% for the relief of bruises, sprains and soft tissue injuries in adults and children aged 6 years and over GSL
Hepatitis A Vaccine POM
Hepatitis B vaccine POM
Hepatyrix vaccine POM
Heplok sol POM
Hepsal sol POM
Hepsera tablets POM
Heptabarbitone CD No Register POM
Herbal Concepts GSL
Herbal Laboratories preps all GSL except comfrey oil
Herbalache P
Herbalhypnos GSL
Herbaloa GSL
Herbulax tabs GSL
Herceptin infusion POM
Heroin see Diamorphine
Herpetad cold sore cream P
Herpid POM
Hespan IV inf POM
Hesperidin Complex GSL
Hewletts cream GSL
Hexachlorophane see Hexachlorophene
Hexachlorophene/Hexachlorophane POM but if external (1) soaps maxi-

mum strength 2.0 per cent; (2) aerosols maximum strength 0.1 per cent; (3) preparations other than soaps and aerosols maximum strength 0.75 per cent, P

Hexalen caps POM

Hexamine phenylcinchoninate POM

Hexetidine, if maximum strength 0.1 per cent (external use only) GSL

Hexobarbitone CD No Register POM

Hexobarbitone sodium CD No Register POM

Hexoestrol POM

Hexoestrol dipropionate POM

Hexopal Forte tablets P

Hexopal suspension P

Hexopal tablets P

Hexyl nicotinate, if maximum strength 2.0 per cent (external use only) GSL

Hexylresorcinol, if external use or internal (pastilles, lozenges, throat tablets maximum strength 2.5mg) GSL

H-F Antidote GSL

Hibicet GSL

Hibiscrub GSL

Hibisol GSL

Hibitane 5% concentrate GSL

Hibitane Obstetric cream GSL

Hill's Balsam Adult expectorant GSL

Hill's Balsam Adult suppressant CD Inv P

Hill's Balsam extra strong 2-in-1 pastilles GSL

Hill's Balsam Junior expectorant GSL

Hill's Balsam pastilles GSL

Hioxyl cream P

Hiprex 1g tabs P

Hirudoid cream P

Hirudoid gel P

Hismanal suspension POM

Histac POM

Histafen POM

Histalix syrup P

Histamine hydrochloride, if maximum strength 0.1 per cent (external use only) GSL

Histergan preps P

L-Histidine hydrochloride POM but if for dietary supplementation, P

Histoacryl tissue adhesive P

Hivid tablets POM

Hollister premium powder POM

Hollister universal remover wipes POM

Hollister skin gel protective dressing wipes POM

Holy Thistle (cnicus benedictus), up to 1.5g (MD) GSL

Homatropine POM but if internal 0.15mg (MD) 0.45mg (MDD); external (except ophthalmic), P

Homatropine hydrobromide POM but if 0.2mg (MD) 0.6mg (MDD), P

Homatropine methylbromide POM but if 2mg (MD) 6mg (MDD), P

Honey, Purified GSL

Honvan preparations POM

Hops (lupulus) GSL

Horehound, white GSL

Hormonin tablets POM

Horse-chestnut (Aesculus), external use only GSL

Horseradish GSL

HRF Ayerst ampoules POM

HRI preparations GSL

Humaject M3 POM

Humaject S POM

Humalog KwikPen POM

Humalog vials and cartridges POM

Human Insulins POM

Humatrope injection CD Anab POM

Humegon injection POM

Humiderm cream P

Humira injection POM

Humulin insulins POM

Hyalase POM

Hyalgan inj POM

Hyaluronidase POM

Hycamtin POM

Hycamtin powder for infusion POM

Hycosan eye drops GSL

Hydergine tablets POM

Hydralazine hydrochloride POM

Hydrangea GSL

Hydrargaphen POM but if for local application to skin, P

Hydrea capsules POM

Hydrex spray GSL

Hydrex surgical scrub GSL

Hydrex peri-operative skin disinfection GSL

Hydrobromic acid POM

Hydrocare protein remover tabs GSL

Hydrochlorothiazide POM

Hydrocodone; its salts CD POM

Hydrocortisone POM but if external for use either alone or in conjunction with crotamiton in irritant dermatitis, contact allergic dermatitis, insect bite reactions, mild to moderate eczema, and either in combination with clotrimazole or miconazole nitrate for athlete's foot and candidal intertrigo or in combination with lignocaine for anal and perianal itch associated with haemorrhoids in adults and children not less than 10 years, maximum strength 1.0 per cent cream, ointment or spray and container or package contains not more than 15g of medicinal product (cream or ointment) or 30ml (spray), P; if in combination with nystatin for intertrigo, in adults and children not less than 10 years with a maximum strength of 0.5 per cent, P; if for external use in combination with lidocaine hydrochloride for the symptomatic relief of anal and perianal itch, irritation and pain associated with external haemorrhoids in adults and children aged 16 years and over, in a non-pressurised spray with a maximum strength of 0.2 per cent and a maximum pack size 30ml of product, GSL; if for external use for the treatment of insect bite and sting reactions only, in adults and children aged 10 years and over, in a cream with maximum strength of 1 per cent and a maximum pack size of 10g of product, GSL

Hydrocortisone 17-butyrate POM

Hydrocortisone acetate POM but if external for use in irritant dermatitis, contact allergic dermatitis, insect bite reactions, mild to moderate eczema, and in combination with one or more of the following: benzyl benzoate, bismuth oxide, bismuth subgallate, Peru Balsam, pramoxine hydrochloride, zinc oxide, for haemorrhoids or in combination with miconazole nitrate for athletes foot and intertrigo in adults and children not less than 10 years, cream, ointment or suppositories, maximum strength equivalent to 1.0 per cent hydrocortisone and container or package contains not more than 15g of medicinal product; in the case of suppositories, container or package containing no more than 12, P

Hydrocortisone butyrate POM

Hydrocortisone caprylate POM

Hydrocortisone cream (Vantage) P

Hydrocortisone hydrogen succinate POM

Hydrocortisone sodium phosphate POM

Hydrocortisone sodium succinate POM but if external for aphthous ulceration of the mouth for adults and children not less than 12 years in the form of pellets, maximum strength equivalent to 2.5mg hydrocortisone and container or package contains

not more than equivalent to 50mg of hydrocortisone, P

Hydrocortistab injection POM

Hydrocortisyl preparations POM

Hydrocortone preparations POM

Hydrocyanic acid POM

Hydroflumethiazide POM

Hydrogen peroxide, external use only GSL

Hydromol preparations GSL

Hydromorphinol; its salts; its esters and ethers; their salts CD POM

Hydromorphone; its salts; its esters and ethers; their salts CD POM

Hydromycin-D ear/eye preparations POM

HydroSaluric tablets POM

Hydrotalcite GSL

Hydrous ointment BP GSL

Hydroxocobalamin POM

4-Hydroxy-n-butyric acid see Gammahydroxy-butyrate (GHB)

Hydroxycarbamide/Hydroxyurea POM

Hydroxychloroquine sulphate POM but if for prophylaxis of malaria, P

Hydroxypethidine; its salts; its esters and ethers; their salts CD POM

Hydroxyprogesterone POM

Hydroxyprogesterone caproate/ Hydroxyprogesterone hexanoate POM

Hydroxyprogesterone enanthate POM

Hydroxyprogesterone hexanoate see Hydroxyprogesterone caproate

N-Hydroxy-tenamfetamine CD Lic

Hydroxyurea see Hydroxycarbamide

Hydroxyzine embonate POM

Hydroxyzine hydrochloride POM but if (1) For the management of pruritis associated with acute or chronic urticaria or atopic dermatitis or contact dermatitis, in adults and in children not less than 12 years, 25mg (MD) 75mg (MDD) and container or package contains not more than 750mg of hydroxyzine hydrochloride; (2) For the management of pruritis associated with acute or chronic urticaria or atopic dermatitis or contact dermatitis, in children not less than 6 years but less than12 years, 25 mg (MD) 50mg (MDD) and container or package contains not more than 750mg of hydroxyzine hydrochloride, P

Hygroton tablets POM

Hymosa biocream GSL

Hyoscine POM, but if internal maximum strength 0.15 per cent; external (except ophthalmic), for the prevention of travel sickness symptoms, for use in adults and children aged 10 years or over, maximum strength 1.5mg per patch, maximum pack size 2 patches, P, please refer to proprietary names for the classification granted under the marketing authorisation (See Scopoderm preparations)

Hyoscine butylbromide POM but if (1) Internal, (a) by inhaler, (b) otherwise than by inhaler 20mg (MD) 80mg (MDD) and container or package contains not more than 240mg of hyoscine butylbromide; (2) External, P

Hyoscine hydrobromide POM but if (1) internal (a) by inhaler, (b)otherwise than by inhaler 300mcg (MD) 900mcg (MDD); (2) external (except ophthalmic), P

Hyoscine methobromide POM but if (1) internal (a) by inhaler (b) otherwise than by inhaler 2.5mg (MD) 7.5mg (MDD); (2) external, P

Hyoscine methonitrate POM but if (1) internal (a) by inhaler (b) otherwise

than by inhaler, 2.5mg (MD) 7.5mg (MDD); (2) external, P

Hyoscyamine POM but if (1) internal (a) by inhaler (b) otherwise than by inhaler 300mcg (MD) 1mg (MDD); (2) external, P

Hyoscyamine hydrobromide POM but if (1) internal (a) by inhaler (b) otherwise than by inhaler, equivalent of 300mcg of hyoscyamine (MD) equivalent of 1mg of hyoscyamine (MDD); (2) external, P

Hyoscyamine sulphate POM but if (1) internal (a) by inhaler (b) otherwise than by inhaler equivalent of 300mcg of hyoscyamine (MD) equivalent of 1mg of hyoscyamine (MDD); (2) external, P

Hypaque inj/bottle POM

Hypaque sodium powder P

Hypericum (St John's wort), external use only GSL

Hypnomidate POM

Hypnovel injection CD No Register POM

Hypolar Retard POM

Hypolar XL POM

Hypophosphorous acid, external use only GSL

Hypotears P

Hypovase tablets POM

Hypromellose eye drops BPC P

Hypurin insulins POM

Hyssop GSL

Hyteneze tabs POM

Hytrin BPH tablets POM

Hytrin tablets POM

I

Ibandronic acid POM

Ibufac tabs POM

Ibufem tabs GSL

Ibugel P

Ibugel Forte POM

Ibuleve preps P

Ibuleve Speed Relief Gel GSL

Ibumousse P

Ibuprofen POM but if for internal use in rheumatic and muscular pain, backache, neuralgia, migraine, headache, dental pain, dysmenorrhoea, feverishness, symptoms of colds and influenza and either a controlled release preparation with md 600mg and mdd 1,200mg or any other internal preparation with md 400mg and mdd 1,200mg P; or if tablets, capsules, powder or granules for internal use with ms 200mg, md 400mg and mdd 1,200mg in individual containers or packages containing no more than 16 tablets or capsules, or 12 sachets for use in adults and children over 12 years GSL; or if liquid preparations for internal use, maximum strength 2.0%, for the treatment of rheumatic or muscular pain, headache, dental pain, feverishness, or symptoms of colds and influenza for use in children aged under 12 years, 200mg(MD), 800mg(MDD), in the case of liquid preparations of ibuprofen, individual unit doses of not more than 5 millilitres each to a maximum of 20 unit doses GSL; ibuprofen oral suspension with a strength of 2% or less supplied in multidose containers of not more than 100 millilitres GSL; or if for external use with ms 5% P; or if for external use with ms 10%, md 125mg, mdd 500mg in a container or package containing not more than 50g of medicinal product P; or if for external use with ms 5%, md 125mg, mdd 500mg and in an individual container or package containing not more than 2.5g, for rheumatic pain, muscular aches and pains, swellings such as strains, sprains and sports injuries for use by adults and children over 12 years GSL

Ibuprofen lysine POM but if for rheumatic and muscular pain, pain of non-serious arthritic conditions, backache, neuralgia, migraine, headache, dental pain, dysmenorrhoea, feverishness, symptoms of colds and influenza, (a) in the case of a prolonged release preparation md 600mg and mdd 1,200mg or (b) in any case md 400mg and mdd 1,200mg P; or if maximum strength equivalent to 200mg ibuprofen, in tablet form, for the treatment of rheumatic or muscular pain, backache, neuralgia, migraine, headache, dental pain, dysmenorrhoea, feverishness or symptoms of colds and influenza in adults and in children aged 12 years and over, (MD) equivalent to 400mg ibuprofen, (MDD) equivalent to 1200mg, in an individual container or package containing not more than 16 tablets GSL

Ibuprofen tablets 12s (Galpharm) GSL
Ibuspray P
Ibutop Cuprofen ibuprofen gel P
Icaps GSL
Iceland Moss GSL
Ichthammol, external use only GSL
Icodextrin POM
Icthaband P
Idarubicin hydrochloride POM
Idoxuridine POM
Idrolax sachets P
Ifosfamide POM
Ignatius Bean POM
Ikorel tablets POM
Iloprost POM
Ilosone preparations POM
Ilube POM
Imatinib POM
Imazin XL tabs P
Imbrilon preparations POM
Imdur tablets P
Imidapril POM
Imiglucerase POM
Imigran preparations POM except Imigran Recovery tablets P
Imipenem hydrochloride POM
Imipramine POM
Imipramine hydrochloride POM
Imipramine ion exchange resin bound salt or complex POM
Imiquimod POM
ImmuCyst POM
Immukin POM
Immunoprin tabs POM
Imo LA POM
Imodium POM except for the treatment of acute diarrhoea P; symptomatic treatment of acute diarrhoea in adults and children aged 12 and over, ms 2mg and 4mg (MD) 12mg (MDD), GSL
Imodium Instants tablets 6s GSL; 12s P
Imodium Plus caplets pack sizes 6s GSL; 12s P
Implanon implant POM
Improvera tablets POM
Imuderm oil GSL
Imunovir tablets POM
Imuran preparations POM
Imuvac POM
Inactivated influenza vaccine POM
Inadine GSL
Increlex POM
Indapamide POM
Indapamide hemihydrate POM
Inderal LA capsules POM
Inderal preparations POM
Inderetic capsules POM
Inderex capsules POM
Indian hemp see Cannabis

Indinavir POM
Indivina tablets POM
Indocid PDA POM
Indocid preparations POM
Indocid-R capsules POM
Indolar SR capsules POM
Indomax capsules POM
Indomax SR capsules POM
Indometacin/Indomethacin POM
Indometacin/Indomethacin sodium POM
Indomethacin see Indometacin
Indomod capsules POM
Indoprofen POM
Indoramin hydrochloride POM
Indotard MR capsules POM
InductOs POM
Inegy tablets POM
Infacol liquid GSL
Infaderm therapeutic body oil GSL
Infadrops P
Infai test POM
Infanrix preparations POM
Infestat susp POM
Inflexal V POM
Infliximab POM
Influenza vaccine POM
Influvac subunit POM
Infukoll POM
Innohep POM
Innovace Melt wafers POM
Innovace tablets POM
Innozide POM
Inosine Pranobex POM
Inositol GSL
Inositol nicotinate P
Inovelon POM
Inoven Caplets P
Inspra tablets POM
Instillagel gel P
Insulatard insulins POM
Insulin POM
Insuman insulins POM
Intal preps POM
Integrilin solution POM
Intelence POM
Intrafusin preps POM
Intralgin gel P
Intralipid POM
Intraval sodium preparations POM
Intrinsa CD Anab POM
Intron A inj POM
Invanz infusion POM
Invirase capsules POM
Invivac vaccine POM
Iocare balanced salt solution P
Iodamide POM
Iodamide meglumine POM
Iodamide sodium POM
Iodine tincture GSL
Iodine10mg (MDD) GSL
Iodoflex dressing P
Iodoform, if maximum strength 10 per cent in paints, or maximum strength 50 per cent in pastes (external use only) GSL
Iodophenol, if internal (pastilles, lozenges, throat tablets) maximum strength 0.2mg or external maximum strength 0.08 per cent GSL
Iodosorb ointment P
Iodosorb powder P
Iohexol POM
Iomeprol POM
Iopamidol POM
Iopentol POM
Iopidine Ophthalmic POM
Iothalamic acid POM
Ioversol POM
Ioxaglic acid POM
Ipecacuanha GSL
Ipecacuanha and morphine mix (conc) CD Inv P
Ipocol tablets POM
Ipramol POM

Ipratropium bromide POM
Iprindole hydrochloride POM
Iproniazid phosphate POM
Irbesartan POM
Irinotecan HCl POM
Ironorm preps P
Irriclens GSL
Irripod P
Isclofen tabs POM
Isib preps tabs P
Isisfen tabs POM
Ismelin preparations POM
Ismo preparations P
Ismo Retard tablets P
Ismo tabs P
Iso-lysergamide CD Lic
Isoaminile POM
Isoaminile citrate POM
Isocarboxazid POM
Isocard spray P
Isoconazole nitrate POM but if external and in the case of vaginal use only external use for the treatment of vaginal candidiasis, P
Isodur preparations P
Isoetharine POM
Isoetharine hydrochloride POM
Isoetharine mesylate POM
Isoflurane POM
Isogel granules GSL
Isoket ampoules POM
Isoket Retard tablets P
Isomethadone CD POM
Isomide CR POM
Isoniazid POM
Isopentane, external use only GSL
Isoprenaline hydrochloride POM
Isoprenaline sulphate POM
Isopropamide iodide POM but if equivalent of 2.5mg of isopropamide ion (MD) equivalent of 5.0mg of iso-propamide ion (MDD), P
Isopropyl alcohol, external use only GSL
Isopropyl myristate, external use only GSL
Isopropyl palmitate, external use only GSL
Isopto Alkaline P
Isopto Atropine POM
Isopto Carbachol POM
Isopto Carpine POM
Isopto Frin P
Isopto Plain P
Isordil tablets P
Isordil Tembids capsules P
Isosorbide dinitrate P
Isosorbide mononitrate P
Isotard preps P
Isotrat tabs P
Isotrate tabs P
Isotretinoin POM
Isotrex gel POM
Isotrexin gel POM
Isovorin injection POM
Ispagel GSL
Ispaghula GSL
Ispaghula Husk GSL
Isradipine POM
Istin tablets POM
Itraconazole POM
Ivabradine POM
Ivemend powder for solution for infusion POM

J

Jaap's GSL
Jaborandi POM but if external, P
Jackson's preparations GSL
Jamaica Dogwood GSL
Januvia POM
Jectofer POM
Jeridin tabs P
Jomethid XL capsules POM
Joyrides P
Juniper GSL
Juniper Oil GSL

K

K/L kaolin poultice P
KL preparations P; except magnesium sulphate paste GSL
Kabiglobulin POM
Kabikinase injections POM
Kabimix POM
Kaletra preparations POM
Kalms sleep GSL
Kalspare tablets POM
Kalten capsules POM
Kaltostat P
Kamillosan digital thermometer dummy/soother GSL
Kamillosan ointment GSL
Kanamycin acid sulphate POM
Kanamycin sulphate POM
Kannasyn preparations POM
Kao-C POM
Kao-C Child's diarrhoea mixture GSL
Kaodene suspension CD Inv P
Kaolin and morphine mixture BPC CD Inv P
Kaolin mixture paediatric BP GSL
Kaolin poultice BPC P
Kaolin, heavy, external use only GSL
Kaolin, light GSL
Kapake preparations CD Inv POM
Kaplon tabs POM
Karvol dropper bottle GSL
Karvol inhalant capsules GSL
Kay-Cee-L syrup P
Kefadim inj POM
Kefadol vials POM
Keflex preparations POM
Keftid capsules POM
Kefzol vials POM
Kelfizine W preparations POM
Keloc SR tablets POM
Kelp GSL
Kemadrin preparations POM
Kemicetine preparations POM
Kenalog injection POM
Kentene caps POM
Kentera POM
Kepivance powder for solution for injection POM
Keppra preparations POM
Keral tablets POM
Keri Therapeutic lotion P
Kerlone tablets POM
Ketalar injections POM
Ketamine CD Benz POM
Ketanodur tabs POM
Ketazolam CD Benz POM
Ketek tablets POM
Ketil caps POM
Ketobemidone; its salts; its esters and ethers; their salts CD POM
Ketocid 200mg caps POM
Ketoconazole POM but if external maximum strength 2.0 per cent (a) for the prevention and treatment of dandruff and seborrhoeic dermatitis of the scalp in the form of a shampoo, maximum frequency of application of once every 3 days and container or package contains not more than 120ml of medicinal product and containing not more than 2,400mg of ketoconazole; (b) for the treatment of the following mycotic infections of the skin: tinea pedis, tinea cruris and candidal intertrigo, please refer to proprietary names for classification granted under the marketing authorisation (see Dandrazol and Nizoral products)
Ketopine 60ml and 100ml GSL; 120ml POM
Ketoprofen POM but if external for rheumatic and muscular pain in adults and children not less than 12 for maximum period of 7 days, maximum strength 2.5 per cent and container or package contains not more than 30g of medicinal product, P

Ketorolac trometamol POM
Ketotard 200XL caps POM
Ketotifen fumarate POM
Ketovail caps POM
Ketovite (Supplement) liquid P
Ketovite tablets POM
Ketozip XL 200mg caps POM
Ketopine shampoo pack sizes 60ml, 100ml GSL; 120ml POM
Ketpron POM
Ketpron XL caps POM
Kiflone preps POM
Kilkof GSL
Kilkof mix GSL
Kineret injection POM
Kinidin Durules POM
Kivexa POM
KL kaolin preparations P
KL magnesium sulphate paste GSL
Klaricid POM
Klaricid IV POM
Klaricid Paediatric POM
Klaricid XL tablets POM
Klean-Prep sachets P
Kliofem tablets POM
Kliovance tablets POM
Kloref tablets P
Kloref-S sachets P
Kogenate Bayer injection POM
Kogenate vials POM
Kola GSL
Kolanticon gel P
Komil 5/40 tablets POM
Konakion ampoules POM
Konakion MM injection POM
Konakion MM Paediatric POM
Konakion tablets POM
Konsyl powder GSL
Kuvan soluble tablets POM
Kwells tablets P
Kytril preparations POM

L

Labetalol hydrochloride POM
Labiton tonic GSL
Labosept pastilles P
Labrador tea, external use only GSL
Lachesine chloride POM
Lacidipine POM
Lacri-Lube ointment P
Lactic acid, external use only GSL
Lacticare GSL
Lactitol P
Lacto-calamine lotion GSL
Lactugal liquid P
Ladropen preps POM
Lady's Mantle GSL
Lamictal POM
Lamictal chewable and dispersible tablets POM
Laminaria GSL
Lamisil AT cream GSL
Lamisil AT gel P
Lamisil AT spray GSL
Lamisil cream POM except OTC 15g GSL
Lamisil Once solution P
Lamisil tablets POM
Lamivudine POM
Lamotrigine POM
Lamprene capsules POM
Lanacane cream GSL
Lanacort cream (PL 3157/0008) P
Lanacort ointment (PL 3157/0011) P
Lanatoside C POM
Lanatoside Complex A, B and C POM
Langdale's tablets GSL
Lanolin BP GSL
Lanoxin preparations POM
Lanoxin-PG preparations POM
Lanreotide POM
Lansoprazole POM
Lantus injection POM
Lanvis tablets POM
Lappa (Burdock) GSL
Laractone tablets POM
Larafen CR caps 200mg POM

Larapam preparations POM
Laratrim preps POM
Largactil Forte suspension POM
Largactil preparations POM
Lariam tablets POM
Laronidase POM
Laryng-O-Jet POM
Lasikal tablets POM
Lasilactone capsules POM
Lasix + K POM
Lasix preparations POM
Lasma tablets P
Lasonil ointment P
Lasoride tablets POM
Latanoprost POM
Latanoprost eye drops POM
Lauromacrogols, external use only GSL
Lauryl alcohol, ethoxylated, external use only GSL
Lavender oil GSL
Laxoberal P
Laxose P
Lecithin, internal use GSL
Ledclair injection POM
Lederfen preparations POM
Lederfolin injection POM
Lederfolin solution POM
Ledermycin capsules POM
Lederspan injections POM
Lefetamine; it salts CD POM
Leflunomide POM
Lemlax (lactulose) P
Lemon GSL
Lemon oil GSL
Lemsip preparations GSL except Cold & Flu sinus 12hr (ibuprofen and pseudoephedrine) P
Lemsip max preparations GSL except Lemsip Max Flu 12hr (ibuprofen and pseudoephedrine) P
Lenium P
Lenograstim see Granocyte
Lentard MC insulin POM
Lentaron depot POM
Lentaron injection POM
Lentizol capsules POM
Lepirudin injection POM
Lercanidipine hydrochloride POM
Lercanidipine tablets POM
Lescol POM
Lescol XL tablets POM
Letrozole POM
Letrozole tablets POM
Lettuce (Lactuca sativa) GSL
Leucomax injection POM
Leucovorin POM
Leukeran tablets POM
Leuprorelin acetate preparations POM
Leustat POM
Levallorphan tartrate POM
Levemir preparations POM
Levetiracetam POM
Levitra tablets POM
Levobunolol hydrochloride POM
Levobupivacaine POM
Levocabastine hydrochloride POM but if maximum strength equivalent of 0.05 per cent levocabastine (1) nasal sprays for the symptomatic treatment of seasonal allergic rhinitis and container or package contains not more than 10ml of medicinal product; (2) aqueous eye drops for the symptomatic treatment of seasonal allergic conjunctivitis and container or package contains not more than 4ml of medicinal product, P
Levocetirizine tablets POM
Levodopa POM
Levofloxacin preparations POM
Levomepromazine/Methotrimeprazine POM
Levomepromazine/Methotrimeprazine maleate POM
Levomethorphan; its salts CD POM
Levomoramide; its salts CD POM
Levonelle 1500 POM
Levonelle One-Step P

Levonorgestrel POM but if maximum strength 1.5mg and for use as an emergency contraceptive in women aged 16 years and over P
Levophed POM
Levophenacylmorphan; its salts, esters and ethers CD POM
Levorphanol; its salts, esters and ethers CD POM
Levothyroxine sodium/thyroxine sodium POM
Lexotan tablets CD Benz POM
Lexpec syrup POM
Lexpec syrup with Iron POM
Lexpec syrup with Iron-M POM
LH see Luteinising Hormone
LH-RH see Gonadorelin
Li-liquid POM
Libanil tablets POM
Liberim HB POM
Liberim T POM
Liberim Z POM
Libetist syrup POM
Librium preparations CD Benz POM
Librofem tablets pack sizes 12s GSL; 24s P
Lidifen tablets POM
Lidocaine/Lignocaine POM but for non-ophthalmic use, P; internal (teething gel maximum strength 0.6 per cent) or external maximum strength 2.0 per cent, except local ophthalmic use, in adults and in children aged 12 years and over, GSL
Lidocaine/Lignocaine hydrochloride POM but if non-ophthalmic use, P; internal (teething gel maximum strength 0.7 per cent) or external (except local ophthalmic use maximum strength 0.7 per cent), or external (except local ophthalmic use for adults and children aged 12 years and over, all preparations except sprays, maximum strength 2.0 per cent) GSL, or external (except local opthalmic use for adults and children aged 16 years and over, in combination with hydrocortisone for symptomatic relief of anal and peri-anal itch, irritation and pain associated with external haemorrhoids, in a non pressurised spray with a maximum strength of 1%) GSL, please refer to proprietary names for the classification granted under the marketing authorisation (See Germoloids HC products)
Lidoflazine POM
Light liquid paraffin, external use only GSL
Lignocaine see Lidocaine
Lignospan POM
Lignostab injection POM
Lignostab-A injection POM
Limclair injection POM
Lime Oil GSL
Lincomycin POM
Lincomycin hydrochloride POM
Lingraine tablets POM
Linseed GSL
Linseed oil, external use only GSL
Linus powder GSL
Lioresal intrathecal POM
Lioresal liquid POM
Lioresal tablets POM
Liothyronine sodium POM
Lipantil capsules POM
Lipantil Micro capsules POM
Lipase POM
Lipiodol Ultra fluid P
Lipitor tablets POM
Lipobase P
Lipobay tablets POM
Lipofundin S POM
Liposic P
Liposomal Daunorubicin POM
Liposomal Doxorubicin Citrate POM
Lipostat tablets POM

Lippes Loop intrauterine contraceptive device POM
Liprinal capsules POM
Liqufruta cough medicines GSL
Liqui-Char P
Liquifilm Tears P
Liquivisc gel P
Liquorice GSL
Liquorice extract deglycyrrhizinised GSL
Lisicostad tablets POM
Lisinopril POM
Liskonum tablets POM
Lisuride/Lysuride maleate POM
Litarex tablets POM
Lithium carbonate POM but if equivalent of 5mg of lithium (MD) equivalent of 15mg of lithium (MDD), P
Lithium citrate POM
Lithium succinate POM
Lithium sulphate POM but if equivalent of 5mg of lithium (MD) equivalent of 15mg of lithium (MDD), P
Lithonate POM
Liver extract GSL
Livial tablets POM
Livostin Direct P
Livostin eye drops POM
Livostin nasal spray POM
Lloyd's cream GSL
Lobelia, up to 65mg (MD) GSL
Lobeline POM but if internal 3mg (MD) 9mg (MDD); external, P
Lobeline hydrochloride POM but if internal equivalent of 3mg of lobeline (MD) equivalent of 9mg of lobeline (MDD); external, P
Lobeline sulphate POM but if internal equivalent of 3mg of lobeline (MD) equivalent of 9mg of lobeline (MDD); external, P
Locabiotal aerosol POM
Loceryl cream POM
Loceryl nail lacquer POM
Locoid C preparations POM
Locoid Crelo POM
Locoid Lipocream POM
Locoid preparations POM
Locorten-Vioform ear drops POM
Lodiar POM
Lodine preparations POM
Lodine SR tablets POM
Lodoxamide trometamol POM but if maximum strength equivalent of 0.1% lodoxamide, for the treatment of ocular signs and symptoms of allergic conjunctivitis, in adults and in children aged 4 years and over P
Loestrin 20 tablets POM
Loestrin 30 tablets POM
Lofensaid preparations POM
Lofentanil; its stereoisomers, salts, esters and ethers CD POM
Lofepramine POM
Lofepramine hydrochloride POM
Lofexidine hydrochloride POM
Logynon ED tablets POM
Logynon tablets POM
Lomefloxacin hydrochloride POM
Lomexin pessaries POM
Lomont POM
Lomotil preparations CD Inv POM
Lomustine POM
Loniten tablets POM
Lopace POM
LoperaGen capsules POM
Loperamide hydrochloride POM but if for treatment of acute diarrhoea, P; symptomatic treatment of acute diarrhoea, in adults and children aged 12 years and over, maximum strength 2mg and 4mg (MD) 12mg (MDD), GSL; or for the symptomatic treatment of acute episodes of diarrhoea associated with irritable bowel syndrome in adults aged 18 years and over following initial diagnosis by a doctor, maximum strength 2mg, 4mg (MD) and 12mg (MDD), GSL

Lopid preparations POM
Lopinavir POM
Lopranol LA POM
Loprazolam CD Benz POM
Lopresor SR tablets POM
Lopresor tablets POM
Loratadine POM; but if 10mg (MDD) P; or if maximum strength 10mg, in tablet form for the symptomatic relief of perennial rhinitis, seasonal allergic rhinitis and idiopathic chronic urticaria, in adults and children aged 2 years and over and weighing 30Kg or more, 10mg (MDD), in an individual container or package containing not more than 7 tablets GSL.
Lorazepam CD Benz POM
Lormetazepam CD Benz POM
Lornoxicam POM
Loron preparations POM
Losartan POM
Losartan potassium POM
Losec preparations POM
Lotemax eye drops POM
Lotriderm cream POM
Loxapac capsules POM
Loxapine succinate POM
LSD see Lysergide
Luborant Saliva P
Lubri-Tears ointment P
Lucentis POM
Lucerne (Alfalfa) GSL
Ludiomil tablets POM
Lumigan eye-drops POM
Lung Surfactant Porcine POM
Lungwort GSL
Lustral tablets POM
Lustys preparations GSL
Luteinising hormone POM
Luveris POM
Luvinsta XL tablets
Lyclear preparations P
Lyflex POM
Lymecycline POM
Lynoestrenol POM
Lypressin POM
Lypsyl preparations GSL
Lyrica capsules POM
Lyrinel XL POM
Lysergamide; its salts CD Lic
Lysergide and other N-alkyl derivatives of lysergamide; their salts CD Lic
Lysine hydrochloride GSL
Lysodren POM
Lysovir capsules POM
Lysuride see Lisuride

M

M&M tulle GSL
Maalox Plus tablets and suspension GSL
Maalox suspension GSL
MabCampath preparations POM
Mabron tablets POM
Mabthera vials POM
Mac Throat lozenges GSL
MacKenzies smelling salts GSL
Macrobid capsules POM
Macrodantin capsules POM
Macrogol P
Macugen injection POM
Madopar CR capsules POM
Madopar preparations POM
Mafenide POM
Mafenide acetate POM
Mafenide hydrochloride POM
Mafenide propionate POM but if eye drops maximum strength 5.0 per cent, P
Magaldrate GSL
Magnapen preparations POM
Magnesia, cream of (Magnesium hydroxide) GSL
Magnesium alginate GSL
Magnesium carbonate, heavy GSL
Magnesium carbonate, light GSL
Magnesium citrate P

Magnesium fluoride POM
Magnesium glycerophosphate GSL
Magnesium hydroxide GSL
Magnesium metrizoate POM
Magnesium oxide, heavy GSL
Magnesium oxide, light GSL
Magnesium phosphate GSL
Magnesium stearate GSL
Magnesium sulphate GSL
Magnesium sulphate paste GSL
Magnesium trisilicate GSL
Magnesium trisilicate compound tablets BPC GSL
Magnesium trisilicate mixture BP GSL
Magnesium trisilicate oral powder BP GSL
Maize GSL
Malarivon syrup POM but if for the prevention of malaria P
Malarone Paediatric tablets POM
Malarone tablets POM
Malathion P
Malix tablets POM
Maloprim tablets POM
Malt Extract GSL
Malted Milk GSL
Maltose GSL
Mandafen ibuprofen suspension P
Mandafen ibuprofen 400mg tablets pack sizes 24s, 48s, 84s P; 250s POM
Mandafen ibuprofen 600mg tablets pack sizes 100s POM
Mandalyn preparations P
Mandanol 6+ suspension SF P
Mandanol caplets blister pack 500mg pack sizes 16s GSL; 32s P
Mandanol infant suspension SF P
Mandanol Plus P
Mandanol tablets 500mg pack sizes 32s PO; 100s POM
Mandanol tablets blister pack 500mg pack sizes 16s GSL; 32s PO
Mandragora Autumnalis POM
Manerix tablets POM
Manevac granules P
Manganese glycerophosphate, if MDD equivalent to 1mg elemental manganese GSL
Manganese sulphate, if MDD equivalent to 1mg elemental manganese GSL
Mannitol injection POM
Mannomustine hydrochloride POM
Manorfen P
Manusept antibacterial hand rub GSL
Maprotiline hydrochloride POM
Marcain injection POM
Marcain Polyamp Steripak POM
Marcain with Adrenaline injection POM
Marevan tablets POM
Marshmallow Root GSL
Marvelon tablets POM
Masculine balance GSL
Masnoderm cream P
Mastaflu POM
Mastic, external use only GSL
Mate GSL
Matricaria (German Chamomile) GSL
Matrifen patches CD POM
Maxalt preparations POM
Maxepa capsules and liquid P
Maxidex eye drops POM
Maximet capsules POM
Maxitrol preparations POM
Maxivent POM
Maxolon preparations POM
Maxolon SR capsules POM
Maxtrex tablets POM
Mazindol CD No Register POM
MCR 50 capsules P
Meadow Sweet GSL
Measles vaccine (live attenuated) POM
Mebanazine POM
Mebendazole POM but for oral use in the treatment of enterobiasis in adults and in children not less than 2 years, 100mg (MD) and container or package contains not more than 800mg of Mebendazole, P

Mebeverine hydrochloride POM but if (a) for the symptomatic relief of irritable bowel syndrome 135mg (MD) 405mg (MDD); (b) for uses other than the symptomatic relief of irritable bowel syndrome 100mg (MD) 300mg (MDD), P
Mebeverine pamoate POM
Mebhydrolin POM
Mebhydrolin napadisylate POM
Mebolazine CD Anab POM
Mecamylamine hydrochloride POM
Mecillinam POM
Meclofenoxate hydrochloride POM
Mecloqualone CD POM
Meclozine P
Medazepam CD Benz POM
Medi-Test preparations GSL
Medical Interporous GSL
Medicinal opium CD POM but if in, (a) any preparations from which the opium cannot be readily recovered in amounts which constitute a risk to health and with ms 0.2% (calculated as anhydrous morphine base) CD Inv POM; (b) if in a powder containing 10% opium, 10 % ipecacuanha root and 80% of another powdered ingredient (not a controlled drug) CD Inv POM; (c) if for nonparenteral use in unit preparations diluted to at least one part in a million (6X) in response to a specific request, CD Inv P; or (d) if for nonparenteral use in unit preparations diluted to at least one part in a million million (6C), CD Inv P

Medicoal GSL
Medicoal granules P
Medicross burn gel sachets GSL
Medijel gel GSL
Medijel pastilles P
Medikinet IR CD POM
Medikinet XL CD POM
Medinex P
Medinol Over 6 P
Medinol Paediatric P
Medinol Under 6 P
Medised suspension P
Medocodene 30/500 capsules CD Inv POM
Medomet preparations POM
Medrone preparations POM
Medroxyprogesterone acetate POM
Mefenamic acid POM
Mefenorex; its salts; its stereoisomers; their salts CD Benz POM
Meflam preparations POM
Mefloquine hydrochloride POM
Mefoxin injection POM
Mefruside POM
Megace tablets POM
Megestrol acetate POM
Meggezones lozenges GSL
Meglumine iothalamate POM
Melaleuca oil, external use only GSL
Melleril preparations POM
Meloxicam POM
Melphalan hydrochloride POM
Meltus adult chesty coughs (original and SF/colour free) GSL
Meltus adult dry coughs P
Meltus baby cough linctus GSL
Meltus decongestant P
Meltus junior chesty coughs GSL
Meltus junior dry coughs P
Meltus adult chesty coughs and congestion P
Meltus family honey & lemon GSL
Memantine POM
Mendys capsules POM
Mengivac (A+C) POM
Meningitec POM
Meningococcal Polysaccharide Vaccine POM
Menitorix POM
Menjugate POM

Menogon POM
Menopur POM
Menorest Transdermal patches POM
Menoring 50 POM
Menotrophin POM
Menthodex mixture GSL
Menthodex original lozenges GSL
Menthol GSL
Menthol and eucalyptus inhalation GSL
Menthol BP GSL
Mentholatum Antiseptic lozenge GSL
Mentholatum Deep Heat max strength 35g GSL
Mentholatum Deep Heat spray GSL
Mentholatum ibuprofen gel pack sizes 50g GSL; 100g P
Mentholatum Rub GSL
Mentholatum Vapour rub GSL
Menthyl valerate up to 100mg (MS), 200mg (MD) GSL
Menyanthes (bogbean, buckbean) GSL
Mepitiostane CD Anab POM
Mepivacaine hydrochloride POM but any use except ophthalmic use, P
Mepradec POM
Mepranix POM
Meprate tablets CD No Register POM
Meprobamate CD No Register POM
Meptazinol POM
Meptid injection POM
Meptid tablets POM
Mepyramine maleate, if external use for the symptomatic relief of insect stings and bites, and nettle stings and jellyfish stings, in adults and children aged two years and over and maximum strength 2.0% in a pack containing no more than 22g of the product GSL
Mequitazine POM
Merbentyl syrup POM
Merbentyl tablets POM
Mercaptamine bitartrate POM
Mercaptopurine POM
Mercilon tablets POM
Merieux vaccine POM
Merional injection POM
Merocaine lozenges P
Merocet lozenges GSL
Merocets Plus GSL
Meronem preparations POM
Meropenem POM
Mersalyl POM
Mersalyl acid POM
Mesabolone CD Anab POM
Mesalazine POM
Mesna POM
Mesocarb CD Benz POM
Mesren MR POM
Mesterolone CD Anab POM
Mestinon preparations POM
Mestranol POM
Metalyse injection POM
Metanium cradle cap cream GSL
Metanium ointment GSL
Metaraminol tartrate POM
Metastron (radioactive isotope) POM
Metatone tonic GSL
Metazocine; its salts; its esters and ethers; their salts CD POM
Meted shampoo P
Metenix 5 tablets POM
Meterfolic tablets P
Metergoline POM
Metformin hydrochloride POM
Methacycline POM
Methacycline calcium POM
Methacycline hydrochloride POM
Methadole see Dimepheptanol
Methadone; its salts CD POM
Methadose diluent POM
Methadose oral concentrate CD POM
Methadyl acetate; its salts CD POM
Methallenoestril POM
Methamphetamine see Methylamfetamine
Methandienone CD Anab POM
Methandriol CD Anab POM

Methaqualone; its salts CD POM
Metharose CD POM
Methcathinone CD Lic
Methenamine hippurate P
Methenolone CD Anab POM
Methenolone enanthate CD Anab POM
Methex CD POM
Methicillin sodium POM
Methixene POM
Methixene hydrochloride POM
Methocarbamol POM
Methocidin POM but if throat lozenges and throat pastilles, P
Methohexital see Methohexitone
Methohexitone sodium POM
Methoin POM
Methoserpidine POM
Methotrexate POM
Methotrexate sodium POM
Methotrimeprazine see Levomepromazine
Methoxamine hydrochloride POM but if nasal sprays or nasal drops not containing liquid paraffin as a vehicle maximum strength 0.25 per cent, P
Methoxymethane, external use only GSL
Methsuximide POM
Methyclothiazide POM
Methyl cellulose GSL
Methyl nicotinate, external use only GSL
Methyl salicylate, if internal (nasal inhalations except aerosols) or internal (pastilles, lozenges, throat tablets maximum strength 1mg) or external GSL
Methylamfetamine; its salts CD POM
4-Methyl-aminorex CD Lic

Methylated spirits industrial, if external use or internal (nasal inhalations to be inhaled from a handkerchief or other soft material) GSL
Methylbenzethonium chloride, external use only GSL
Methylcysteine P
Methyldesorphine; its salts; its esters and ethers; their salts CD POM
Methyldihydromorphine (6-methyldihydromorphine); its salts; its esters and ethers; their salts CD POM
Methyldihydromorphinone see Metopon
Methyldopa POM
Methyldopate hydrochloride POM
Methylephedrine hydrochloride POM but if 30mg (MD) 60mg (MDD), P
2-Methyl-3-morpholino-1,1-diphenyl-propanecarboxylic acid; its salts, ethers and esters CD POM
Methylphenidate; its salts CD POM
Methylphenobarbital/Methylphenobarbitone CD No Register POM
Methylphenobarbitone see Methylphenobarbital
1-Methyl-4-phenylpiperidine-4-carboxylic acid CD POM
Methylprednisolone POM
Methylprednisolone acetate POM
Methylprednisolone sodium succinate POM
Methyltestosterone CD Anab POM
Methylthiouracil POM
Methyprylone CD No Register POM
Methysergide maleate POM
Metipranolol POM
Metirosine POM
Metoclopramide hydrochloride POM
Metoject POM
Metolazone POM
Metomidate hydrochloride POM
Metopirone capsules POM
Metopon; its salts; its esters and ethers; their salts CD POM
Metoprolol fumarate POM

Metoprolol succinate POM
Metoprolol tartrate POM
Metosyn FAPG cream POM
Metosyn FAPG ointment POM
Metosyn ointment POM
Metosyn scalp lotion POM
Metribolone CD Anab POM
Metrodin High Purity POM
Metrogel POM
Metrolyl preparations POM
Metronidazole POM
Metronidazole benzoate POM
Metrosa POM
Metrotop gel POM
Metrozol IV inf POM
Metsol POM
Metvix cream POM
Metyrapone POM
Mexenone, external use only GSL
Mexiletine hydrochloride POM
Mexitil POM
Mezlocilin sodium POM
Miacalcic injection POM
Mianserin hydrochloride POM
Mibolerone CD Anab POM
Micanol cream 1 per cent P
Micanol cream 3 per cent POM
Micardis tablets POM
MicardisPlus tablets POM
Micolette Micro-enema P
Miconazole POM but if external and in the case of vaginal use only external use for the treatment of vaginal candidiasis, P; in the case of creams or powders, including spray powders for the treatment of tinea pedis (athlete's foot) only maximum strength 2.0% (for spray powders this shall be weight for weight excluding any propellants) GSL
Miconazole nitrate POM but if external and in the case of vaginal use only external use for the treatment of vaginal candidiasis, P
Micralax Micro-enema P
Microcrystalline wax, external use only GSL
Microgynon 30 tablets POM
Microgynon ED tablets POM
Micronor HRT tablets POM
Micronor tablets POM
Micropirin P
Microval tablets POM
Mictral granules POM
Midazolam CD No Reg POM
Midrid capsules pack sizes 15s P; 30s POM
Mifegyne tablets POM
Mifepristone POM
Migard tablets POM
Miglitol POM
Miglustat POM
Migrafen tablets P
Migraleve pack sizes 12s, 24s CD Inv P; 48s CD Inv POM
Migramax sachets POM
Migranal nasal spray POM
Migravess forte tablets POM
Migravess tablets POM
Migril tablets POM
Mildison Lipocream POM
Milk of Magnesia liquid GSL
Milk of Magnesia tablets GSL
Milpar P
Milrinone POM
Milrinone lactate POM
Mimpara tablets POM
Min-I-Jet preparations POM except Min-I-Jet morphine CD POM
Minalka GSL
Minihep ampoules POM
Minihep-Calcium injection POM
Minims amethocaine hydrochloride POM
Minims artificial tears P
Minims atropine sulphate POM
Minims benoxinate (oxybuprocaine) hydrochloride POM

Minims chloramphenicol POM
Minims cyclopentolate hydrochloride POM
Minims dexamethasone POM
Minims ephedrine hydrochloride P
Minims fluorescein sodium P
Minims gentamicin POM
Minims homatropine hydrobromide POM
Minims hyoscine hydrobromide POM
Minims lidocaine and fluorescein POM
Minims metipranolol POM
Minims neomycin sulphate POM
Minims oxybuprocaine POM
Minims phenylephrine hydrochloride P
Minims pilocarpine nitrate POM
Minims prednisolone POM
Minims proxymetacaine POM
Minims proxymetacaine and fluorescein POM
Minims Rose Bengal P
Minims sodium chloride P
Minims tetracaine POM
Minims tetracaine hydrochloride POM
Minims tropicamide POM
Minitran patches P
Minocin MR capsules POM
Minocin tablets POM
Minocycline POM
Minocycline hydrochloride POM
Minodiab tablets POM
Minoxidil POM; but (1) if for external use, maximum strength 5%, for the treatment of alopecia androgenetica in men aged 18 to 65 (but not women) P; (2) if for external use, maximum strength 2% P; (3) if for external use for the treatment of alopecia androgenetica in men and women aged between 18 and 65 years, in a solution or gel with a maximum strength 2% and a maximum pack size of 60ml, GSL, please refer to proprietary names for classification granted under the marketing authorisation (see Regaine products)
Mintec capsules GSL
Mintezol tablets POM
Minulet tablets POM
Miochol E POM
Mirapexin tablets POM
Mirena intrauterine system POM
Mirtazapine POM
Misoprostol POM
Mistamine tablets POM
Mitobronitol POM
Mitomycin POM
Mitomycin C Kyowa POM
Mitomycin injection POM
Mitotane POM
Mitoxana injection POM
Mitoxantrone/Mitozantrone hydrochloride POM
Mitozantrone see Mitoxantrone
Mivacron injection POM
Mivacurium chloride POM
Mixtard insulins POM
Mizolastine POM
Mizollen tablets POM
MMR II vaccine POM
Mobic preparations POM
Mobiflex tablets POM
Mobiflex vials POM
Mobigel spray gel POM
Moclobemide POM
Modafinil POM
Modalim tablets POM
Modaplate POM
Modecate concentrate injection POM
Modecate injection POM
Modern Herbals preparations GSL
Modisal LA preparations P
Modisal XL tablets P
Moditen preparations POM
Modrasone cream, and ointment POM
Modrenal capsules POM
Moducren tablets POM
Moduret 25 POM

Moduretic solution POM
Moduretic tablets POM
Moexipril POM
Mogadon preparations CD Benz POM
Moisture-eyes P
Molcer ear drops P
Molgramostim POM
Molindone hydrochloride POM
Molipaxin preparations POM
Mometasone furoate POM
Monit LS tablets P
Monit SR tablets P
Monit tablets P
Monit XL tablets P
Mono-Cedocard 10 tablets P
Mono-Cedocard 20 tablets P
Mono-Cedocard 40 tablets P
Monoclate-P injection POM
Monocor tablets POM
Monodur tabs POM
Monoethanolamine oleate POM
Monomax SR capsules P
Monomax XL tablets P
Monomil POM
Mononine POM
Monoparin preparations POM
Monosorb XL 60 tablets POM
Monotard insulins POM
Monotrim preparations POM
Monovent preparations POM
Monozide 10 tablets POM
Monphytol P
Montelukast POM
Moorland GSL
Moracizine hydrochloride POM
Moraxen suppositories POM
Morazone hydrochloride POM
Morcap SR capsules CD POM
Morhulin ointment POM
Morpheridine; its salts CD POM
Morphgesic SR CD POM
Morphine; its salts; its esters and ethers; their salts; its pentavalent nitrogen derivatives; their esters and ethers CD POM; but for morphine salts if in, (a) any preparations from which the morphine cannot be readily recovered in amounts which constitute a risk to health and with ms 0.2% (calculated as anhydrous morphine base) CD Inv POM; (b) if for non-parenteral use in unit preparations diluted to at least one part in a million (6X) in response to a specific request, CD Inv P; or (c) if for non-parenteral use in unit preparations diluted to at least one part in a million million (6C), CD Inv P
Morphine acetate see Morphine
Morphine and ipecacuanha mixture BPC CD Inv P
Morphine hydrochloride see Morphine
Morphine methobromide, morphine N-oxide and other pentavalent nitrogen morphine derivatives CD POM
Morphine N-oxide; its esters and ethers CD POM
Morphine sulphate Rapiject CD POM
Morphine sulphate see Morphine
Morphine tartrate see Morphine
Morpholinoethylnorpethidine see Morpheridine
Motens tablets POM
Motherwort GSL
Motherwort compound tabs GSL
Motifene capsules POM
Motilium 10 tablets P
Motilium suppositories POM
Motilium suspension POM
Motilium tablets POM
Motipress tablets POM
Motival tablets POM
Motrin tablets POM
Movelat preparations P
Movicol Paediatric plain sachets POM
Movicol Sachets P
Movicol-Half sachets P
Moviprep P

Moxifloxacin POM
Moxisylyte/Thymoxamine POM
Moxisylyte/Thymoxamine hydrochloride POM
Moxonidine POM
MST Continus tablets CD POM
MST suspension CD POM
Mucaine POM
Mucodyne preparations POM
Mucogel suspension GSL
Mucron tablets P
Multibionta infusion POM
Multiload IUDs POM
Multiparin injection POM
Mumpsvax vaccine POM
Mupirocin POM
Mupirocin calcium POM
Murine P
Muscinil tablets POM
Muse system POM
Mustard oil, volatile, if maximum strength 0.1 per cent (external use only) GSL
Mustine see Chlormethine
MXL capsules CD POM
Mycamine POM
Mycardol tablets P
Mycifradin preparations POM
Mycil Gold P
Mycil preparations GSL
Mycobutin capsules POM
Mycophenolate mofetil POM
Mycophenolic acid POM
Mycota preparations GSL
Mydriacyl eye drops POM
Mydrilate eye drops POM
Myelobromol tablets POM
Myfortic tablets POM
Myleran tablets POM
Myocet POM
Myocrisin injections POM
Myotonine chloride tablets POM
Myrophine; its salts CD POM
Myrrh GSL
Myrrh tincture BPC GSL
Mysoline preparations POM

N

Nabilone POM
Nabumetone POM
Nadolol POM
Nafarelin acetate POM
Naftidrofuryl oxalate POM
Naftifine hydrochloride POM
Nalbuphine hydrochloride POM
Nalcrom capsules POM
Nalidixic acid POM
Nalorex tablets POM
Nalorphine hydrobromide POM
Naloxone hydrochloride POM
Naltrexone hydrochloride POM
Nandrolone CD Anab POM
Nandrolone decanoate CD Anab POM
Nandrolone laurate CD Anab POM
Nandrolone phenylpropionate CD Anab POM
Naphazoline hydrochloride POM but if nasal sprays or nasal drops not containing liquid paraffin as a vehicle, maximum strength 0.05 per cent; eye drops maximum strength 0.015 per cent, P
Naphazoline nitrate POM but if nasal sprays or nasal drops not containing liquid paraffin as a vehicle maximum strength 0.05 per cent, P
Napratec tablets POM
Naprosyn preparations POM
Naprosyn SR tablets POM
Naproxen POM but if for the treatment of primary dysmenorrhoea in women aged between 15 and 50 years, maximum strength 250mg, 500mg (MD), 750mg (MDD), for a maximum of 3 days treatment, in a maximum pack size of 9 tablets, P
Naproxen sodium POM

Napsalgesic tablets CD Inv POM
Naramig tablets POM
Naratriptan POM
Narcan ampoules POM
Narcan Neonatal ampoules POM
Nardil tablets POM
Naropin preparations POM
Narphen preparations CD POM
Nasacort spray POM
Naseptin cream POM
Nasivin GSL
Nasobec aqueous spray POM
Nasobec Hayfever P
Nasofan allergy POM
Nasonex aqueous nasal spray POM
Natalizumab POM
Natamycin POM
Natecal D3 tablets P
Nateglinide POM
Natracalm tabs GSL
Natramid POM
Natrasleep GSL
Natravene GSL
Natrilix SR tablets POM
Natrilix tablets POM
Navelbine injection POM
Navidrex tablets POM
Navispare tablets POM
Navoban preparations POM
Nebcin vials POM
Nebido solution for injection CD Anab POM
Nebilet tablets POM
Nebivolol hydrochloride POM
Nedocromil sodium POM but if for the prevention, relief and treatment of seasonal and perennial allergic conjunctivitis maximum strength 2.0 per cent and container or package contains not more than 3ml of medicinal product, P
Nefazodone hydrochloride POM
Neflinavir POM
Nefopam hydrochloride POM
Negaban powder for solution for injection/infusion POM
Negram preparations POM
NeisVac-C POM
Nelfinavir POM
Nelsons preparations GSL
Neo-Bendromax POM
Neo-Cantil preparations POM
Neo-Cortef preparations POM
Neo-Cytamen injection POM
Neo-Mercazole tablets POM
Neo-NaClex tablets POM
Neo-NaClex-K POM
Neo-planotest 200 P
Neoclarityn oral solution 0.5mg/ml POM
Neoclarityn syrup POM
Neoclarityn tablets POM
Neofel XL POM
Neogest tablets POM
Neomycin POM
Neomycin oleate POM
Neomycin palmitate POM
Neomycin sulphate POM
Neomycin undecanoate POM
Neoral capsules POM
Neoral oral solution POM
NeoRecormon preparations POM
Neosporin eye drops POM
Neostigmine bromide POM
Neostigmine methylsulphate POM
Neotigason capsules POM
Neotren MR POM
Nephril tablets POM
Nerisone Forte preparations POM
Nerisone preparations POM
Nestargel powder P
Netillin injection POM
Netilmicin sulphate POM
Nettle (Urtica dioica) GSL
Neulactil preparations POM
Neulasta injection POM
Neupogen injection POM
Neupogen Singleject POM

Neupro transdermal patch POM
Neurobloc injection POM
Neurontin preparations POM
Neutrogena dermatological cream GSL
Nevirapine POM
New Era preparations GSL
Nexavar POM
Nexium preparations POM
Niaspan tablets POM
Nicam gel P
Nicardipine hydrochloride POM
Nice 'n Clear head lice lotion GSL
Nicef caps POM
Nicergoline POM
Niceritrol POM
Nicobrevin caps GSL
Nicocodine CD POM but if for non parenteral use and: (a) in undivided preparations with ms 2.5% (calculated as base) CD Inv POM; or (b) in single dose preparations with ms per dosage unit 100mg (calculated as base) CD Inv POM
Nicodicodine (6-nicotinoyldihydrocodeine) CD POM but if for non parenteral use and: (a) in undivided preparations with ms 2.5% (calculated as base) CD Inv POM; or (b) in single dose preparations with ms per dosage unit 100mg (calculated as base) CD Inv POM
Nicomorphine; its salts CD POM
Nicorandil POM
Nicorette gum (all flavours and pack sizes) GSL
Nicorette inhalator P
Nicorette InvisiPatch GSL
Nicorette microtab P and GSL
Nicorette nasal spray P
Nicorette patches GSL
Nicotinamide tablets BP GSL
Nicotinamide, up to 300mg (MDD) GSL; or 4% topical gel for treatment of mild to moderate acne vulgaris GSL
Nicotine GSL if for the relief of nicotine withdrawal symptoms as an aid to smoking cessation only, chewing gum maximum strength 4mg, lozenges maximum strength 4mg, sublingual tablets maximum strength 2mg, transdermal patches for continuous application to the skin for a period of 16 hours maximum strength 25mg in 16hrca, transdermal patches for continuous application to the skin for a period of 24 hours maximum strength 21mg in 24 hrca, inhalation cartridge for oromucosal use maximum strength 10mg per cartridge; if for the relief of nicotine withdrawal symptoms as an aid to smoking reduction with the aim of cessation, chewing gum maximum strength 4mg, inhalation cartridge for oromucosal use maximum strength 10mg per cartridge GSL; if nicotine nasal spray delivering 0.5mg nicotine per spray as an aid to smoking cessation for adults and children over 12 years of age GSL
Nicotinell preparations GSL
Nicotinic acid POM but any use, except for the treatment of hyperlipidaemia 600mg (MDD), P 100mg (MDD), GSL
Nicotinyl alcohol P
Nicoumalone see Acenocoumarol
Nicrondil POM
Niddaryl tablets POM
Nifedipine POM
Nifedipress MR POM
Nifedotard 20MR POM
Nifelease tablets POM
Nifenazone POM
Niferex preparations P
Nifopress retard tabs POM
Nifopress MR POM
Night Nurse preparations P
Night time formula P

Nightcalm tablets P
Nikethamide POM
Nilutamide POM
Nimbex Forte injection POM
Nimbex injection POM
Nimetazepam CD Benz POM
Nimodipine POM
Nimodrel XL POM
Nimotop preparations POM
Nindaxa 2.5 POM
Niopam POM
Nipent vials POM
NiQuitin CQ preparations GSL
Niridazole POM
Nirolex preparations P
Nisoldipine POM
Nitrados tablets CD Benz POM
Nitrazepam CD Benz POM
Nitrendipine POM
Nitro-dur P
Nitrocine POM
Nitrofurantoin POM
Nitrofurazone POM
Nitrolingual spray P
Nitromin P
Nitronal injection POM
Nitropatch POM
Nitroprusside POM
Nitroxoline POM
Nivaquine injection POM
Nivaquine syrup and tablets POM but when supplied for the prevention of malaria, P
Nivaten Retard POM
Nivemycin tablets POM
Nix pencil GSL
Nizatidine POM but if for the prevention and treatment of the symptoms of food-related heartburn and meal-induced indigestion in adults and children not less than 16 years 75mg (MD) 150mg (MDD) for a maximum period of 14 days, P
Nizoral Anti-dandruff shampoo 60ml P
Nizoral Cream POM
Nizoral shampoo 120ml POM
Nizoral shampoo 100ml P
Nizoral suspension POM
Nizoral tablets POM
Nocutil nasal spray POM
Nolvadex-D POM
Nomifensine maleate POM
Non-human chorionic gonadotrophin CD Anab POM
Nonivamide, if maximum strength 0.1 per cent (external use only) GSL
Nonoxinols, external use only GSL
Nootropil preparations POM
Noracymethadol; its salts CD POM
Noradran syrup P
Noradrenaline POM
Noradrenaline acid tartrate POM
19-Nor-4-androstene-3,17-dione CD Anab POM
19-Nor-5-androstene-3,17-diol CD Anab POM
Norboletone CD Anab POM
Norclostebol CD Anab POM
Norcodeine CD POM but if for non parenteral use and: (a) in undivided preparations with ms 2.5% (calculated as base) CD Inv POM; or (b) in single dose preparations with ms per dosage until 100mg (calculated as base) CD Inv POM
Norcuron injection POM
Nordazepam CD Benz POM
Norditropin injection CD Anab POM
Norditropin SimpleXx CD Anab POM
Norelgestromin POM
Norepinephrine see Noradrenaline
Norethandrolone CD Anab POM
Norethisterone POM
Norethisterone acetate POM
Norethisterone enanthate POM
Norethynodrel POM
Norfloxacin POM
Norgalax P

Norgestimate POM
Norgeston tablets POM
Norgestrel POM
Noriday tablets POM
Norimin tablets POM
Norimode tabs POM
Norinyl-1 tablets POM
Noristerat injection POM
Norit GSL
Noritate cream POM
Norlevorphanol; its salts; its esters and ethers; their salts CD POM
Normacol Plus preparations GSL
Normacol preparations GSL
Normaloe P
Normasol P
Normax preparations POM
Normegon injection POM
Normethadone; its salts CD POM
Normorphine; its salts; its esters and ethers; their salts CD POM
Normosang infusion POM
Norphyllin preparations POM
Norpipanone; its salts CD POM
Norplant implant POM
Norprolac tablets POM
Nortriptyline hydrochloride POM
Norvir capsules POM
Norvir oral solution POM
Norzol POM
Noscapine POM
Noscapine hydrochloride POM
Novantrone injection POM
Novaprin P
Novobiocin calcium POM
Novobiocin sodium POM
Novofem POM
Novolizer budesonide POM
NovoMix 30 preparations POM
NovoNorm tablets POM
Novorapid injections POM
Novoseven POM
Nowax GSL
Noxafil POM
Noxyflex S vials P
Noxytiolin P
Nozinan POM
Nu-Hope prolapse overbelt P
Nu-Seals Aspirin 300mg pack sizes 100s POM
Nu-Seals Aspirin 75mg pack sizes 56s P
Nubain injection POM
Nucare 300mg aspirin pack sizes 32s P; 100s POM
Nucare co-codamol 8/500 pack size 32s P
Nucare dispersible aspirin 75mg pack size 100s P
Nucare dispersible aspirin 300mg pack size 32s P
Nucare ibuprofen preparations P
Nucare paracetamol caplets pack size 16s GSL
Nucare rehydration sachets GSL
Nucare Sigma Codeine linctus P
Nucare Sigma Paracetamol paediatric P
Nucare Sigma Paracetamol suspension 6 plus P
Nucare Sigma Pholcodine linctus P
Nucare Sigma Simple linctus P
Nucare Sigma Simple linctus paediatric P
Nuelin preparations P
Nulacin tablets GSL
Numark allergy eye drops P
Numark allergy relief and hayfever tablets GSL
Numark allergy relief syrup P
Numark anti-dandruff shampoo GSL
Numark antihistamine oral solution P
Numark baby cream GSL
Numark chloramphenicol 0.5% antibiotic eye-drops P
Numark cold remedy night time P
Numark cold sore cream P
Numark constipation relief GSL
Numark cough mixture adult chesty P/GSL (depending on ingredients)

Numark cough mixture adult dry P
Numark cystitis relief GSL
Numark diarrhoea & dehydration relief GSL
Numark flu relief capsules GSL
Numark flu strength all-in-one P
Numark heartburn relief tablets POM
Numark herbal constipation relief GSL
Numark loratadine liquid P
Numark max strength cold and flu sachets GSL
Numark medicated pastilles GSL
Numark muscle rub GSL
Numark muscle spray GSL
Numark sleep aid 50mg P
Nupercainal P
Nurofen Advance tablets P
Nurofen back pain capsules P
Nurofen Caplets pack sizes 12s, 16s GSL; 24s P
Nurofen Cold and Flu tablets P
Nurofen extra strength P
Nurofen for Children singles sachets GSL
Nurofen for Children oral suspension 3 mths to 9 yrs GSL
Nurofen for Children sugar-free suspension 100ml, 150ml P
Nurofen Gel Maximum Strength P
Nurofen ibuprofen gel 5% 35g GSL
Nurofen liquid capsules pack sizes 10s, 16s GSL; 30s P
Nurofen Long Lasting capsules P
Nurofen Meltlets GSL
Nurofen Micro Granules P
Nurofen migraine pain caplets P
Nurofen migraine pain tablets GSL
Nurofen mobile tablets GSL
Nurofen Muscular pain relief gel GSL
Nurofen Plus tablets CD Inv P
Nurofen recovery GSL
Nurofen tablets 200mg pack sizes 12s, 16s GSL; 24s, 48, 96s P
Nurofen tension headache GSL
Nurse Harvey's gripe mixture GSL
Nurse Sykes bronchial balsam GSL
Nurse Sykes powders pack sizes 4s, 8s GSL
Nutmeg GSL
Nutmeg Oil GSL
Nutracel preparations POM
Nutraplus cream P
NuTRIflex preparations POM
Nutrizym 10 P
Nutrizym 22 P
Nutrizym GR capsules P
NutropinAq CD Anab POM
Nuvaring POM
Nuvelle Continuous tablets POM
Nuvelle tablets POM
Nuvelle TS patches POM
Nux Vomica Seed POM
Nycopren tablets POM
Nylax with senna tablets pack sizes 10s GSL; 30s PO
Nyogel eye gel POM
Nyspes pessaries POM
Nystadermal preparations POM
Nystaform preparations POM
Nystaform-HC preparations POM
Nystamont oral suspension POM
Nystan preparations POM
Nystatin POM
Nytol Caplets P
Nytol herbal tablets GSL
Nytol One-a-Night P
Nytol tablets P

O

Oak Bark GSL
Occlusal P
Octacosactrin POM
Octagam POM
Octaphonium chloride, external use only GSL
Octim injection POM
Octim nasal spray POM

Octreotide POM
Ocufen ophthalmic solution POM
Oculotect eye drops P
Ocusert preparations POM
Ocuvite tablets GSL
Ocuvite lutein GSL
Odrik capsules POM
Oestradiol see Estradiol
Oestrifen tablets POM
Oestriol see Estriol
Oestrogel POM
Oestrogen POM
Oestrogenic Substances Conjugated POM
Oestrone see Estrone
Ofloxacin POM
Oftaquix POM
Oilatum cream GSL
Oilatum emollient GSL
Oilatum gel GSL
Oilatum junior cream 500ml GSL
Oilatum junior emollient bath additive GSL
Oilatum cream pump dispenser GSL
Oilatum Plus GSL
50:50 ointment P
Okacyn eye-drops POM
Olanzapine POM
Olbas inhaler sticks GSL
Olbas oil GSL
Olbas pastilles GSL
Olbetam capsules POM
Old tuberculin POM
Oleic acid, external use only GSL
Oleyl alcohol, external use only GSL
Olive Oil GSL
Olmesartan medoxomil POM
Olmetec tablets POM
Olmetex Plus tablets POM
Olopatadine POM
Olsalazine sodium POM
Omacor capsules P
Omalizumab powder and solvent for injection POM
Omeprazole POM but if for the relief of reflux-like symptoms (eg heartburn) in sufferers aged 18 and over please refer to proprietary names for the classification granted under the marketing authorisation (see Omeprazole 10mg Gastro-resistant Tablets [Galpharm])
Omeprazole 10mg gastro-resistant tablets (Galpharm) P
Omnic MR POM
Omnikan preparations POM
Omniscan vials POM
Oncovin vials POM
Ondansetron hydrochloride POM
Ondemet preparations POM
One-Alpha capsules POM
One-Alpha injection POM
One-Alpha solution POM
Onkotrone injection POM
Opas preparations GSL
Opatanol eye-drops POM
Opazimes CD Inv P
Ophthaine solution POM
Opilon preparations POM
Opium, raw CD Lic
Opizone tablets POM
Oprisine tablets POM
Opticrom Allergy eyedrops P
Opticrom eye drops POM
Optil preparations POM
Optilast eye drops POM
Optimax tablets POM
Optimine syrup P
Optimine tablets P
Optipen Pro 1 Green POM
Optrex allergy eye drops P
Optrex infected eyes eye drops P
Optrex red eyes eye drops P
Optrex sore eyes eye drops P
Opumide tablets POM
Orabet tablets POM
Orajel dental gel GSL
Orajel mouth gel P

Orajel extra strength dental gel P
Oral B sensitive toothpaste GSL
Oral gel 15g P
Oral gel 80g P
Oraldene GSL
Oramorph Concentrated oral solution CD POM
Oramorph oral solution CD Inv POM
Oramorph SR tablets CD POM
Oramorph vials 100mg/5ml CD POM
Oramorph vials 10mg/5ml CD Inv POM
Oramorph vials 30mg/5ml CD POM
Orange GSL
Orap tablets POM
Oraquix periodontal gel POM
Orbifen oral suspension pack sizes 100ml P; 500ml POM
Orbifen oral suspension sachets GSL
Orciprenaline sulphate POM
Orelox POM
Orelox suspension POM
Orencia injection POM
Orgafol injection POM
Orgalutran POM
Organon injection POM
Orimeten tablets POM
Orlept preparations POM
Orlistat POM
Orovite 7 sachets GSL
Orovite tablets GSL
Orphenadrine citrate POM
Orphenadrine hydrochloride POM
Ortho Gyne-T intrauterine copper contraceptive device POM
Ortho-Creme GSL
Ortho-Gynest cream POM
Ortho-Gynest pessaries POM
Ortho-Novin preparations POM
Orthoforms pessaries GSL
Orudis capsules POM
Orudis suppositories POM
Oruvail capsules POM
Oruvail gel pack sizes 100g POM
Oruvail gel pack sizes 30g P
Oruvail IM injection POM
Oseltamivir POM
Ossopan granules P
Ossopan tablets P
Ostex Plus GSL
Ostram sachets P
OTC Concepts preparations GSL
Otex ear drops P
Otodex GSL
Otomize ear spray POM
Otosporin ear drops POM
Otrivine antistin drops P
Otrivine Mu-Cron tablets P
Otrivine preparations GSL
Ovandrotone CD Anab POM
Ovarian Gland Dried POM
Ovestin cream POM
Ovestin tablets POM
Ovex P
Ovitrelle injection CD anab POM
Ovran 30 tablets POM
Ovran tablets POM
Ovranette tablets POM
Ovysmen tablets POM
Oxabolone CD Anab POM
Oxactin POM
Oxamniquine POM
Oxandrolone CD Anab POM
Oxantel embonate POM
Oxaprozin POM
Oxatomide POM
Oxazepam CD Benz POM
Oxazolam CD Benz POM
Oxcarbazepine POM
Oxedrine tartrate POM
Oxerutins P
Oxetacaine/Oxethazaine POM but if 10mg (MD) 30mg (MDD) container or package contains not more than 400mg of oxethazaine, P
Oxethazaine see Oxetacaine
Oxis turbohaler POM
Oxitropium bromide POM
Oxivent inhaler POM

Oxolinic acid POM
Oxpentifylline see Pentoxifylline
Oxprenolol hydrochloride POM
Oxy Daily cleanser GSL
Oxy daily face wash GSL
Oxy in the shower GSL
Oxy on the spot GSL
Oxy wipeout pads GSL
Oxy 10 P
Oxy-gen products GSL
Oxybuprocaine hydrochloride POM but if non-ophthalmic use, P
Oxybutynin hydrochloride POM
Oxycodone; its salts; its esters and ethers; their salts CD POM
Oxycontin tablets CD POM
Oxydon tablets POM
Oxygen GSL
Oxymesterone CD Anab POM
Oxymetazoline hydrochloride, if non-oily nasal sprays and nasal drops maximum strength 0.05 per cent GSL
Oxymetazoline, if non-oily nasal sprays and nasal drops maximum strength 0.05 per cent GSL
Oxymetholone CD Anab POM
Oxymorphone; its salts; its esters and ethers; their salts CD POM
Oxymycin tablets POM
Oxynorm preparations CD POM
Oxypertine POM
Oxypertine hydrochloride POM
Oxyphenbutazone POM
Oxyphencyclimine hydrochloride POM
Oxyphenonium bromide POM but if 5mg (MD) 15mg (MDD), P
Oxysept 1-step neutralising tablets GSL
Oxysept saline 90ml GSL
Oxytetracycline POM
Oxytetracycline calcium POM
Oxytetracycline dihydrate POM
Oxytetracycline hydrochloride POM
Oxytetramix tablets POM
Oxytocin, natural POM
Oxytocin, synthetic POM

P

P2S POM
Pabal injections POM
Pabrinex injections POM
Pacifene Maximum Strength tablets P
Pacifene tablets 200mg pack sizes 12s GSL; 24s, 48s, 96s P
Paclitaxel POM
Padimate 0, external use only GSL
Paedo-Sed syrup POM
Paeony (Peony), external use only GSL
Palacos LV POM
Palacos R POM
Palfermin POM
Palfium preparations CD POM
Palivizumab POM
Palladone capsules CD POM
Palladone SR capsules CD POM
Palonosetron POM
Paludrine P
Paludrine/avloclor travel packs P
Pamergan P100 injection CD POM
Pamidronate disodium POM
Pamine tablets POM
Panadeine CD Inv P
Panadol Actifast pack sizes 8s, 16s GSL; 30s P; compack GSL
Panadol capsules pack sizes 16s GSL
Panadol elixir P
Panadol Extra Soluble pack sizes 24s GSL
Panadol Extra tablets pack sizes 12s, 16s GSL; 32s P
Panadol Night tablets P
Panadol Soluble tablets pack sizes 12s, 24s GSL
Panadol tablets pack sizes 12s, 16s GSL; 32s P
Panadol Ultra tablets 20s CD Inv P
Pancrease capsules P

Pancrease HL POM
Pancreatin POM but if capsules maximum strength 21,000 European Pharmacopoeia units of lipase per capsule; powder maximum strength 25,000 European Pharmacopoeia units of lipase per gram, P
Pancrex granules P
Pancrex V preparations P
Pancuronium bromide POM
Panoxyl preparations P
Pantaprazole sodium POM
Pantoprazole POM
Pantothenic acid GSL
Papain GSL
Papaveretum see Medicinal opium
Papaverine POM but if (1) by inhaler; (2) otherwise than by inhaler 50mg (MD) 150mg (MDD), P
Papaverine hydrochloride POM but if (1) by inhaler; (2) otherwise than by inhaler equivalent of 50mg of papaverine (MD) equivalent of 150mg of papaverine (MDD), P
Papulex P
Paracetamol tablets, capsules, powders, granules, liquid preparations, see tables pp65-66
Paracetamol suppositories pack size 10s P
Paracets capsules pack size 16s GSL
Paracets Plus capsules GSL
Paracets powders pack size 5s GSL
Paracodol capsules CD Inv P
Paracodol soluble tablets CD Inv P
Paradote pack sizes 24s P; 96s POM
Paraffin white & yellow soft BP, external use only GSL
Paraffin, hard, external use only GSL
Paraffin, liquid, all preparations except nasal drops, nasal sprays, nasal inhalations and oral laxatives GSL
Parake tablets CD Inv POM
Paraldehyde POM
Paramax sachets POM
Paramax tablets POM
Paramed GSL
Paramethadione POM
Paramethasone acetate POM
Paramol tablets CD Inv P
Paranorm P
Paraplatin injection POM
Parathyroid Gland POM
Pardelprin MR capsules POM
Parecoxib POM
Paregoric BP CD Inv POM
Pargyline hydrochloride POM
Pariet tablets POM
Parlodel preparations POM
Parmid preparations POM
Parnate tablets POM
Paromomycin sulphate POM
Paroven capsules P
Paroxetine hydrochloride POM
Parsley GSL
Parsley piert GSL
Parstelin tablets POM
Partobulin POM
Partobulin SDF POM
Parvolex injection POM
Passiflora GSL
Patent Blue VE131 GSL
Pavacol-D pack sizes 150ml P; 300ml CD Inv P
Pavulon ampoules POM
Paxene concentrate POM
Paxidorm tablets P
Paxoran POM
Pecilocin POM
Pectin GSL
Pediacel vaccine POM
Peditrace POM
Peg-Intron POM
Pegaptanib POM
Pegasys injection POM
Pegfilgrastim POM
Peginterferon alfa POM
Pegvisomant POM

Pellitory GSL
Pemetrexed POM
Pemoline CD Benz POM
Penamecillin POM
Penbritin preparations POM
Penbutolol sulphate POM
Penciclovir POM; but if for external use for the treatment of herpes simplex virus infections of the lips and face (Herpes labialis) in adults and children aged 12 or more; maximum strength 1%; maximum pack size 2g, P
Pendramine tablets POM
Penicillamine POM
Penicillamine hydrochloride POM
Penicillin POM
Pennsaid topical solution POM
Pentacarinat POM
Pentamidine injection BP POM
Pentamidine isethionate POM
Pentasa enemas POM
Pentasa sachets POM
Pentasa suppositories POM
Pentasa Sustained Release tablets POM
Pentaspan IV infusion POM
Pentazocine CD No Register POM
Penthienate bromide POM but if 5mg (MD) 15mg (MDD), P
Pentobarbitone CD No Register POM
Pentobarbitone sodium CD No Register POM
Pentolinium tartrate POM
Pentostam injection POM
Pentostatin POM
Pentoxifylline/Oxpentifylline POM
Pentrax shampoo P
Pep tablets GSL
Pepcid AC indigestion tablets GSL
Pepcid PM tablets POM
Pepcid tablets POM
Pepcidtwo chewable tablets GSL
Peppermint GSL
Peppermint oil GSL
Peptac liquid PO
Peptimax tablets POM
Pepto-bismol P
Peralvex P
Percutaneous Bacillus Calmette-Guerin vaccine POM
Percutol ointment P
Perdix tablets POM
Perfalgan POM
Perfan injection POM
Perfluamine POM
Pergolide mesylate POM
Pergonal injection POM
Perhexiline maleate POM
Periactin tablets P
Pericyazine POM
Perinal spray (0173/0049) P
Perindopril POM
Perindopril erbumine POM
Perio.aid GSL
Periostat tablets POM
Permethrin cream (Sandoz) P
Permitabs P
Peroxyl GSL
Perphenazine POM
Persantin ampoules POM
Persantin Retard tablets POM
Persantin tablets POM
Pertussis vaccine POM
Peru, balsam of, external use only GSL
Pethidine-scopolamine CD POM
Pethidine; its salts CD POM
Pevaryl P
Pevaryl TC cream POM
Pharmalgen Venom vaccines POM
Pharmaton capsules GSL (100 pack size P and GSL)
Pharmorubicin Rapid Dissolution injection POM
Pharmorubicin Solution for Injection POM
Phasonit LA 50 P
Phenacetin POM but if maximum strength 0.1 per cent, P

Phenadone see Methadone
Phenadoxone; its salts CD POM
Phenampromide; its salts CD POM
Phenazocine; its salts; its esters and ethers; their salts CD POM
Phenazone POM but if external P
Phenazone salicylate POM
Phenbutrazate hydrochloride POM
Phencyclidine; its salts; its esters; their salts CD POM
Phendimetrazine; its salts CD No Register POM
Phenelzine sulphate POM
Phenergan elixir P
Phenergan injection POM
Phenergan Nightime tablets P
Phenergan tablets P
Phenethicillin potassium POM
Phenethylamine derivatives formed by substitution in the ring to any extent with alkyl, alkoxy, alkylenedioxy or halide substituents, whether or not further substituted in the ring by one or more other univalent substituents, also derivatives formed by such substitution of the following (except methoxyphenamine); N-alkylphenethylamines, alpha-methylphenethylamine, N-alkyl-alpha-methylphenethylamine, alpha-ethylphenethylamine, or N-alkyl-alpha-ethylphenethylamine; their salts; their esters and ethers; their salts CD Lic
Phenformin hydrochloride POM
Phenglutarimide hydrochloride POM
Phenindamine tartrate POM
Phenindione POM
Phenmetrazine hydrochloride CD POM
Phenmetrazine theoclate CD POM
Phenmetrazine; its salts CD POM
Phenobarbital/Phenobarbitone CD No Register POM Note: emergency supply at request of patient not permitted except for use in the treatment of epilepsy
Phenobarbital/Phenobarbitone sodium CD No Register POM Note: emergency supply at request of patient not permitted except for use in the treatment of epilepsy
Phenobarbitone see Phenobarbital
Phenol, if internal (except smelling salts) maximum strength 1.0 per cent, or smelling salts maximum strength 5.0 per cent or external maximum strength 2.5 per cent GSL
Phenolphthalein POM
Phenomorphan; its salts; its esters and ethers; their salts CD POM
Phenoperidine; its salts; its esters and ethers; their salts CD POM
Phenoxybenzamine hydrochloride POM
Phenoxymethylpenicillin POM
Phenoxymethylpenicillin calcium POM
Phenoxymethylpenicillin potassium POM
Phenprocoumon POM
Phensic original tablets pack sizes 12s GSL; 24s P
Phensuximide POM
Phentanyl see Fentanyl
Phentermine CD No Register POM
Phentolamine hydrochloride POM
Phentolamine mesylate POM
Phenylbutazone POM
Phenylbutazone sodium POM
Phenylephrine hydrochloride, if internal (all preparations except nasal drops, nasal sprays and nasal inhalations equivalent to 10 mg phenylephrine [MD]) GSL
Phenylephrine injection BP POM
Phenylmethylbarbituric acid CD No Register POM
4-Phenylpiperidine-4-carboxylic acid ethyl ester CD POM

Paracetamol legal status: Tablets, capsules, powders and granules (*see* Note 1)

Product	Container size	Legal status	Where it can be sold	Maximum that can be sold to a person at any one time (*see* Note 2)
Non-effervescent tablets and capsules				
Paracetamol (non-effervescent) tablets and capsules up to 120mg (*see* Note 3)	Up to 16	GSL (for the treatment of children aged less than 6 years)	Pharmacies and non-pharmacy retail outlets	Not more than 100 tablets or capsules (*see* Note 4)
Paracetamol (non-effervescent) tablets and capsules up to 250mg	Up to 16	GSL (for the treatment of children aged 6 years and over)	Pharmacies and non-pharmacy retail outlets	Not more than 100 tablets or capsules (*see* Note 4)
Paracetamol (non-effervescent) tablets and capsules up to 250mg	Between 17 and 32 inclusive	P (if wholly or mainly for children aged less than 12 years)	Pharmacies only	Not more than 100 tablets or capsules (*see* Note 4)
Paracetamol (non-effervescent) tablets and capsules up to 500mg (*see* Note 3)	Up to 16	GSL (for the treatment of adults)	Pharmacies and non-pharmacy retail outlets	Not more than 100 tablets or capsules (*see* Note 4)
Paracetamol (non-effervescent) tablets and capsules up to 500mg	Between 17 and 32 inclusive	If wholly or mainly for adults and children not less than 12 years, *see* Note 6(i)	Pharmacies only	Not more than 100 tablets or capsules (see Note 4)
Paracetamol (non-effervescent) tablets and capsules up to 500mg	Greater than 32	POM	Pharmacies only	To be sold or supplied only in accordance with a prescription
Effervescent tablets (*see* Note 5)				
Paracetamol (effervescent) tablets up to 120mg (*see* Note 3)	Up to 30	GSL (for children aged less than 6 years)	Pharmacies and non-pharmacy retail outlets	No legal limit
Paracetamol (effervescent) tablets up to 120mg (*see* Note 3)	Greater than 30	For children aged less than 6 years, *see* Note 6(ii)	Pharmacies only	No legal limit
Paracetamol (effervescent) tablets up to 250mg	Up to 30	GSL (for children aged 6 and over	Pharmacies and non-pharmacy retail outlets	No legal limit
Paracetamol (effervescent) tablets up to 250mg	Greater than 30	For children aged 6 and over, *see* Note 6(i)	Pharmacies only	No legal limit
Paracetamol (effervescent) tablets up to 500mg (*see* Note 3)	Up to 30	GSL (for the treatment of adults)	Pharmacies and non-pharmacy retail outlets	No legal limit
Paracetamol (effervescent) tablets up to 500mg (*see* Note 3)	Greater than 30	For the treatment of adults, *see* Note 6(i)	Pharmacies only	No legal limit
Powders and granules				
Paracetamol powders and granules up to 240mg (see Note 3)	Up to 10	GSL (for the treatment of children)	Pharmacies and non-pharmacy retail outlets	No legal limit
Paracetamol powders and granules up to 1000mg (see Note 3)	Up to 10	GSL (for the treatment of adults)	Pharmacies and non-pharmacy retail outlets	No legal limit

Note 1: When paracetamol is in combination with a pharmacy medicine (eg, low-strength codeine) or a prescription-only medicine (eg, dextropropoxyphene), the more stringent legal category applies

Note 2: While several products have no legal limit for the amount that may be sold or supplied, pharmacists are expected to exercise professional control to limit the amount of paracetamol which may be stored in a patient's home

Note 3: For product containing paracetamol except when combined with methionine DL

Note 4: The quantity of non-effervescent tablets, capsules or a combination of both, sold or supplied to a person at any one time shall not exceed 100

Note 5: Effervescent preparations in relation to a tablet, means containing not less than 75 per cent, by weight of the tablet, of ingredients included wholly or mainly for the purpose of releasing carbon dioxide when the tablet is dissolved or dispersed in water

Note 6: Strictly speaking, paracetamol is classified as a POM or a GSL product, but is limited to sale through pharmacies under certain conditions and exemptions. Products marked 6(i) would be P medicines and 6(ii) GSL medicines, unless specific products are otherwise licensed

Paracetamol legal status: Liquids (*see* Note 1)

Product	Container size	Legal status	Where it can be sold	Maximum that can be sold to a person at any one time (*see* Note 2)
Liquids				
Paracetamol liquid preparations, up to 2.4 per cent (*see* Note 3)	In unit doses of not more than 5ml and no more than 20 unit doses (100ml)	GSL (for children under 12 years) MD 480mg, MDD 1,920mg	Pharmacies and non-pharmacy retail outlets	No legal limit
Paracetamol liquid preparations, up to 2.4 per cent (*see* Note 3)	In multidose containers of not more than 100ml	GSL (for children under 12 years) MD 480mg, MDD 1,920mg	Pharmacies and non-pharmacy retail outlets	No legal limit
Paracetamol liquid preparations, up to 2.5 per cent (*see* Note 3)	Up to 160ml	GSL (for the treatment of adults and children aged 12 years and over)	Pharmacies and non-pharmacy retail outlets	No legal limit
Paracetamol liquid preparations, up to 2.5 per cent (*see* Note 3)	Greater than 160ml	*see* Note 6(i)	Pharmacies only	No legal limit
Paracetamol liquid preparations, up to 5 per cent	In unit doses of not more than 5ml and no more than 12 unit doses	GSL (for persons aged 6 years and over)	Pharmacies and non-pharmacy retail outlets	No legal limit
Paracetamol liquid preparations, up to 5 per cent	In multidose containers of not more than 80ml	GSL (for persons aged 6 years and over)	Pharmacies and non-pharmacy retail outlets	No legal limit
Paracetamol liquid preparations, up to 5 per cent	Up to 160ml	GSL (for the treatment of adults and children aged 12 years and over)	Pharmacies and non-pharmacy retail outlets	No legal limit

Note 1: When paracetamol is in combination with a pharmacy medicine (eg, low-strength codeine) or a prescription-only medicine (eg, dextropropoxyphene), the more stringent legal category applies

Note 2: While several products have no legal limit for the amount that may be sold or supplied, pharmacists are expected to exercise professional control to limit the amount of paracetamol which may be stored in a patient's home

Note 3: For product containing paracetamol except when combined with methionine DL

Note 4: The quantity of non-effervescent tablets, capsules or a combination of both, sold or supplied to a person at any one time shall not exceed 100

Note 5: Effervescent preparations in relation to a tablet, means containing not less than 75 per cent, by weight of the tablet, of ingredients included wholly or mainly for the purpose of releasing carbon dioxide when the tablet is dissolved or dispersed in water

Note 6: Strictly speaking, paracetamol is classified as a POM or a GSL product, but is limited to sale through pharmacies under certain conditions and exemptions. Products marked 6(i) would be P medicines and 6(ii) GSL medicines, unless specific products are otherwise licensed

---

Phenylpropanolamine hydrochloride POM but if internal (1) all preparations except prolonged release capsules, nasal sprays and nasal drops, 25mg (MD) 100mg (MDD); (2) prolonged release capsules 50mg (MD) 100mg (MDD); (3) nasal sprays and nasal drops maximum strength 2.0 per cent, P

Phenytoin POM

Phenytoin sodium POM

Phillips preparations GSL

Phillips Milk of Magnesia GSL

Phimetin POM

Pholcodine CD POM but if for non-parenteral use and (a) in undivided preparations with ms 2.5% (calculated as base) CD Inv POM; or (b) in single dose preparations with ms per dosage unit 100mg (calculated as base) CD Inv POM; or (c) in unit preparations diluted to at least one part in a million (6X) in response to a specific request, CD Inv P; or (d) in unit preparations diluted to at least one part in a million million (6C), CD Inv P

Pholcodine citrate see Pholcodine

Pholcodine tartrate see Pholcodine

Phor Pain pack sizes 30g, 50g GSL; 100g P

Phor Pain Forte P

Phortinea paint P

Phosex tablets POM

Phosphate-Sandoz tablets P

Phospholine iodide POM

Photofrin injection POM

Phthalylsulphathiazole POM

Phyldrox tablets CD No Register POM

Phyllocontin Continus tablets P

Phyllocontin Forte Continus tablets P

Phyllocontin Paediatric Continus tablets P

Physeptone preparations CD POM

Physiotens tablets POM

Physostigmine POM

Physostigmine aminoxide salicylate POM

Physostigmine salicylate POM

Physostigmine sulphate POM

Phytex P

Phytomenadione POM but any use except the prevention or treatment of haemorrhagic disorders, P

Pickles foot ointment P

Pickles soothake toothache gel and tincture GSL

Picolax powder P

Picrotoxin POM

Pilewort GSL

Pilocarpine POM

Pilocarpine hydrochloride POM

Pilocarpine nitrate POM

Pilogel POM

Pimecrolimus POM

Pimento Oil GSL

Piminodine; its salts CD POM

Pimozide POM

Pinadone mixture CD POM

Pinazepam CD Benz POM

Pindolol POM

Pinefeld XL POM

Pini silvestris oil, if external use or inhalant capsules [maximum strength 9mg], or pastilles, lozenges, throat tablets [maximum strength 6mg], or cough syrups [maximum strength 0.05mg/5ml] GSL

Pioglitazone POM

Pipenzolate bromide POM but if 5mg (MD) 15mg (MDD), P

Piperacillin sodium POM

Piperacillin/tazobactam powder for solution for injection or infusion POM

Piperazine estrone/Oestrone sulphate POM

Piperidolate hydrochloride POM but if 50mg (MD) 150mg (MDD), P

Piperonal GSL

Piportil Depot injection POM

Pipothiazine see Pipotiazine

Pipotiazine/Pipothiazine palmitate POM

Pipradol; its salts CD No Register POM

Pipril injection POM

Piracetam POM

Pirbuterol acetate POM

Pirbuterol hydrochloride POM

Pirenzepine dihydrochloride monohydrate POM

Pirenzepine hydrochloride POM

Piretanide POM

Piriject injection POM

Piriteze Allergy tablets pack sizes 7s GSL; 30s P

Piriteze allergy syrup GSL

Piriton Allergy tablets P

Piriton Duolets P

Piriton injection POM

Piriton syrup P

Piritramide; its salts CD POM

Piroflam POM

Piroxicam POM but if external for the relief of rheumatic pain, pain of non-serious arthritic conditions and muscular aches, pains and swellings such as strains, sprains and sports injuries for use in adults and children not less than 12 years for maximum period of 7 days maximum strength 0.5 per cent and container or package containing not more than 30g of medicinal product, P

Piroxicam beta-cyclodextrin POM

Pirozip capsules POM

Pitressin injection POM

Pituitary anterior lobe POM

Pituitary Gland (Whole Dried) POM but if by inhaler, P

Pituitary Powdered (Posterior Lobe) POM but if by inhaler, P
Pivampicillin POM
Pivampicillin hydrochloride POM
Pivmecillinam POM
Pivmecillinam hydrochloride POM
Pizotifen POM
Pizotifen malate POM
Placidex liquid P
Plague vaccine POM
Plaquenil tablets POM
Platinex POM
Plavix tablets POM
Plendil POM
Plesmet syrup P
Pletal tablets POM
Pleurisy root GSL
Plicamycin POM
Pneumococcal vaccine (bacterial antigen) POM
Pneumovax vaccine POM
Pnu-imune vaccine POM
Pnu-Imune vials POM
Podophyllin paint, compound BP POM
Podophyllotoxin POM
Podophyllum POM
Podophyllum Indian POM
Podophyllum resin POM but if external ointment or impregnated plaster maximum strength 20.0 per cent, P
Poke root (Phytolacca), if external use or internal 120mg (MD) GSL
Poldine methylsulphate POM but if 2mg (MD) 6mg (MDD), P
Polidexide POM
Poliomyelitis vaccine (inactivated) POM
Poliomyelitis vaccine (oral) POM
Poliomyelitis vaccine, live (oral) BP POM
Pollenase preparations P
Pollenshield hayfever 7s GSL; 30 P
Pollinex POM
Pollon-eze tablets POM
Poloxamer POM
Polyestradiol phosphate POM
Polyethoxyethanol, external use only GSL
Polyfax ointment POM
Polyfax ophthalmic ointment POM
Polyfax preparations POM
Polygeline P
Polyhexedrine POM
Polymyxin B sulphate POM
Polynoxylin P
Polyoestradiol phosphate POM
Polytar preparations GSL
Polytar AF GSL
Polytar Plus GSL
Polythiazide POM
Polytrim preparations POM
Polyvidone P
Pondocillin preparations POM
Ponstan forte POM
Ponstan preparations POM
Poplar (Aspen) GSL
Poppy capsule POM
Poractant alfa POM
Poregon injection POM
Porfimer sodium POM
Pork insulin POM
Posalfilin ointment P
Posiject POM
PostMI preparations P
Potaba preparations P
Potassium acid tartrate GSL
Potassium aminobenzoate P
Potassium arsenite POM but if 0.0127 per cent, P
Potassium benzoate P
Potassium bicarbonate GSL
Potassium bromide POM
Potassium canrenoate POM
Potassium carbonate GSL
Potassium chloride and sodium chloride injection POM
Potassium chloride, if external use, or internal use for the treatment of

acute diarrhoea, maximum strength 0.15 per cent
Potassium citrate GSL
Potassium citrate mixture BP GSL
Potassium clavulanate POM
Potassium clorazepate see Dipotassium clorazepate
Potassium edetate, external use only GSL
Potassium gluconate GSL
Potassium glycerophosphate GSL
Potassium hydroxide, external use only GSL
Potassium hydroxyquinoline sulphate, if maximum strength 0.6 per cent (external use only) GSL
Potassium iodide, if MDD equivalent to 10mg iodine GSL
Potassium molybdate, if MDD equivalent to 200mcg elemental molybdenum GSL
Potassium nitrate, up to 100mg (MD) GSL
Potassium perchlorate POM
Potassium phosphate POM
Potassium sulphate GSL
Potassium thiocyanate, external use only GSL
Potters day and night P
Potters decongestant GSL
Potters Gees linctus CD Inv P
Potter's Herbal supplies all GSL except cleansing herbs, cough remover, malt extracts, skin lotion and ointment and tabritis rubbing oils
Potters pholcodine CD Inv P
Povidone P
Povidone-iodine, all preparations for external use, except those for vaginal use or for use in surgical operations GSL
Powergel POM
PR spray GSL
Practolol POM
Pradaxa capsules POM
Pragmatar ointment P
Pralenal tablets POM
Pralidoxime chloride POM
Pralidoxime iodide POM
Pralidoxime mesylate POM
Pramipexole hydrochloride POM
Prandin POM
Prasterone CD Anab POM
Pravastatin sodium POM
Praxilene preparations POM
Prazepam CD Benz POM
Prazosin hydrochloride POM
Preconceive tablets GSL
Precortisyl tablets POM
Pred Forte eye drops POM
Predenema POM
Predfoam POM
Prednesol tablets POM
Prednisolone POM
Prednisolone 21-steaglate POM
Prednisolone acetate POM
Prednisolone butylacetate POM
Prednisolone hexanoate POM
Prednisolone metasulphobenzoate POM
Prednisolone metasulphobenzoate sodium POM
Prednisolone pivalate POM
Prednisolone sodium phosphate POM
Prednisolone steaglate POM
Prednisone POM
Prednisone acetate POM
Predsol eye/ear drops POM
Predsol preparations POM
Predsol-N eye/ear drops POM
Pregabalin POM
Pregaday tablets P
Pregnyl injections CD Anab POM
Prelude GSL
Premarin preparations POM
Premique Cycle tablets POM
Premique Low Dose tablets POM
Premique tablets POM
Premjact P

Prempak POM
Prempak-C tablets POM
Prenalterol hydrochloride POM
Prenylamine lactate POM
Preotact POM
Prepadine tablets POM
Preparation H preparations GSL
Prepidil gel POM
Prepulsid Quicklet tablets POM
Prepulsid suspension POM
Prepulsid tablets POM
Prescal tablets POM
Preservex tablets POM
Presinex nasal spray POM
Pressimmune injection POM
Prestim tablets POM
Prevenar vaccine POM
Prexige tablets POM
Prezista POM
Priadel preparations POM
Prialt POM
Prickly Ash Bark (Zanthoxylum clava-herculis) GSL
Prilocaine hydrochloride POM but if non-ophthalmic use, P
Primacor injection POM
Primalan tablets POM
Primaquine phosphate tablets (ICI) P
Primaxin infusion POM
Primaxin Monovial POM
Primene POM
Primidone POM
Primolut N tablets POM
Primoteston Depot CD Anab POM
Primperan preparations POM
Primula Rhizome Extract GSL
Prioderm cream shampoo P
Prioderm lotion P
Priorix MMR vaccine POM
Pripsen preparations P
Pro-Banthine preparations POM
Pro-Epanutin POM
Pro-Epanutin concentrate for injection POM
ProPlus GSL
Pro-Viron tablets CD Anab POM
Probenecid POM
Probeta-LA capsules POM
Probucol POM
Procainamide hydrochloride POM
Procaine benzylpenicillin/Procaine penicillin POM
Procaine hydrochloride POM but if non-ophthalmic use, P
Procaine penicillin see Procaine benzylpenicillin
Procarbazine hydrochloride POM
Prochlorperazine POM
Prochlorperazine edisylate POM
Prochlorperazine maleate POM but buccal tablets for the treatment of nausea and vomiting in cases of previously diagnosed migraine only. For use in persons aged 18 years and over, with MDD 12mg, in a container or package containing not more than 8 tablets P
Prochlorperazine mesylate POM
Procorolan tablets POM
Proctocream HC P
Proctofoam HC aerosol POM
Proctosedyl preparations POM
Procyclidine hydrochloride POM
Profasi injection CD Anab POM
Proflavine hemisulphate, external use only GSL
Proflex cream 100g P
Proflex cream 30g GSL
Progesterone POM
Prograf capsules POM
Proguanil P
Progynova preparations POM
Proheptazine; its salts CD POM
Prolactin POM
Proladone preparations CD POM
Proleukin infusion POM
Proligestone POM
Prolintane hydrochloride POM

Proluton Depot injection POM
Promazine embonate POM
Promazine hydrochloride POM
Prominal tablets CD No Register POM
Promixin powder for nebuliser solution POM
Pronestyl preparations POM
Prontosan GSL
Propaderm preparations POM
Propafenone POM
Propafenone hydrochloride POM
Propain Caplets pack sizes 16s, 32s CD Inv P
Propain Plus CD Inv P
Propamidine P
Propanidid POM
Propanix SR capsules POM
Propantheline bromide POM but if 15mg (MD) 45mg (MDD), P
Propecia tablets POM
Properidine; its salts CD POM
Propess pessaries POM
Propetandrol CD Anab POM
Propicillin potassium POM
Propine eye drops POM
Propiram; its salts CD POM but if in preparations containing, per dosage unit, not more than 100mg of propiram (calculated as base) and compounded with at least the same amount of methylcellulose CD Inv POM
Propiverine hydrochloride POM
Propofol POM
Propranolol hydrochloride POM
Propress RS POM
Propylene glycol, external use only GSL
Propylene phenoxetol, external use only GSL
Propylthiouracil POM
Proquazone POM
Prosaid POM
Proscar tablets POM
Prosparol emulsion P
Prostaglandin F2 alpha tromethamine POM
Prostap 3 depot injection POM
Prostap SR injection POM
Prostin preparations POM
Prosulf ampoules POM
Protamine sulphate POM
Protease POM
Protelos granules POM
Prothiaden preparations POM
Prothionamide see Protionamide
Protionamide/Prothionamide POM
Protirelin POM
Protium IV vials POM
Protium tablets POM
Protopic ointment POM
Protriptyline hydrochloride POM
Provera tablets POM
Provigil tablets POM
Proxymetacaine hydrochloride POM but if non-ophthalmic use, P
Prozac preparations POM
Proziere tablets POM
Prozit POM

Pseudoephedrine hydrochloride POM but if internal (a) In the case of a prolonged release preparation 120mg (MD) 240mg (MDD) (b) in any other case 60mg (MD) 240mg (MDD), P
Pseudoephedrine sulphate POM but if 60mg (MD) 180mg (MDD), P
Psilocin; its salts; its esters and ethers; their salts CD Lic
Psoriderm preparations P
Psorigel P
Psorin preparations P
Psyllium GSL
Pulmicort preparations POM
Pulmo Bailly CD Inv P
Pulmozyme POM
Pulsatilla GSL
Pulvinal beclometasone dipropionate dry powder inhaler POM

Pulvinal salbutamol dry powder inhaler POM
Pumilio Pine Oil GSL
Pump-Hep injection POM
Pure Health aspirin dispersible tablets P
Pure Health saline nasal drops GSL
Puregon POM
Puri-Nethol tablets POM
Pylobactell POM
Pylorid tablets POM
Pyralvex solution P
Pyrantel embonate POM but if (a) For the treatment of enterobiosis, in adults and children not less than 12 years 750mg MDD (as a single dose) and container or package contains not more than 750mg of pyrantel embonate; (b) For the treatment of enterobiosis, in children less than 12 years but not less than 6 years 500mg MDD (as a single dose) and container or package contains not more than 750mg of pyrantel embonate; (c) For the treatment of enterobiosis in children less than 6 years but not less than 2 years 250mg MDD (as a single dose) and container or package contains not more than 750mg of pyrantel embonate, P
Pyrantel tartrate POM
Pyrazinamide POM
Pyrethrum (Chrysanthemum), external use only GSL
Pyridostigmine bromide POM
Pyridoxine hydrochloride GSL
Pyrimethamine POM
Pyrithione zinc, external use only GSL
Pyrogastrone preparations POM
Pyrovalerone; its salts; its stereoisomers; their salts CD Benz POM
Pyroxylin P

Q

Qlaira film-coated tablets POM
Quassia GSL
Queen's Delight, up to 320mg (MD) GSL
Quellada M preparations P
Questran POM
Questran Light POM
Quetiapine fumarate POM
Quiet Life GSL
Quinaband P
Quinagolide POM
Quinalbarbitone see Secobarbital
Quinapril POM
Quinapril hydrochloride POM
Quinbolone CD Anab POM
Quinestradol POM
Quinestrol POM
Quinethazone POM
Quingestanol POM
Quinicardine tablets POM
Quinidine POM
Quinidine bisulphate POM
Quinidine polygalacturonate POM
Quinidine sulphate POM
Quinil POM
Quinine POM but if 100mg (MD) 300mg (MDD), P; quinine base 35mg (MD), GSL
Quinine and urea hydrochloride POM
Quinine bisulphate POM but if equivalent of 100mg of quinine (MD) equivalent of 300mg of quinine (MDD), P
Quinine cinchophen POM but if equivalent of 100mg of quinine (MD) equivalent of 300mg of quinine (MDD), P
Quinine dihydrochloride POM but if equivalent of 100mg of quinine (MD) equivalent of 300mg of quinine (MDD), P

Quinine ethyl carbonate POM but if equivalent of 100mg of quinine (MD) equivalent of 300mg of quinine (MDD) P
Quinine glycerophosphate POM but if equivalent of 100mg of quinine (MD) equivalent of 300mg of quinine (MDD), P
Quinine hydrobromide POM but if equivalent of 100mg of quinine (MD) equivalent of 300mg of quinine (MDD), P
Quinine hydrochloride POM but if equivalent of 100mg of quinine (MD) equivalent of 300mg of quinine (MDD), P
Quinine in combination with urea hydrochloride POM
Quinine iodobismuthate POM but if equivalent of 100mg of quinine (MD) equivalent of 300mg of quinine (MDD), P
Quinine phosphate POM but if equivalent of 100mg of quinine (MD) equivalent of 300mg of quinine (MDD), P
Quinine salicylate POM but if equivalent of 100mg of quinine (MD) equivalent of 300mg of quinine (MDD), P
Quinine sulphate POM but if equivalent of 100mg of quinine (MD) equivalent of 300mg of quinine (MDD), P; equivalent to 35 mg quinine (MD), GSL
Quinine tannate POM but if equivalent of 100mg of quinine (MD) equivalent of 300mg of quinine (MDD), P
Quinocort cream POM
Quinoderm cream P
Quinoderm Lotio-Gel P
Quinoped cream P
Quinupristin POM
Qvar POM

R

Rabeprazole POM
Rabies vaccine POM
Rabipur POM
Racemethorphan; its salts CD POM
Racemoramide; its salts CD POM
Racemorphan; its salts; its esters and ethers; their salts CD POM
Radian-B preparations GSL
Ralgex preparations GSL
Raloxifine hydrochloride POM
Raltitrexed POM
Ramipril POM
Ramysis POM
Ranace POM
Ranclav POM
Ranexa prolonged release tablets POM
Ranflutin POM
Ranitic POM
Ranitidine 75mg tablets, for short term symptomatic relief of heartburn, dyspepsia, acid indigestion and hyperacidity, mdd 150mg GSL
Ranitidine hydrochloride POM but if for the short term symptomatic relief of heartburn, dyspepsia, indigestion, acid indigestion and hyperacidity or the prevention of these symptoms when associated with consuming food and drink, equivalent to 75mg of ranitidine (MD) equivalent to 300mg of ranitidine (MDD) for a maximum period of 14 days, P
Ranitil POM
Rantec POM
Ranvera MR POM
Ranzac 7s GSL
Ranzolont POM
Rap-eze tablets GSL
Rapamune oral solution POM

Rapamune tablets POM
Rapifen injection CD POM
Rapifen Intensive Care injection CD POM
Rapilysin POM
Rapitil eye drops POM
Rapolyte GSL
Rappell pump spray GSL
Rapranol SR POM
Raptiva POM
Rapydan medicated plasters POM
Rasagiline POM
Rasburicase POM
Rasilex POM
Raspberry GSL
Rastinon preparations POM
Ratiograstim POM
Raudixin tablets POM
Rautrax tablets POM
Rauwiloid + Veriloid tablets POM
Rauwiloid tablets POM
Rauwolfia Serpentina POM
Rauwolfia Vomitoria POM
Raxar tablets POM
Razoxane POM
RBC cream GSL
Rebetol capsules POM
Rebetol 40mg/ml oral solution POM
Rebif injection POM
Reboxetine mesilate POM
Recombinate POM
Rectogesic rectal ointment POM
Rectubes CD Benz POM
Redoxon tablets GSL
Reductil capsules POM
Refacto injection POM
Refludan vials POM
Refolinon POM
Refolion preparations POM
Refresh P
Regaine Extra Strength P
Regaine gel for men GSL
Regaine hair supplements for women GSL
Regaine Regular Strength topical solution GSL
Regaine Regular Strength for Women GSL
Regranex gel POM
Regulan sachets GSL
Regulose P
Regurin tablets POM
Rehidrat sachets P
Relaxit P
Relaxyl capsules P
Relcofen tablets P
Relefact LH-RH ampoules POM
Relenza inhalation powder POM
Relestat eye-drops POM
Relifex preparations POM
Relistor POM
Relpax tablets POM
Remedeine preparations CD Inv POM
Remegel chewy squares GSL
Remegel tablets GSL
Remegel Wind Relief tablets GSL
Remicade infusion POM
Remifentanil CD POM
Reminyl preparations POM
Remnos tablets CD Benz POM
Remoxipride hydrochloride POM
Renagel preparations POM
Rennie Deflatine GSL
Rennie Duo preparations PO
Rennie Fruit GSL
Rennie preparations GSL
Rennie soft chews GSL
ReoPro POM
Repaglinide POM
Repevax vaccine POM
Replenate POM
Replenine POM
Replens GSL
Reproterol hydrochloride POM
Requip tablets POM
Rescinnamine POM
Rescue flow infusion POM
Reserpine POM

Resolve Extra sachets GSL
Resolve granules GSL
Resonium A P
Respacal syrup POM
Repaglinide POM
Respontin nebules POM
Resorcinol P
Resprin POM
Restandol capsules CD Anab POM
Retcin tablets POM
Reteplase POM
Retin-A preparations POM
Retinova cream POM
Retrovir preparations POM
Revanil tablets POM
Revasc injection POM
Revatio tablets POM
Revaxis vaccine POM
Reviparin POM
Rexocaine POM
Reyataz capsules POM
Rheomacrodex preparations POM
Rheumacin LA capsules POM
Rheumatac Retard POM
Rheumox preparations POM
Rhinacort Aqua POM
Rhinolast Allergy P
Rhinolast Hayfever P
Rhinolast nasal spray POM
Rhophylac 300 POM
Rhubarb rhizome GSL
Rhumalgan tablets POM
Rhumalgan SR capsules POM
Rhumalgan XL capsules POM
Riamet tablets POM
Ribavirin/Tribavirin POM
Riboflavin/Riboflavine GSL
Riboflavin/Riboflavine sodium phosphate GSL
Riboflavine see Riboflavin
Ricola herb cough lozenges GSL
Ridaura tablets POM
Rideril POM
Rifabutin POM
Rifadin preparations POM
Rifamide POM
Rifampicin POM
Rifampicin sodium POM
Rifamycin POM
Rifater tablets POM
Rifinah tablets POM
Rilutek tablets POM
Riluzole POM
Rimacillin POM
Rimactane preparations POM
Rimactazid tablets POM
Rimafen POM
Rimapam tablets POM
Rimapurinol tablets POM
Rimexolone POM
Rimiterol hydrobromide POM
Rimonabant POM
Rimoxacillin preparations POM
Rimso-50 POM
Rinatec inhaler POM
Rinatec nasal spray POM
Ringer's injection POM
Rinstead gel P
Rinstead pastilles GSL
Risedronate sodium POM
Risperdal preparations POM
Risperidone POM
Ritalin CD POM
Ritodrine hydrochloride POM
Ritonavir POM
Rituximab POM
Rivastigmine POM
Rivotril preparations CD Benz POM
Rizatriptan POM
Roaccutane capsules POM
Robaxin 750 tablets POM
Robaxin Injectable POM
Robinul injection POM
Robinul-Neostigmine injection POM
Robitussin Chesty Cough 100ml PO
Robitussin Chesty Cough with Congestion P
Robitussin Dry Cough P

Robitussin dry cough pastilles P
Robitussin Junior P
Robitussin Night-Time P
Rocaltrol capsules POM
Rocephin vials POM
Rocuronium POM
Roferon prefilled syringes POM
Roferon-A POM
Rogitine ampoules POM
Rohypnol tablets CD No Register POM
Rolicyclidine CD Lic
Rolitetracycline nitrate POM
Rommix preparations POM
Rondomycin preparations POM
Ronicol tablets P
Ronicol Timespan tablets P
Ropinirole hydrochloride POM
Ropivacaine POM
Rose Fruit GSL
Rosemary GSL
Rosemary Oil GSL
Rosiglitazone POM
Rosuvastatin POM
Rotarix POM
Rotigotine POM
Rovamycin preparations POM
Rowachol POM
Rowatinex POM
Roxibolone CD Anab POM
Rozex gel POM
Rubella vaccine (live attenuated) POM
Rubella, mumps, measles vaccine POM
Rubellin GSL
Rue, if maximum strength 0.1 per cent
    (external use only) GSL
Rusyde POM
Rynacrom preparations P
Rythmodan preparations POM

S

Sabadilla POM
Sabril tablets POM
Sage GSL
Sage Oil GSL
Saizen injection CD Anab POM
Salactol P
Salagen tablets POM
Salamol CFC-Free inhaler POM
Salamol Easi-Breathe POM
Salapin syrup POM
Salatac gel P
Salazopyrin preparations POM
Salazosulphadimidine POM
Salbutamol POM
Salbutamol sulphate POM
Salcatonin see Calcitonin (Salmon)
Salicylic acid if (1) internal: maximum
    strength 0.06 per cent antiseptic liq-
    uid, pastilles, lozenges, throat tablets
    GSL (2) external: corn plasters GSL
    (3) external: all other preparations
    for treatment of corns and calluses
    maximum strength 12.5 per cent
    GSL (4) external: dusting powder
    maximum strength 3.0 per cent GSL
    (5) external: cream, ointment or gel
    maximum strength 2.0 per cent GSL
    (6) external: medicated pads maxi-
    mum strength 0.5 per cent in the
    impregnating solution GSL (7) exter-
    nal: antiseptic liquid maximum
    strength 0.06 per cent GSL (8) exter-
    nal liquids neither for the treatment
    of corns or callouses, nor antiseptic
    liquids maximum strength 0.05 per
    cent GSL (9) external: soap maxi-
    mum strength 3.0 per cent GSL (10)
    external: wart plasters GSL
Salmefamol POM
Salmeterol xinafoate POM
Salofalk preparations POM
Salonpas medicated plaster GSL
Salsalate POM
Saluric tablets POM

Salzone P
Sambucus GSL
Sanderson's throat specific GSL
Sandimmun preparations POM
Sando-K effervescent tablets P
Sandocal effervescent tablets P
Sandoglobulin POM
Sandostatin POM
Sandostatin LAR POM
Sandrena gel POM
Sanomigran preparations POM
Saquinavir POM
Saralasin acetate POM
Sarsaparilla GSL
Savene POM
Saventrine tablets POM
Savlon antiseptic cream GSL
Savlon antiseptic wipes GSL
Savlon bites & stings gel GSL
Savlon blister plasters GSL
Savlon concentrated liquid GSL
Savlon disinfectant liquid GSL
Savlon Dry GSL
Savlon First Aid kit GSL
Savlon Liquid antiseptic GSL
Savlon Nappy Rash cream GSL
Savlon wound wash GSL
Saw Palmetto GSL
Scandonest POM
Schering PC4 tablets POM
Scheriproct preparations POM
Schick control POM
Schick test toxin POM
Scholl's athletes foot range GSL
Scholl's callous removal pads GSL
Scholl's corn & callous removal liquid -
    GSL
Scholl's corn and callous salve P
Scholl's corn removal pads GSL
Scholl's corn removal plasters GSL
Scholl's polymer gel corn removers GSL
Scholl's verruca removal gel seal & heal
    GSL
Scholl's verruca removal system - GSL
Scoline injection POM
Scopoderm TTS POM
Scopoderm1.5mg Patch P
Scullcap GSL
Sea-legs tablets P
Seatone 500mg capsules GSL
Sebco GSL
Sebomin capsules POM
Sebren MR POM
Secadrex tablets POM
Secbutobarbitone CD No Register POM
Secbutobarbitone sodium CD No
    Register POM
Secobarbital/Quinalbarbitone CD POM
Secobarbital/Quinalbarbitone sodium
    CD POM
Seconal sodium capsules CD POM
Secron suspension P
Sectral preparations POM
Securon preparations POM
Securopen injection POM
Sedonium tablets P
Select-A-Jet Dopamine POM
Selegiline hydrochloride POM
Selenase POM
Selenium sulphide P
Selexid POM
Selsun P
Semi-Daonil tablets POM
Semisodium valproate POM
Semprex capsules POM
Senega GSL
Senna fruit GSL
Senna leaf GSL
Sennosides A and B, up to 15mg (MD)
    GSL
Senokot direct relief suppositories GSL
Senokot dual relief tablets GSL
Senokot granules PO
Senokot hi-fibre GSL
Senokot max strength tablets GSL
Senokot syrup 150ml GSL
Senokot tablets pack sizes 20s, 40s GSL;
    60s, 100s PO

Sensodyne total care toothpaste gel
    75ml GSL
Sential cream POM
Sential E cream P
Seominal tablets CD No Register POM
Septex cream No.1 P
Septex cream No.2 POM
Septopal Chains POM
Septrin preparations POM
Sera and antisera: Botulin antitoxin
    POM Diphtheria antitoxin POM;
    Gas-gangrene antitoxin (oedema-
    tiens) POM; Gas-gangrene antitoxin
    (perfringens) POM; Gas-gangrene
    antitoxin (septicum) POM; Mixed
    gas-gangrene antitoxin POM;
    Leptospira antiserum POM; Rabies
    antiserum POM; Scorpion venom
    antiserum POM; Snake venom anti-
    serum POM; Tetanus antitoxin POM
Seractil tablets POM
Serc POM
Serdolect tablets POM
Serenace preparations POM
Seretide Accuhaler POM
Seretide Evohaler POM
Serevent preparations POM
Sermorelin POM
Serophene tablets POM
Seroquel tablets POM
Serotulle dressing P
Seroxat preparations POM
Sertindole POM
Sertraline POM
Serum gonadotrophin POM
Setlers hearburn and indigestion liquid
    GSL
Setlers tablets GSL
Setlers Tums GSL
Sevelamer POM
Seven Seas cod liver oil GSL
Seven Seas cod liver oil & orange syrup
    GSL
Seven Seas cod liver oil capsules GSL
Seven Seas One a Day Pure cod liver oil
    capsules GSL
Seven Seas vitamin & mineral tonic GSL
Sevoflurane POM
Sevredol concentrated oral solution CD
    POM
Sevredol oral solution CD Inv POM
Sevredol tablets CD POM
Shark liver oil, if maximum strength
    3.0g for suppositories, or all prepara-
    tions for external use except supposi-
    tories (external use only) GSL
Shepherd's Purse GSL
Siberian fir oil, external use only GSL
Sibutramine POM
Silandrone CD Anab POM
Sildenafil POM
Silkis POM
Silver sulfadiazine/sulphadiazine POM
Simeco tablets P
Simple eye ointment P
Simple linctus BP GSL
Simple linctus paed BP GSL
Simplene eye drops POM
Simpson's foot ointment GSL
Simulect infusion POM
Simvador POM
Simvastatin POM, but where maximum
    strength 10mg, maximum daily dose
    10mg and maximum pack size 28
    tablets, P, please refer to proprietary
    names for the classification granted
    under the marketing authorisation
    (see Zocor Heart-Pro preparations)
Simzal POM
Sinemet preparations POM
Sinepin POM
Sinequan capsules POM
Singulair Paediatric granules POM
Singulair Paediatric tablets POM
Singulair tablets POM
Sinthrome tablets POM
Sinutab tablets P
Siopel cream GSL

Sirolimus POM
Sissomicin POM
Sissomicin sulphate POM
Sitaxentan POM
Skelid tablets POM
Skin traction kit GSL
Skinoren cream POM
Skintex GSL
Skunk Cabbage (Symplocarpus) GSL
Slippery Elm powdered bark GSL
Slippery Elm tabs GSL
Slocinx XL POM
Slo-Indo POM
Slo-phyllin capsules P
Slofedipine XL tablets POM
Slofenac POM
Sloprolol capsules POM
Slow Sodium tablets GSL
Slow-Fe Folic tablets POM
Slow-Fe tablets P
Slow-K tablets P
Slow-Trasicor tablets POM
Slozem capsules POM
Smallpox vaccine POM
Snake Venoms POM
Sno Phenicol eye drops POM
Sno Tears P
Sno-Pilo preparations POM
Snowfire Healing tablet GSL
Snufflebabe vapour rub GSL
Snug GSL
Sodiofolin POM
Sodium acetrizoate POM
Sodium acid phosphate GSL
Sodium acid pyrophosphate, external
    use only GSL
Sodium alginate GSL
Sodium alkylsulphoacetate P
Sodium amidiatrizoate preparations
    POM except powder P
Sodium aminosalicylate POM
Sodium amytal preparations CD No
    Register POM
Sodium antimonylgluconate POM
Sodium arsanilate POM
Sodium arsenate POM
Sodium arsenite POM but if 0.013 per
    cent, P
Sodium ascorbate GSL
Sodium aurothiomalate POM
Sodium bicarbonate GSL
Sodium bromide POM
Sodium calcium edetate POM
Sodium carbonate GSL
Sodium chloride GSL
Sodium chloride and dextrose injection
    POM
Sodium chloride BP tablets GSL
Sodium chloride injection POM
Sodium citrate GSL
Sodium citrate oral solution 0.3M
    (Viridian Pharma) POM
Sodium clodronate POM
Sodium cromoglicate/Sodium cromogly-
    cate POM but if (a) for nasal admin-
    istration; (b) for the treatment of
    acute seasonal allergic conjunctivitis
    or perennial allergic conjunctivitis in
    the form of aqueous eye drops maxi-
    mum strength 2.0 per cent and con-
    tainer or package contains not more
    than 10ml of medicinal product; (c)
    for the treatment of acute seasonal
    allergic conjunctivitis in the form of
    an eye ointment maximum strength
    4.0 per cent and container or pack-
    age contains not more than 5g of
    medicinal product, P; or (d) for the
    relief and treatment of eye symptoms
    of hayfever, in the form of aqueous
    eye drops maximum strength 2.0 per
    cent and container or package con-
    tains not more than 10ml of medici-
    nal product, GSL
Sodium cromoglycate see Sodium cro-
    moglicate
Sodium ethacrynate POM
Sodium feredate P

Sodium fluoride POM but if tablets or drops for prevention of dental caries with mdd 2.2mg P; external use, if maximum strength 0.33 per cent dentifrice or 0.05 per cent daily use mouth rinses for prevention of dental caries, or 0.2 per cent mouth rinses for other than daily use for the prevention of dental caries, GSL

Sodium fusidate POM

Sodium glycerophosphate GSL

Sodium hydroxide, if maximum strength 12.0 per cent (external use only) GSL

Sodium iodide, if MDD equivalent to 10mg iodine GSL

Sodium lactate, external use only GSL

Sodium lauryl ether sulphate, external use only GSL

Sodium lauryl ether sulphosuccinate, external use only GSL

Sodium metrizoate POM

Sodium monofluorophosphate POM but if dentifrice maximum strength 1.14 per cent, GSL (external use only)

Sodium nitrite POM

Sodium oxidronate POM

Sodium para-aminohippurate vials (MSD) POM

Sodium phenylbutyrate POM

Sodium phosphate GSL

Sodium picosulfate/Sodium picosulphate, for adults and children aged 10 years and over maximum stren GSL

Sodium picosulphate see Sodium picosulfate

Sodium potassium tartrate GSL

Sodium pyrophosphate, external use only GSL

Sodium pyrrolidone carboxylate, external use only GSL

Sodium salicylate GSL

Sodium selenite, internal use GSL

Sodium stibocaptate/Stibocaptate POM

Sodium stibogluconate POM

Sodium sulphate GSL

Sodium tetradecyl sulphate POM

Sodium valproate POM

Sofradex preparations POM

Soframycin preparations POM

Soft soap, external use only GSL

Solaquin P

Solarcaine preparations P

Solareze gel POM

Solian tablets POM

Solifenacin POM

Solivito-N vials POM

Soloc tablets POM

Solpadeine Headache preparations GSL

Solpadeine Max CD Inv P

Solpadeine Migraine CD Inv P

Solpadeine Plus CD Inv P

Solpadol preparations CD Inv POM

Solpaflex tablets CD Inv P

Soltamox oral solution POM

Solu-Cortef injection POM

Solu-Medrone vials POM

Solvazinc tablets P

Somatorelin acetate POM

Somatotropin CD Anab POM

Somatrem CD Anab POM

Somatropin CD Anab POM

Somatuline Autogel POM

Somatuline LA POM

Somavert injection POM

Sominex Herbal GSL

Sominex tablets P

Somnite preparations CD Benz POM

Somnwell POM

Sonata capsules POM

Sondate 200EC POM

Soneryl tablets CD No Register POM

Soothake gel GSL

Soothelip cold sore cream P

Sorafenib POM

Soraway P

Sorbichew tablets P

Sorbid SA tablets P

Sorbitol GSL

Sorbitrate tablets P

Sotacor preparations POM

Sotalol hydrochloride POM

Sotol tablets GSL

Southern Wood, external use only GSL

Soya oil GSL

Spasmonal P

Spasmonal Forte capsules P

Spatone GSL

Spectinomycin POM

Spectinomycin hydrochloride POM

SpectraBAN lotion 25 GSL

Spinach GSL

Spiramycin POM

Spiramycin adipate POM

Spiretic tablets POM

Spiriva inhalation capsules POM

Spiro-Co tablets POM

Spiroctan preparations POM

Spiroctan-M injection POM

Spirolone tablets POM

Spironolactone POM

Spirospare tablets POM

Sporanox IV infusion POM

Sporanox preparations POM

Sprilon GSL

Sprycel POM

Squalane, external use only GSL

Squaw Vine GSL

Squill linctus, opiate BPC CD Inv P

Squill Vinegar GSL

Squill, Indian GSL

Squill, White GSL

St. James balm GSL

St Mary's Thistle GSL

Stafoxil capsules POM

Stalevo tablets POM

Stamaril vaccine POM

Stannous fluoride POM but if (a) dentifrice maximum strength 0.62 per cent; (b) dental gels for use in the prevention and treatment of dental caries and decalcification of the teeth maximum strength 0.4 per cent, P

Stanolone CD Anab POM

Stanozolol CD Anab POM

Stantar P

Starch GSL

Staril tablets POM

Starlix tablets POM

Starpax balsam GSL

Stavudine POM

STD injection POM

Stearyl alcohol, ethoxylated, external use only GSL

Stelara solution for injection POM

Stelazine preparations POM

Stemetil preparations POM

Stenbolone CD Anab POM

Ster-Zac preparations GSL

Sterculia GSL

Sterets P

Sterets H P

Steri-Neb Ipratropium POM

Steri-Neb Salamol POM

Stericlens GSL

Steriflex injections POM

Sterillium GSL

Steripaste P

Steripod chlorhexidine/cetrimide P

Steripod topical wound cleanser (sodium chloride 0.9%) P

Steripoules POM

Stesolid rectal tubes CD Benz POM

Stibocaptate see Sodium stibocaptate

Stibophen POM

Stiedex lotion POM

Stiedex LP 0.05% POM

Stiemycin POM

Stilboestrol see Diethylstilbestrol

Stilline POM

Stilnoct tablets CD Benz POM

Stimlor capsules POM

Stingose GSL

Stone root GSL

Stop 'N Grow GSL

Storax GSL

Strattera capsules POM

Strefen lozenges P

Strepsils preparations GSL

Streptase injection POM

Streptodornase POM but if external, P

Streptokinase POM but if external, P

Streptomycin POM

Streptomycin sulphate POM

Stressless GSL

Striant SR tablets CD Anab POM

Stromba preparations CD Anab POM

Stronazon MR capsules POM

Strontium acetate, if dentifrice (external use only) GSL

Strontium chloride hexahydrate, if dentifrice (external use only) GSL

Strontium ranelate POM

Strychnine POM

Strychnine arsenate POM

Strychnine hydrochloride POM

Strychnine nitrate POM

Stud 100 Desensitising spray for men P

Stugeron Forte capsules P

Stugeron tablets P

Stump GSL

Styramate POM

Subcuvia injection POM

Subgam POM

Sublimaze injection CD POM

Suboxone CD No Reg POM

Subutex tablets CD No Register POM

Succinylsulphathiazole POM

Sucralfate POM

Sucrose GSL

Sucrose Octa-acetate GSL

Sudafed Congestion cold & flu tablets P

Sudafed Congestion Relief capsules, non-drowsy GSL

Sudafed decongestant elixir P

Sudafed Dual Relief Max tablets, non-drowsy P

Sudafed Elixir P

Sudafed expectorant P

Sudafed linctus P

Sudafed nasal spray GSL

Sudafed non-drowsy 12-hour tablets P

Sudafed non-drowsy childrens syrup P

Sudafed non-drowsy dual relief capsules 16s GSL

Sudafed Plus preparations P

Sudafed tablets P

Sudafed-Co tablets pack sizes 12s P

Sudocrem preparations GSL

Sufentanil ; its salts; its esters and ethers; their salts CD POM

Sulazine EC tablets POM

Sulbactam Sodium POM

Sulbenicillin POM

Sulbenicillin sodium POM

Sulconazole nitrate POM but if external (except vaginal), P

Suleo-C lotion POM

Suleo-M lotion P

Sulfabenz POM

Sulfabenzamide POM

Sulfacetamide/Sulphacetamide POM

Sulfacetamide/Sulphacetamide sodium POM

Sulfacytine POM

Sulfadiazine/Sulphadiazine POM

Sulfadiazine/Sulphadiazine sodium POM

Sulfadicramide POM

Sulfadimidine/Sulphadimidine POM

Sulfadimidine/Sulphadimidine sodium POM

Sulfadoxine POM

Sulfamerazine POM

Sulfamerazine sodium POM

Sulfamethoxazole/Sulphamethoxazole POM

Sulfametopyrazine POM

Sulfamonomethoxine POM

Sulfapyrazole POM

Sulfapyridine/Sulphapyridine POM

Sulfapyridine/Sulphapyridine sodium POM

Sulfasalazine/Sulphasalazine POM

Sulfathiazole/Sulphathiazole POM

Sulfathiazole/Sulphathiazole sodium POM

Sulfinpyrazone/Sulphinpyrazone POM

Sulindac POM

Sulparex tablets POM

Sulphabromomethazine POM

Sulphacetamide see Sulfacetamide

Sulphachlorpyridazine POM

Sulphadiazine see Sulfadiazine

Sulphadimethoxine POM

Sulphadimidine see Sulfadimidine

Sulphafurazole POM

Sulphafurazole diethanolamine POM

Sulphaguanidine POM

Sulphaloxic acid POM

Sulphamethizole POM

Sulphamethoxazole see Sulfamethoxazole

Sulphamethoxydiazine POM

Sulphamethoxypyridazine POM

Sulphamethoxypyridazine sodium POM

Sulphamoxole POM

Sulphanilamide POM

Sulphaphenazole POM

Sulphapyridine see Sulfapyridine

Sulphasalazine see Sulfasalazine

Sulphathiazole see Sulfathiazole

Sulphatriad preparations POM

Sulphaurea POM

Sulphinpyrazone see Sulfinpyrazone

Sulphur POM

Sulpiride POM

Sulpitil tablets POM

Sulpor oral solution POM

Sultamicillin POM

Sultamicillin tosylate POM

Sulthiame POM

Sultrin cream POM

Sumatriptan POM; but if tablets for oral use, for the acute relief of migraine attacks, with or without aura, in patients who have a stable well established pattern of symptoms, for adults aged 18 to 65 years, for a maximum period of 1 day, max strength 50mg, max dose 50mg, max daily dose 100mg and with a max pack size of 2 tablets, P

Sumatriptan succinate POM

Sunerven tablets GSL

Sunflower oil GSL

Sunitinib POM

Supralip tablets POM

Suprane POM

Suprax paediatric suspension POM

Suprax suspension POM

Suprax tablets POM

Suprecur injection POM

Suprecur nasal spray POM

Suprefact injection and nasal spray POM

Suprofen POM

Sure-amp ampoules POM

Sure-Lax GSL

Surgam SA capsules POM

Surgam tablets POM

Surmontil preparations POM

Survanta POM

Suscard Buccal tablets P

Sustac tablets P

Sustamycin capsules POM

Sustanon ampoules CD Anab POM

Sustiva preparations POM

Sutent POM

Sutoprofen POM

Suxamethonium bromide POM

Suxamethonium chloride POM

Suxethonium bromide POM

Swarm GSL

Sweet Birch oil GSL

Symbicort Turbohaler POM

Symmetrel preparations POM

Synacthen ampoules POM

Synacthen Depot POM

Synagis injection POM

Synalar C preparations POM

Synalar N preparations POM

Synalar preparations POM
Synandone preparations POM
Synarel nasal spray POM
Synastone injection CD POM
Syndol tablets CD Inv P
Synercid infusion POM
Syner-Kinase POM
Synflex capsules POM
Synphase tablets POM
Syntaris nasal spray POM
Syntex Menophase POM
Synthamin 7S injection POM
Synthamin injections POM
Synthamix POM
Syntocinon preparations POM
Syntometrine ampoules POM
Syntopressin nasal spray POM
Synuretic tablets POM
Syprol oral solution POM
Syscor MR tablets POM
Sytron elixir P

T

T-Zone clear pore body spray GSL
T-Zone clear & restore night gel patches GSL
T-Zone daily skin balancing moisturiser GSL
T/Gel shampoo GSL
Tabphyn MR POM
Tacalcitol monohydrate POM
TachoSil medicated sponge P
Tacrine hydrochloride POM
Tacrolimus POM
Tadalafil POM
Tagamet 100 P
Tagamet Dual Action liquid P
Tagamet preparations POM
Talampicillin POM
Talampicillin hydrochloride POM
Talampicillin napsylate POM
Talc, external use only GSL
Tambocor preparations POM
Tamiflu capsules POM
Tamiflu powder for oral suspension POM
Tamofen tablets POM
Tamoxifen POM
Tamoxifen citrate POM
Tampovagan N pessaries POM
Tampovagan pessaries POM
Tamsulosin POM
Tamsulosin hydrochloride POM
Tanatril tablets POM
Tannic acid, if internal (pastilles, lozenges, throat tablets maximum strength 5mg) or external GSL
Tar, external use only GSL
Tarceva tablets POM
Tarcortin cream POM
Targinact prolonged release tablets CD POM
Targocid injection POM
Targretin capsules POM
Tarivid preparations POM
Tarka capsules POM
Tarodent GSL
Tartaric acid GSL
Tasigna capsules POM
Tasmar tablets POM
Taumasthman tablets POM
Tavanic IV POM
Tavanic tablets POM
Tavegil elixir P
Tavegil tablets P
Taxol concentrate for solution for infusion POM
Taxotere POM
Taxotere for infusion POM
Tazarotene POM
Tazobactam sodium POM
Tazocin POM
TCP antiseptic cream GSL
TCP cool menthol lozenge GSL
TCP First Aid cream GSL
TCP Liquid Antiseptic GSL
TCP ointment GSL

TCP Sore Throat lozenges GSL
Tea tree & witch hazel cream GSL
Tears Naturale P
Teclothiazide potassium POM
Tegretol preparations POM
Tegretol Retard POM
Teicoplanin POM
Telfast preparations POM
Telithromycin POM
Telmisartan POM
Telzir preparations POM
Temazepam CD No Register POM
Temazepam Gelthix CD No Register POM
Temcapril hydrochloride POM
Temgesic injection CD No Register POM
Temgesic sublingual tablets CD No Register POM
Temocillin sodium POM
Temodal POM
Temoporfin POM
Temozolomide POM
Tenben capsules POM
Tenecteplase POM
Tenif capsules POM
Tenkicin tablets POM
Tenkorex POM
Tenocyclidine CD Lic
Tenofovir POM
Tenoret 50 tablets POM
Tenoretic tablets POM
Tenormin preparations POM
Tenoxicam POM
Tensipine MR tablets POM
Tensium tablets CD Benz POM
Tensopril tablets POM
Teoptic eye drops POM
Terazosin hydrochloride POM
Terbinafine POM but if for external use for the treatment of tinea pedis, tinea cruris and tinea corporis in the form of a gel with maximum strength 1.0%, and in a container or package containing not more than 30g of medicinal product P
Terbinafine hydrochloride POM but (a) preparations, other than spray solutions, for external use of the treatment of tinea pedis and tinea cruris, maximum strength 1.0%, and in a container or package containing not more than 15g of medicinal product, P, but please refer to proprietary names for classification granted under the marketing authorisation (see Lamisil products) ; (b) spray solutions for external use for the treatment of tinea corporis, tinea cruris and tinea pedis, maximum strength 1%, in a container containing not more than 30ml of medicinal product, P, but please refer to proprietary names for classification granted under the marketing authorisation (see Lamisil products); (c) creams, for external use for the treatment of tinea pedis and tinea cruris, maximum strength 1%, in a container containing not more than 15g of medicinal product, GSL, but please refer to proprietary names for classification granted under the marketing authorisation (see Lamisil products) ; (d) sprays for external use for the treatment of tinea pedis and tinea cruris, maximum strength 1%, in a container containing not more than 30ml of medicinal product, GSL, but please refer to proprietary names for classification granted under the marketing authorisation (see Lamisil products).
Terbutaline POM
Terbutaline sulphate POM
Tercolix CD Inv POM
Terebene (Terepene), external use only GSL
Terfenadine POM

Terfinax tablets POM
Teril CR tablets POM
Teriparatide POM
Terlipressin POM
Terodiline hydrochloride POM
Terpineol GSL
Terpoin CD Inv POM
Terra-Cortil Nystatin cream POM
Terra-Cortil preparations POM
Terramycin preparations POM
Tertroxin tablets POM
Testim gel CD Anab POM
Testoderm patches CD Anab POM
Testogel gel CD Anab POM
Testosterone CD Anab POM
Tetabulin POM
Tetanus and pertussis vaccine POM
Tetanus vaccine POM
Tetrabenazine POM
Tetracaine/Amethocaine POM but if non-ophthalmic use P
Tetracaine/Amethocaine gentisate POM but if non-ophthalmic use P
Tetracaine/Amethocaine hydrochloride POM but if non-ophthalmic use P
Tetrachel preparations POM
Tetracosactide/Tetracosactrin POM
Tetracosactide/Tetracosactrin acetate POM
Tetracosactrin see Tetracosactide
Tetracycline POM
Tetracycline hydrochloride POM
Tetracycline phosphate complex POM
Tetrahydrocannabinol see Cannabinol derivatives
Tetralysal preparations POM
Tetrazepam CD Benz POM
Tetroxoprim POM
Teveten tablets POM
Thallium acetate POM
Thallous chloride POM
THC see Cannabinol derivatives
Thebacon; its salts CD POM
Thebaine; its salts CD POM
Thelin POM
Theo-dur tablets P
Thephorin tablets P
Thiabendazole see Tiabendazole
Thiambutosine POM
Thiamine hydrochloride GSL
Thiamine mononitrate GSL
Thiazamide tablets POM
Thiethylperazine malate POM
Thiethylperazine maleate POM
Thiocarlide POM
Thioguanine see Tioguanine
Thiomesterone CD Anab POM
Thiopental/Thiopentone sodium POM
Thiopentone see Thiopental
Thiopropazate hydrochloride POM
Thioproperazine mesylate POM
Thioridazine POM
Thioridazine hydrochloride POM
Thiosinamine POM
Thiosinamine and ethyl iodide POM
Thiostrepton POM
Thiotepa POM
Thiothixene POM
Thiouracil POM
Throaties antibacterial pastilles GSL
Thurfyl salicylate, external use only GSL
Thyme GSL
Thyme Oil GSL
Thymol GSL
Thymoxamine see Moxisylyte
Thyrogen POM
Thyroid POM
Thyrotrophin POM
Thyrotrophin releasing hormone POM
Thyroxine sodium see Levothyroxine sodium
Tiabendazole/Thiabendazole POM
Tiagabine POM
Tiamulin fumarate POM
Tiaprofenic acid POM
Tibolone POM
Ticarcillin sodium POM
Ticlid tablets POM

Ticlopidine hydrochloride POM
Tiger Balm GSL
Tigloidine hydrobromide POM
Tilade aerosol POM
Tilarin nasal spray POM
Tildiem LA tablets POM
Tildiem Retard POM
Tildiem tablets POM
Tilia (Lime Flowers) GSL
Tilidate its salts; its esters and ethers; their salts CD POM
Tilofyl CD POM
Tiloket POM
Tilolec POM
Tiloryth capsules POM
Tiludronate disodium POM
Tiludronic acid POM
Timecef injection POM
Timentin injection POM
Timodine cream POM
Timolol maleate POM
Timonil Retard tablets POM
Timoptol POM
Timoptol LA ophthalmic solutions POM
Timpron tablets POM
Tinaderm cream GSL
Tinaderm Plus powder GSL
Tinaderm-M cream POM
Tinazaparin POM
Tinidazole POM
Tinzaparin POM
Tioconazole POM but if external (except vaginal) maximum strength 2.0 per cent; (2) vaginal for treatment of vaginal candidiasis, P
Tioguanine/Thioguanine POM
Tiotropium POM
Tipranavir capsules POM
Tirofiban POM
Titanium dioxide GSL
Titanium peroxide, external use only GSL
Titanium salicylate, external use only GSL
Titralac tablets GSL
Tixycolds cold and allergy nasal drops GSL
Tixycolds cold and hayfever inhalant capsules GSL
Tixylix baby syrup GSL
Tixylix Catarrh syrup P
Tixylix Chesty Cough syrup GSL
Tixylix Cough and Cold linctus CD Inv P
Tixylix Daytime linctus CD Inv P
Tixylix dry cough P
Tixylix Night-time linctus CD Inv P
Tixymol suspension P
Tixyplus suspension P
Tizanidine POM
Tobi nebuliser solution POM
Tobradex eye drops POM
Tobramycin POM
Tobramycin sulphate POM
Tocainide hydrochloride POM
Tocopheryl acetate GSL
Toepodo cream P
Tofenacin hydrochloride POM
Tofranil preparations POM
Tofranil with promazine capsules POM
Tolanase tablets POM
Tolazamide POM
Tolazoline hydrochloride POM but if external, P
Tolbutamide POM
Tolbutamide sodium POM
Tolcapone POM
Tolfenamic acid POM
Tolmetin sodium POM
Tolnaftate, external use only GSL
Tolperisone POM
Tolterodine tartrate POM
Tolu Balsam GSL
Tolu-flavour solution GSL
Tomudex POM
Topal tablets GSL

Topamax Sprinkle capsules POM
Topamax tablets POM
Topicycline solution POM
Topiramate POM
Topotecan POM
Toradol injection POM
Toradol tablets POM
Torasemide POM
Torbetol GSL
Torem tablets POM
Toremifene POM
Torisel POM
Totamol tablets POM
Totaretic tablets POM
Toviaz prolonged release tablets POM
Tracleer tablets POM
Tracrium injection POM
Tractocile preparations POM
Tradorec XL POM
Tramacet tablets POM
Tramadol hydrochloride POM
Tramake capsules POM
Tramake Insts sachets POM
Tramazoline POM
Trandate preparations POM
Trandolapril POM
Tranexamic acid POM
Trangina XL POM
Tranquax capsules POM
Tranquilyn tablets CD POM
Transiderm-Nitro P
Transtec transdermal patches CD No
    Register POM
Transvasin cream GSL
Transvasin Heat spray GSL
Tranxene capsules CD Benz POM
Tranylcypromine sulphate POM
Trasicor preparations POM
Trasidrex tablets POM
Trastuzumab POM
Trasylol injection POM
Travasept 100 P
Travatan eye-drops POM
Traveleeze pastilles P
Travogyn vaginal tablets POM
Travoprost POM
Traxam gel POM
Traxam Pain Relief gel P
Traxam Quick Break foam POM
Trazodone hydrochloride POM
Treacle GSL
Trenbolone CD Anab POM
Trental preparations POM
Treosulfan POM
Tretamine POM
Tretinoin POM
TRH-Roche preparations POM
Tri-Adcortyl Otic ointment POM
Tri-Adcortyl preparations POM
Tri-Minulet tablets POM
Triacetyloleandomycin POM
Triadene POM
Triam-Co tablets POM
Triamax-Co tablets POM
Triamcinolone POM

Triamcinolone acetonide POM but if (1)
    for the treatment of common mouth
    ulcers maximum strength 0.1% and
    container or package contains not
    more than 5g of medicinal product,
    or (2) in the form of a pressurised
    nasal spray, for the treatment of
    symptoms of seasonal allergic rhini-
    tis in persons aged 18 years and over,
    110mcg per nostril (MD) 110mcg per
    nostril (MDD) for a maximum period
    of 3 months, in a container or pack-
    age containing not more than
    3.575mg of triamcinolone acetonide
    P
Triamcinolone diacetate POM
Triamcinolone hexacetonide POM
Triamterene POM
Triapin Mite tablets POM
Triapin tablets POM
Triazolam CD Benz POM
Tribavirin see Ribavirin

Trichlorofluoromethane (Propellant 11),
    external use only GSL
Triclofos sodium POM
Triclosan, external use only GSL
Tricyclamol chloride POM
Tridene POM
Tridestra tablets POM
Trientine POM
Trientine dihydrochloride POM
Trifluoperazine POM
Trifluoperazine hydrochloride POM
Trifluperidol POM
Trifluperidol hydrochloride POM
Trifyba GSL
Trihexyphenidyl/Benzhexol hydrochlo-
    ride POM
Triiodothyronine injection POM
Trileptal oral suspension POM
Trileptal tablets POM
Trilostane POM
Triludan tablets POM
Trimeperidine; its salts CD POM
Trimeprazine see Alimemazine
Trimetaphan camsylate POM
Trimetazidine POM
Trimetazidine hydrochloride POM
Trimethoprim POM
Trimetrexate glucuronate POM
Trimipramine maleate POM
Trimipramine mesylate POM
Trimogal tablets POM
Trimopan suspension POM
Trimopan tablets POM
Trimovate preparations POM
Trimustine hydrochloride POM
Trinordiol tablets POM
Trinovum ED tablets POM
Trinovum tablets POM
Trintek patches P
Triogesic tablets P
Triominic tablets P
Triprimix tablets POM
Triprolidine P
Triptafen preparations POM
Triptorelin POM
Trisenox POM
Trisequens Forte POM
Trisequens tablets POM
Trisodium edetate POM
Tritace capsules POM
Tritace tablets POM
Trivax vaccine POM
Trivax-AD vaccine POM
Trivax-Hib POM
Trizivir tablets POM
Trobicin vials POM
Tropergen tablets POM
Tropicamide POM
Tropisetron hydrochloride POM
Tropium preparations CD Benz POM
Trosyl nail solution POM
Troxidone POM
Trusopt ophthalmic solution POM
Truvada POM
Tryptizol preparations POM
L-Tryptophan POM but if (1) oral
    dietary supplementation (2) external,
    P
Trypure POM
Tuberculin purified protein derivative
    POM
Tubocurarine chloride POM
Tuinal capsules CD POM
Tulobuterol POM
Tulobuterol hydrochloride POM
Tums tablets GSL
Tunes GSL
Turpentine oil, if internal (vapour
    inhalations except preparations to be
    applied topically), or external or
    internal (vapour inhalations from
    products to be applied topically max-
    imum strength 5%) GSL
Twinrix Adult vaccine POM
Twinrix paediatric POM
Tybamate POM
Tygacil solution for infusion POM
Tylex capsules CD Inv POM

Tylex effervescent CD Inv POM
Tylosin POM
Tylosin phosphate POM
Tylosin tartrate POM
Typherix vaccine POM
Typhim Vi vaccine POM
Typhoid and tetanus vaccine POM
Typhoid vaccine POM
Typhoid-paratyphoid A and B cholera
    vaccine POM
Typhoid-paratyphoid A and B tetanus
    vaccine POM
Typhoid-paratyphoid A and B vaccine
    POM
Typhus vaccine POM
Tyrothricin POM but if throat lozenges
    or throat pastilles, P
Tyrozets lozenges P
Tysabri POM
Tyverb film coated tablets POM

U

Ubretid preparations POM
Ucerax preparations POM
Ucine tablets POM
Uftoral capsules POM
Ukidan injection POM
Ultec tablets POM
Ultiva injection CD POM
Ultra Chloraseptic P
Ultrabase GSL
Ultralanum plain preparations POM
Ultramol soluble tablets CD Inv P
Ultraproct preparations POM
Ultratard insulins POM
Undecenoic acid, external use only GSL
Unguentum M cream GSL
Unichem allergy relief syrup P
Unichem allergy relief tablets P
Unichem bronchial mixture GSL
Unichem childs diarrhoea mixture GSL
Unichem cold relief capsules GSL
Unichem cold relief powders hot lemon
    flu strength GSL
Unichem cystitis relief sachets GSL
Unichem diarrhoea relief capsules 2mg
    GSL
Unichem Hayfever & Allergy non-
    drowsy tablets GSL
Unichem heartburn relief tablets P
Unichem junior paracetamol suspension
    P
Unichem pain relief capsules long last-
    ing P
Unichem Rehydration Treatment GSL
Unichem rehydration treatment sachets
    P
Unichem sleep aid capsule P
Unichem sleep aid extra capsules P
Unichem throat lozenges GSL
Unicorn Root False GSL
Uniflor tablets P
Uniflu with gregovite C CD Inv P
Unigest tablets P
Unihep injection POM
Uniparin injection POM
Uniphyllin Continus tablets P
Unipine XL POM
Uniroid HC preparations POM
Unisept solution P
Univer capsules POM
Uorazepam CD Benz POM
Uprima sublingual tablets POM
Uracil POM
Uramustine POM
Urdox tablets POM
Urea hydrogen peroxide, external use
    only GSL
Urea Stibamine POM
Urea, external use only GSL
Urethane POM
Uriben preparations POM
Uridine 5'-triphosphate POM
Uriflex-G P
Uriflex-R P
Uriflex-S P
Uriflex-SP P

Uriflex-W P
Urispas tablets POM
Urofollitrophin see Urofollitropin
Urofollitropin/Urofollitrophin POM
Urokinase POM
Uromitexan injection POM
Uromitexan tablets POM
Urotainer chlorhexidine 1:5000 P
Ursodeoxychoic Acid POM
Ursofalk capsules POM
Ursofalk suspension POM
Ursogal tablets and capsules POM
Utinor tablets POM
Utovlan tablets POM
Uva Ursi (Bearberry) GSL
Uvacin GSL

V

Vaccine: Bacillus Salmonella Typhi POM
Vaccine: Poliomyelitis (Oral) POM
Vadarex rub GSL
Vagifem vaginal tablets POM
Vaginyl tablets POM
Vagisil cream GSL
Valaciclovir POM
Valclair CD Benz POM
Valcyte powder for oral solution
    50mg/ml POM
Valcyte tablets POM
Valdecoxib POM
Valderma GSL
Valerian GSL
Valerian tabs GSL
Valerina tablets GSL
Valganciclovir POM
Valium preparations CD Benz POM
Vallergan Forte syrup POM
Vallergan preparations POM
Vallestril tablets POM
Valoid injection POM
Valoid tablets P
Valonorm P
Valpeda GSL
Valpiform POM
Valproic acid POM
Valsartan POM
Valtrex tablets POM
Vamin preparations POM
Vaminolact POM
Vanair cream P
Vancocin preparations POM
Vancomycin hydrochloride POM
Vaniqa cream POM
Vantage Allergy relief preparations P
Vantage Baby cream GSL
Vantage Clearsore cold sore cream P
Vantage clotrimazole cream P
Vantage co-codamol tablets P
Vantage constipation relief tablets P
Vantage cough syrups P
Vantage cystitis relief sachets GSL
Vantage Flu-strength all-in-one P
Vantage haemorrhoid cream GSL
Vantage hayfever relief nasal spray P
Vantage heartburn relief tablets P
Vantage hydrocortisone cream P
Vantage ibuprofen suspension P
Vantage loperamide tablets P
Vantage paracetamol preparations P
Vantage sleep aid tablets P
Vantage thrush treatment capsule P
Vaqta injection POM
Vaqta Paediatric vaccine POM
Vardenafil POM
Varenicline POM
Varicella vaccine POM
Varidase preparations POM
Varilrix vaccine POM
Varivax injection POM
Vascace tablets POM
Vascalpha tablets POM
Vasculit tablets P
Vasodon-A eye drops POM
Vasogen GSL
Vasopressin POM
Vasopressin injection POM
Vasopressin tannate POM

Vasosulf eye drops POM
Vasoxine injection POM
Vectavir cold sore cream POM
Vectibix POM
Vecuronium bromide POM
Veganin tablets pack sizes 10s, 30s CD Inv P
Vegetable laxative tablets BPC 1963 POM
Velbe POM
Velcade injection POM
Velosef preparations POM
Velosulin insulins POM
Venaxx XL modified release capsules POM
Venlafaxine POM
Veno's Dry cough mixture GSL
Veno's Expectorant cough mixture GSL
Veno's for Kids GSL
Veno's Honey & Lemon cough mixture GSL
Venofer injection POM
Venofundin POM
Ventavis POM
Ventide inhaler POM
Ventmax POM
Ventolin preparations POM
Vepesid preparations POM
Vera-til SR POM
Veracur gel GSL
Verapamil hydrochloride POM
Verapress MR tablets POM
Veratrine POM
Veratrum, Green POM
Veratrum, White POM
Verbena GSL
Veripaque P
Vermox preparations POM
Verrugon P
Versatis POM
Vertab SR POM
Verteporfin POM
Vesagex cream GSL
Vesanoid capsules POM
Vesicare tablets POM
Vexol ophthalmic suspension POM
Vfend powder for oral suspension POM
Vfend tablets and infusion POM
Viagra tablets POM
Viatim vaccine POM
Viazem XL capsules POM
Vibramycin preparations POM
Vibramycin-D tablets POM
Vicks Action P
Vicks Coldcare P
Vicks First Defence GSL
Vicks inhaler GSL
Vicks Medinite P
Vicks Sinex preparations GSL
Vicks Ultra chloraseptic throat spray P
Vicks VapoRub GSL
Vicks Vaposyrup Chesty Cough GSL
Vicks Vaposyrup Chesty Cough & Congestion P
Vicks Vaposyrup Childrens Dry Cough P
Vicks Vaposyrup Dry Cough & Nasal Congestion P
Vidarabine POM
Vidaza powder for suspension for injection POM
Videne preparations P
Videx EC capsules POM
Videx tablets POM
Vidopen preparations POM
Vielle lubricant GSL
Vielle menopause kit GSL
Vigabatrin POM
Vigam liquid POM
Vigam S POM
Vigranon B syrup P
Vikonon GSL
Viloxazine hydrochloride POM
Vinblastine sulphate POM
Vincristine sulphate POM
Vindesine sulphate POM
Vinorelbine tartrate POM
Vioform-hydrocortisone preparations POM

Viomycin pantothenate POM
Viomycin sulphate POM
Vioxx preparations POM
VioxxAcute tablets POM
Viracept tablets POM
Viraferon injection POM
Viraferonpeg injection POM
ViraferonPeg prefilled pens POM
Viralief P
Viramune preparations POM
Virasorb cold sore cream GSL
Virazid powder for aerosol POM
Virazole POM
Viread tablets POM
Virgan eye gel POM
Virginiamycin POM
Viridal Duo injection POM
Viridal injection POM
Viroflu vaccine POM
Virormone injections CD Anab POM
Virovir tablets POM
Visclair tablets P
Viscotears liquid gel P
Viscotears single dose units P
Viskaldix tablets POM
Visken tablets POM
Vista-Methasone drops POM
Vista-Methasone-N drops POM
Vistabel POM
Visthesia Intercameral P
Visthesia Light Intercameral P
Vistide solution POM
Visudyne infusion POM
Vitacoll Extra GSL
Vitacoll Gold GSL
Vitalux Plus capsules P
Vitamin A POM but if (1) external, P; (2) internal 7,500iu (2,250mcg retinol equivalent) (MDD), GSL
Vitamin A acetate POM but if (1) external, P; (2) internal equivalent to 7,500iu Vitamin A (2,250mcg retinol equivalent) (MDD), GSL
Vitamin A palmitate POM but if (1) external, P; (2) internal equivalent to 7,500iu Vitamin A (2,250mcg retinol equivalent) (MDD), GSL
Vitamin D (calciferol), up to 400iu (10mcg cholecalciferol) (MDD) GSL
Vitlipid Adult POM
Vitlipid Infant POM
Vitlipid N POM
Vitravene injection POM
Vitrimix KV POM
Vivabec P
Vivacor POM
Vivadone POM
Vivaglobin POM
Vivalan tablets POM
Vivazide POM
Vivicrom eye-drops P
Vividrin eye drops POM
Vividrin nasal spray P
Vivioptal capsules P
Vivotif vaccine POM
Vivpryl tablets POM
Viz-on eyedrops POM
Vocalzone throat pastilles GSL
Volmax tablets POM
Volplex POM
Volraman tablets POM
Volsaid Retard tablets POM
Voltarol Emulgel P 30g and 50g P
Voltarol Optha POM
Voltarol Paineze Emulgel GSL
Voltarol preparations POM
Voltarol Rapid tablets POM
Voluven POM
Voriconazole POM

W

Wahoo (Euonymus atropurpureus) GSL
Wala pillules all PO except Apis/Levisticum, Belladonna/Chamomilla, Chamomilla/Nicotiana, Silicea Comp and Valeriana Comp GSL

Warfarin POM
Warfarin sodium POM
Wartex ointment (Pickles) P
Warticon preparations POM
Warticon Fem POM
Waspeze aerosol for stings P
Waspeze bites & stings spray GSL
Wate-On P
Water GSL
Water Balance tablets GSL
Water for injection ampoules POM
Watercress GSL
Wax-Aid P
Waxsol GSL
Weleda Aconite/Bryonia drops PO
Weleda Antimony ointment PO
Weleda Apatite 6X Comp tablets PO
Weleda Arnica ointment GSL
Weleda Arnica 6X tablets GSL
Weleda Avena Sativa compound GSL
Weleda Balsamicum ointment PO
Weleda Bidor tablets GSL
Weleda Bolus Eucalypti compound PO
Weleda Calendolon ointment GSL
Weleda Catarrh cream PO
Weleda Chamomilla 3X drops GSL
Weleda Choleodoron drops PO
Weleda Cinnabar 20X/Pyrites 3X tablets PO
Weleda Combudoron ointment GSL
Weleda Combudoron spray GSL
Weleda Conchae 5% compound tablets PO
Weleda Copper ointment GSL
Weleda Cough drops PO
Weleda Cough drops compound PO
Weleda Cratageus Comp drops PO
Weleda Dermatodoron ointment PO
Weleda Digestodoron drops PO
Weleda Digestodoron tablets PO
Weleda Dulcamara/Lysamachia drops PO
Weleda Erysidoron drops PO
Weleda Ferrum phosphate Co. pillules POM
Weleda Ferrum Siderum 6X tablets PO
Weleda Feverfew 6X drops GSL
Weleda Feverfew 6X tablets GSL
Weleda Fragador tablets GSL
Weleda Fragaria/Urtica drops PO
Weleda Fragaria/Vitis tablets PO
Weleda Frost cream PO
Weleda Gencydo ointment PO
Weleda granules GSL
Weleda homoeopathic medicines tablets GSL
Weleda Hypericum/Calendula ointment GSL
Weleda Infludo drops POM
Weleda juices & elixirs GSL
Weleda Larch resin ointment GSL
Weleda Laxadoron tablets GSL
Weleda lotions GSL
Weleda Mandragora Comp drops PO
Weleda massage balms GSL
Weleda medicinal gargle GSL
Weleda Melissa compound GSL
Weleda Menodoron drops PO
Weleda Mercurius Cyanat 4X POM
Weleda mini medicines massage balm GSL
Weleda mini medicines ointments GSL
Weleda nasal spray GSL
Weleda Nausyn tablets POM
Weleda Oleum Rhinale drops PO
Weleda Onopordon Comp A drops PO
Weleda Onopordon Comp B drops PO
Weleda Pertudoron 1 drops POM
Weleda Pertudoron 2 drops PO
Weleda Phosphorus/Tart POM
Weleda Pyrites 3X tablets PO
Weleda Rheumadoron 1 drops POM
Weleda Rheumadoron 102A drops PO
Weleda Rheumadoron 2 drops PO
Weleda Rheumadoron ointment PO
Weleda Rhus Tox ointment GSL
Weleda Ruta ointment GSL
Weleda Scleron tablets PO

Weleda Vitis Comp tablets PO
Weleda W.C.S. dusting powder PO
Welldorm preparations POM
Wellferon POM
Wellvone suspension POM
Wellvone tablets POM
Wheat GSL
Whita preparations GSL
Wild Cherry GSL
Wild Indigo GSL
Wild Lettuce GSL
Willow White GSL
Wilzin POM
Wind-Eze products GSL
Windcheaters capsules GSL
Windsetlers GSL
WinRho SDF POM
Witch Doctor skin treatment gel GSL
Witch Doctor hydrating gel GSL
Witch Doctor radiance serum GSL
Wood Betony GSL
Woodward's gripe water GSL
Woodwards teething gel GSL
Wool alcohols, acetylated, external use only GSL
Wool alcohols, external use only GSL
Wool fat, external use only GSL
Wright's vaporiser blocks P
Wright's vaporising fluid P

X

Xagrid tablets POM
Xalacom eye-drops POM
Xalantan eye drops POM
Xamiol gel POM
Xamoterol fumarate POM
Xanax tablets CD Benz POM
Xanthan gum GSL
Xanthomax POM
Xarelto POM
Xatral SR tablets POM
Xatral tablets POM
Xatral XL tablets POM
Xefo tablets and injection POM
Xeloda tablets POM
Xenazine 25 tablets POM
Xenical capsules POM
Xepin cream POM
Xigris infusion POM
Xipamide POM
Xismox XL POM
Xolair POM
Xylocaine 4% topical P
Xylocaine antiseptic gel P
Xylocaine eye drops POM
Xylocaine gel P
Xylocaine injections POM
Xylocaine ointment P
Xylocaine spray P
Xylocaine with adrenaline injections POM
Xylocard injections POM
Xylometazoline hydrochloride, if non-oily nasal sprays and nasal drops maximum strength 0.1 per cent GSL
Xyloproct preparations POM
Xylotox injections POM
Xyrem oral solution CD Benz POM
Xyzal tablets POM

Y

Yariba GSL
Yarrow GSL
Yasmin tablets POM
Yeast GSL
Yeast-Vite GSL
Yellow Dock GSL
Yellow fever vaccine POM
Yentreve capsules POM
Yohimbine hydrochloride POM
Yomesan tablets P
Yondelis POM
Yutopar preparations POM

Z

Z Span Spansules P
Z-Span P
Zacin cream POM
Zaditen capsules POM
Zaditen elixir POM
Zaditen eye-drops POM
Zaditen tablets POM
Zadstat preparations POM
Zaedoc tablets POM
Zafirlucast POM
Zalcitabine POM
Zaleplon POM
Zamadol 24hr tablets POM
Zamadol Melt tablets POM
Zamadol preparations POM
Zamadol SR capsules POM
Zanaflex tablets POM
Zanamivir POM
Zanidip tablets POM
Zanprol tablets P
Zantac 75 P
Zantac 75 Dissolve P
Zantac 75 Relief GSL
Zantac 75 Relief Dissolve GSL
Zantac preparations POM
Zanza GSL
Zapain capsules CD Inv POM
Zaponex tablets POM
Zarontin preparations POM
Zavedos capsules POM
Zavedos injection POM
Zavesca capsules POM
Zeasorb powder P
Zeffix preparations POM
Zelapar tablets POM
Zemon XL tablets POM

Zemplar injection POM
Zemtard XL capsules POM
Zenalb solution POM
Zenapax infusion POM
Zenoxone cream (PL 0181/0033) P
Zerit capsules POM
Zerobase GSL
Zestoretic tablets POM
Zestril tablets POM
Zevalin POM
Ziagen preparations POM
Zibor preparations POM
Zida-Co tablets POM
Zidoval vaginal gel POM
Zidovudine POM
Zileze tablets POM
Zimbacol XL tablets POM
Zimeldine hydrochloride POM
Zimovane POM
Zimovane LS POM
Zinacef preparations POM
Zinamide tablets POM

Zinc carbonate, external use only GSL
Zinc citrate trihydrate, if dentifrice, external use only GSL
Zinc gluconate, if MDD equivalent to 5mg elemental zinc GSL
Zinc oleate, external use only GSL
Zinc oxide, if MDD equivalent to 5mg elemental zinc GSL
Zinc stearate, external use only GSL
Zinc sulphate, if internal equivalent to 5mg elemental zinc (MDD) or external maximum strength 1.0 per cent GSL
Zinc undecenoate, external use only GSL

Zincaband P
Zindaclin gel POM
Zineryt application POM
Zinga capsules POM
Zinnat preparations POM
Zipeprol CD POM
Zipzoc P
Zirtek Allergy relief tablets pack sizes 7s GSL
Zirtek Allergy solution pack sizes 70ml GSL; 150ml P; 200ml P
Zirtek allergy tablets pack sizes 21s P; 30s P
Zispin SolTabs POM
Zispin tablets POM
Zita tablets POM
Zithromax preparations POM
Ziz Forte P
Ziz tablets P
Zocor Heart-Pro tablets P
Zocor tablets POM
Zofran Flexi-Amps POM
Zofran preparations POM
Zoladex injection POM
Zoledronic acid POM
Zoleptil tablets POM
Zolmitriptan POM
Zolpidem CD Benz POM
Zolpidem tartrate CD Benz POM
Zolvadex LA Depot injection POM
Zolvera oral solution POM

Zomacton CD Anab POM
Zomepirac sodium POM
Zometa infusion POM
Zomig nasal spray POM
Zomig nasal spray POM
Zomig Rapimelt tablets POM

Zomig tablets POM
Zomorph capsules CD POM
Zonegran capsules POM
Zonisamide POM
Zonivent Aquanasal spray POM
Zopiclone POM
Zorac gel POM
Zotepine POM
Zoton preparations POM
Zovirax 5% pump GSL
Zovirax cold sore cream GSL
Zovirax cream POM
Zovirax dispersible tablets POM
Zovirax Double Strength suspension POM
Zovirax IV POM
Zovirax ophthalmic ointment POM
Zovirax suspension POM
Zoxin capsules POM
Zoxycil capsules POM
Zubes lozenges GSL
Zuclopenthixol acetate POM
Zuclopenthixol decanoate POM
Zuclopenthixol dihydrochloride POM
Zumenon tablets POM
Zuvogen POM

Zyban tablets POM
Zydol preparations POM
Zydol SR tablets POM
Zydol XL tablets POM
Zyloric 300 tablets POM
Zyloric tablets POM
Zyomet gel POM
Zyprexa IntraMuscular POM
Zyprexa tablets POM
Zyprexa Velotab tablets POM
Zyvox preparations POM

1.4 Non-medicinal poisons

A "non-medicinal poison," or simply a "poison," is a substance that is included in the poisons list made under the Poisons Act 1972, as amended. A reference to a poison includes substances containing that poison. Other substances, no matter how toxic, are not poisons under this Act.

A comprehensive fact sheet on poisons is now available from the Legal and Ethical Advisory Service (*see* p146).

Some substances in the poisons list (eg, arsenic, mercuric oxide) also have medicinal uses. When sold as medicines such substances are controlled by the Medicines Act 1968, as amended, but when sold for non-medicinal purposes they are subject to the Poisons Act 1972, as amended.

The poisons list is divided into two parts. In general, substances included in **Part I** of the list (ie, Part I poisons) may be sold only by persons lawfully conducting retail pharmacy businesses. Such sales <u>must be conducted at a registered pharmacy under the supervision of a pharmacist</u>.

Part II of the list (ie, Part II poisons) may be sold both by persons lawfully conducting a retail pharmacy business and by listed sellers of Part II poisons, that is, by persons whose names appear in a list of sellers maintained by a local authority. A listed seller may nominate one or two deputies who also may effect the sale of Schedule 1 poisons.

Listed sellers may only sell Part II poisons in prepacked containers and sales must be mde on the listed premises.

Certain Part II poisons may be sold only by listed sellers if the poison is in a specified form, and some of these poisons may only be sold to persons engaged in the trade or business of horticulture, agriculture or forestry and for the purposes of that trade or business.

Apart from these matters, the requirements for the sale of Part II poisons are substantially the same for listed sellers as for persons lawfully conducting retail pharmacy businesses.

NB: Since 1 September 2006, strychnine no longer has approval for purchase or use for mole control, from the Pesticides Safety Directorate (PSD).

1.4.1 Poisons schedules

The Poisons Rules 1982, as amended, apply or relax the restrictions imposed by the Act in particular circumstances. There are eight schedules to the Rules and they are described, briefly, below (more detailed reference is made to some of them later):

Schedule 1 A list of poisons to which special restrictions apply relating to storage, conditions of sale and keeping of records of sales. The restrictions do not apply to articles which contain barium carbonate or to alpha-chloralose and zinc phosphide when they are prepared for the destruction of rats and mice as described in the individual entries in the alphabetical list (see *Medicines, Ethics and Practice*, Section 1.5).

Schedule 4 A list of articles exempted from control as poisons. There are two groups. Group I comprises classes of articles which contain poisons which are totally exempt from the requirements of the Poisons Act 1972, as amended, and the Poisons Rules 1982, as amended, eg, builders' materials. Group II lists exemptions for certain poisons when in specified articles or substances, eg, sulphuric acid in accumulators.

Schedule 5 Some Part II poisons may be sold by listed sellers only in certain forms. The details are given in this schedule which also specifies certain poisons which may be sold by listed sellers only to persons engaged in the trade or business of agriculture, horticulture or forestry and for the purpose of that trade or business. In any other circumstances the sale of Schedule 5 poisons is restricted to pharmacies.

Schedule 8 Form of application for inclusion in local authority's list of sellers of Part II poisons.

Schedule 9 Form of the list of listed sellers of Part II poisons kept by a local authority.

Schedule 10 Certificate for the purchase of a non-medicinal poison.

Schedule 11 Form of entry to be made in poisons book on sale of Schedule 1 poison.

Schedule 12 Restriction of sale and supply of strychnine and other substances. Forms of authority required for certain of these poisons.

Schedules 2, 3, 6 and 7 were deleted by a Poisons Rules Amendment Order in 1985.

1.4.2 Sales of poisons

Sales of Schedule 1 poisons

There are certain requirements that must be fulfilled for the lawful sale of Schedule 1 poisons (and no other poisons). These requirements are concerned with record keeping and having knowledge, or confirmation of the identity by way of certification, of the purchaser.

Knowledge of the purchaser

The purchaser of a Schedule 1 poison must be either:

(a) certified in writing in the prescribed manner by a householder to be a person to whom the poison may properly be sold (*see Figure 1.1*). If the householder is not known to the seller to be a responsible person of good character, the certificate must be endorsed by a police officer in charge of a police station. It must be retained by the seller; or,

(b) known by the seller, or by a pharmacist employed by the seller at the premises where the sale is effected, to be a person to whom the poison may properly be sold.

If the purchaser is known by the person in charge of the premises on which the poison is sold, or of the department of the business in which the sale is effected, then the requirement as to knowledge of the purchaser by the seller is deemed to be satisfied in the case of (a) sales made by listed sellers of Part II poisons, and (b) sales exempted by Section 4 of the Act (*see* p77).

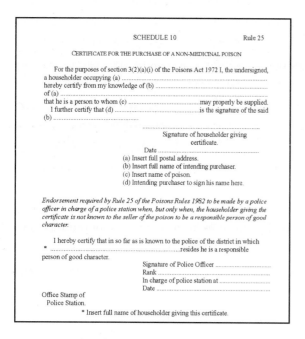

Figure 1.1: Certificate for the purchase of a non-medicinal poison

The requirements as to knowledge of the purchaser, entry in the poisons book and signature (or signed order) by the purchaser do not apply to:

(a) the sale of poisons to be exported to purchasers outside the United Kingdom;
(b) the sale of any article by its manufacturer or by a person carrying on a business in the course of which poisons are regularly sold by way of wholesale dealing, if
(i) the article is sold to a person carrying on a business in the course of which poisons are sold or regularly used in the manufacture of other articles; and
(ii) the seller is reasonably satisfied that the purchaser requires the article for the purpose of that business.

The requirements which apply to the sale of Schedule 1 poisons apply also to the supply of such poisons in the form of commercial samples. The requirement that the person supplied must be known to the seller is satisfied, for the supply of commercial samples, if the person to be supplied is known by the person in charge of the department of the business through which the sale is made.

Records

The seller must not deliver a Schedule 1 poison until he has made the required entry in the poisons book and the purchaser has signed it. The particulars to be recorded are:

(a) the date of the sale;
(b) the name and quantity of poison supplied;
(c) the name and address of the purchaser;
(d) the business, trade or occupation of the purchaser;
(e) the purpose for which it is stated by the purchaser to be required;
(f) the name and address of the householder, if any, by whom a certificate was given and the date of the certificate.

Entries in the poisons book must be made in the manner prescribed in the Poisons Rules 1982, as amended. The book must be retained for two years from the date on which the last entry was made.

A signed order may be accepted in lieu of the purchaser's signature in the circumstances described below.

The Poisons Rules 1982, as amended, require any authority or certificate to be retained by the seller of the poison to which the authority or certificate relates. As the poisons register must be retained for two years after the date of the last entry, the authority or certificate must also be retained for at least two years.

There is no requirement under the legislation to make an entry of receipts of poisons. Only records of supplies are legally required.

Signed orders

A signed order in writing may be accepted from a person who requires a Schedule 1 poison for the purpose of his trade, business or profession. The seller must be reasonably satisfied that the purchaser carries on the trade, business or profession stated, and that the signature is genuine. In addition to the signature of the purchaser the order must state:

(a) his name and address;
(b) his trade, business or profession;
(c) total quantity to be purchased;
(d) the purpose for which the poison is required.

A signed order is required to be dated. The entry made in the poisons book before delivery of the poison must be dated. The date of the signed order and the words "signed order" must be recorded in place of the signature and be identified by a reference number. In an emergency the seller may deliver the poison on receiving an undertaking that a signed order will be furnished within the next 72 hours. Failure to comply with an undertaking, or the making of false statements to obtain a Schedule 1 poison without a signed order, are contraventions of the Poisons Rules.

Labelling of poisons

Substances in the Poisons List are also subject to the legislation concerned with Chemicals and must be labelled accordingly (*see* p83).

Containers for poisons

Substances in the Poisons List are subject to the legislation concerned with Chemicals and must be supplied in an appropriate container (*see* p84).

Storage of Schedule 1 poisons

Schedule 1 poisons in any retail shop, or premises used in connection with such a shop, must be stored in one of the following ways:

(a) in a cupboard or drawer reserved solely for the storage of poisons; or
(b) in a part of the premises which is partitioned off or otherwise separated from the remainder of the premises and to which customers are not permitted to have access; or
(c) on a shelf reserved solely for the storage of poisons, and no food is kept directly under the shelf.

If the poison is to be used in agriculture, horticulture or forestry then:

(a) it must not be stored on any shelf or any part of the premises where food is kept; and

(b) it may only be stored in a cupboard or drawer which is reserved for poisons used in agriculture, horticulture or forestry.

The Control of Substances Hazardous to Health Regulations 1994, as amended, made under the Health and Safety at Work Act imposes duties on employers to protect employees and other persons who may be exposed to substances hazardous to health. For this reason a COSSH risk assessment would have to be carried out by a pharmacist before storing and selling poisons.

Schedule 1 poisons subject to special restrictions

Some Schedule 1 poisons are subject to special restrictions on sale or supply as detailed in Schedule 12 of the Poisons Rules 1982, as amended. They may only be sold:

(a) by way of wholesale dealing,

(b) for export to purchasers outside the United Kingdom, or

(c) to persons or institutions concerned with scientific education or research or chemical analysis for the purpose of that education, research or analysis.

Sale or supply of these poisons is also permitted in the circumstances indicated below:

(1) Fluoroacetic acid its salts or fluoroacetamide may be sold:
To a person producing a certificate, in form "A" or form "B" as provided in Schedule 12, which has been issued within the preceding three months. The certificate must specify the quantity of the poison to be used as a rodenticide and identify the places where it is to be used, which may be:

(a) ships or sewers as indicated in the certificate; or

(b) drains identified in the certificate, being drains situated in restricted areas and wholly enclosed and inaccessible when not in use; or

(c) warehouses identified in the certificate which are in restricted dock areas and kept securely locked and barred when not in use.

The proper officer of health of a local authority or port health authority may issue forms "A" to employees of the authority for the purpose of purchasing rodenticide for use as in (a), (b) or (c) above.

The proper officer of health of a local authority or port health authority may issue forms "B" to persons carrying on the business of pest control, or to their employees for the purpose of purchasing rodenticide for use as in (a) or (b) above.

For the purchase of rodenticide for use as in (a) or (b) above form "B" may also be issued, in England, by a person duly authorised by the Department for Environment, Food and Rural Affairs (DEFRA), or in Scotland a person authorised by the Scottish Ministers, or in Wales a person authorised by the National Assembly for Wales (NAW), certifying that the substance is required for use by their officers.

(2) Strychnine
Strychnine is no longer approved for purchase or use for the killing of moles, but there is provision for the supply of strychnine for the purpose of killing foxes in an infected area within the meaning of the Rabies (Control) Order 1974, as amended. A request under these circumstances is very unlikely, as there have been no requests for this use in recent years, but would have to be in accordance with a written authority, as detailed in the Poisons Rules.

The sale and supply of thallium salts, potassium and sodium arsenites,and zinc phosphide are also restricted to certain circumstances but no longer have Pesticides Safety Directorate (PSD) approval.

The sale and supply of calcium, potassium and sodium cyanide are also restricted and also no longer have PSD approval.

Sales exempted by Section 4

Section 4 of the Poisons Act 1972, as amended, exempts certain categories of sales of poisons from the provisions of Section 3(1) and 3(2) of the Act, except as provided by the Poisons Rules 1982, as amended. The principal effect is that exempted transactions of any Part 1 poison may be made without the supervision of a pharmacist, provided the sales are not made by a shopkeeper on premises connected with his retail business. The requirements as to signed orders and poisons book records in respect of Schedule 1 poisons also apply.

The exempted categories are:

(1) Sales of poisons by way of wholesale dealing, that is, sales made to a person who buys for the purpose of selling again.

(2) The sale of an article to a doctor, dentist, veterinary surgeon or veterinary practitioner for the purpose of his profession.

(3) The sale of an article for use in or in connection with any hospital infirmary or dispensary or similar institution approved by an order, whether general or special of the Secretary of State.

(4) The sale of an article by a person carrying on a business in the course of which poisons are regularly sold either by way of wholesale dealing or for use by the purchasers in their trade or business to:

(a) a government department or an officer of the Crown requiring the article for the purposes of the public service, or any local authority, requiring the article in connection with the exercise by the authority, of any statutory powers; or

(b) a person or institution concerned with scientific education or research, if the article is required for the purposes of that education or research; or

(c) a person who requires the article for the purpose of enabling him to comply with any requirements with respect to the medical treatment of persons employed by that person in any trade or business carried on by him; or

(d) a person who requires the article for the purpose of his trade or business. A person can be said to be carrying on a business if he engages in full-time or part-time commercial activity with a view to profit.

Sales of poisons to be exported to purchasers outside the United Kingdom are also listed as exempted categories. However, these types of transaction are exempted from the provisions of Section 3(1) and 3(2) of the Act and the Rules requiring signed orders and poisons book records etc.

Wholesale dealing to a shopkeeper

"Sale by way of wholesale dealing" means sale to a person who buys for the purpose of selling again.

It is not lawful to sell by way of wholesale dealing any poison included in Part I of the Poisons List to a person carrying on a business of shopkeeping unless the seller:

(a) has reasonable grounds for believing that the purchaser is a person lawfully conducting a retail pharmacy business; or

(b) has received a statement signed by the purchaser or by a person authorised by him on his behalf to the effect that the purchaser does not intend to sell the poison on any premises used for or in connection with his retail business.

1.5 Alphabetical list of non-medicinal poisons

Acetarsol P1; S1 except substances containing less than the equivalent of 0.0075% arsenic (P1 only)

Acetarsone P1; S1 except substances containing less than the equivalent of 0.0075% arsenic (P1 only)

Aldicarb P2; S1; S5 listed sellers of poisons permitted to sell only if in preparations for use in agriculture, horticulture or forestry and such sales are restricted to these trade or business users

Alpha-chloralose see Chloralose

Aluminium phosphide P1; S1

Ammonia P2; S4 in substances, not being solutions of ammonia or preparations containing solutions of ammonia, in substances containing less than 10% w/w ammonia, in refrigerators

Ammonium bifluoride P2

Ammonium fluoride P2

Antimony barium tartrate P1; S1

Arecoline-acetarsol P1; S1 except substances containing less than the equivalent of 0.0075% arsenic (P1 only)

Arsanilic acid P1; S1 except substances containing less than the equivalent of 0.0075% arsenic (P1 only); S4 in reagent kits or reagent devices, supplied for medical or veterinary purposes, substances containing less than 0.1% w/w arsanilic acid

Arsenates, except copper arsenates and lead arsenates P1; S1 except substances containing less than the equivalent of 0.0075% arsenic (P1 only)

Arsenic P1; S1 except substances containing less than the equivalent of 0.0075% arsenic (P1 only)

Arsenic, halides of P1; S1 except substances containing less than the equivalent of 0.0075% arsenic (P1 only)

Arsenic, organic compounds of P1; S1 except substances containing less than the equivalent of 0.0075% arsenic (P1 only)

Arsenic, oxides of P1; S1

Arsenic, oxides of P1; S1 except substances containing less than the equivalent of 0.0075% arsenic (P1 only)

Arsenic sulphides P1; S1 except substances containing less than the equivalent of 0.0075% arsenic (P1 only)

Arsenic tribromide P1; S1 except substances containing less than the equivalent of 0.0075% arsenic (P1 only)

Arsenic trichloride P1; S1 except substances containing less than the equivalent of 0.0075% arsenic (P1 only)

Arsenic triiodide P1; S1 except substances containing less than the equivalent of 0.0075% arsenic (P1 only)

Arsenic trioxide P1; S1 except substances containing less than the equivalent of 0.0075% arsenic (P1 only)

Arsenious acid P1; S1 except substances containing less than the equivalent of 0.0075% arsenic (P1 only)

Arsenious anhydride P1; S1 except substances containing less than the equivalent of 0.0075% arsenic (P1 only)

Arsenious iodide P1; S1 except substances containing less than the equivalent of 0.0075% arsenic (P1 only)

Arsenious oxide P1; S1 except substances containing less than the equivalent of 0.0075% arsenic (P1 only)

Arsenites, except calcium arsenites and copper arsenites P1; S1 except substances containing less than the equivalent of 0.0075% arsenic (P1 only)

Arsenobenzene P1; S1 except substances containing less than the equivalent of 0.0075% arsenic (P1 only)

Arsenobenzol P1; S1 except substances containing less than the equivalent of 0.0075% arsenic (P1 only)

Arsenophenolamine P1; S1 except substances containing less than the equivalent of 0.0075% arsenic (P1 only)

Arsphenamine, silver P1; S1 except substances containing less than the equivalent of 0.0075% arsenic (P1 only)

Azinphos-methyl see Phosphorus compounds

B

Barium antimonyltartrate P1; S1

Barium carbonate P2; S1; S4 in witherite, other than finely ground witherite, when bonded to charcoal for case hardening, in sealed smoke generators containing not more than 25% barium carbonate; S5 listed sellers of poisons permitted to sell only for use in preparations for the destruction of rats or mice, but such sales are not restricted to trade or business users

Barium chloride P1; S1; S4 in fire extinguishers containing barium chloride

Barium, salts of, other than barium sulphate P1; S1

Barium silicofluoride P2; S1

Barium sulphide P1; S1

Bismuth glycollylarsanilate P1; S1 except substances containing less than the equivalent of 0.0075% arsenic (P1 only)

Bromomethane P1; S1; S4 in fire extinguishers

C

Calcium arsenate P1; S1 except substances containing less than the equivalent of 0.0075% arsenic (P1 only)

Calcium arsenites P2; S1 except substances containing less than the equivalent of 0.0075% arsenic (P2 only); S5 listed sellers of poisons permitted to sell only for use as agricultural, horticultural and forestal insecticides or fungicides and such sales are restricted to these trade or business users

Calcium cyanide* P1; S1 except substances containing less than the equivalent of 0.1% w/w hydrogen cyanide (P1 only), and except in the case of a sale exempted by Section 4 of the Poisons Act 1972 it is not lawful to sell or supply calcium cyanide

Carbarsone P1; S1 except substances containing less than the equivalent of 0.0075% arsenic (P1 only)

Carbofuran P2; S1; S4 in granular preparations; S5 listed sellers of poisons permitted to sell only if in preparations for use in agriculture, horticulture or forestry and such sales are restricted to these trade or business users

Chloralose P2; S5 listed sellers of poisons permitted to sell only if in preparations intended for indoor use in the destruction of rats or mice and containing not more than 4% w/w chloralose, preparations intended for indoor use in the destruction of rats or mice and containing not more than 8.5% w/w chloralose, where the preparation is contained in a bag or sachet which is itself attached to the inside of a device in which the preparation is intended to be so used and the device contains not more than 3 grams of the preparation, but such sales are not restricted to trade or business users

Chlorfenvinphos see Phosphorus compounds

Chloropicrin P1; S1

Copper acetoarsenite P2; S1 except substances containing less than the equivalent of 0.0075% arsenic (P2 only); S5 listed sellers of poisons permitted to sell only for use as agricultural, horticultural and forestal insecticides or fungicides, and such sales are restricted to these trade or business users

Copper arsenates P2; S1 except substances containing less than the equivalent of 0.0075% arsenic (P2 only); S5 listed sellers of poisons permitted to sell only for use as agricultural, horticultural and forestal insecticides or fungicides and such sales are restricted to these trade or business users

Copper arsenites P2; S1 except substances containing less than the equivalent of 0.0075% arsenic (P2 only); S5 listed sellers of poisons permitted to sell only for use as agricultural, horticultural and forestal insecticides or fungicides and such sales are restricted to these trade or business users

Cyanides (metal) other than ferrocyanides and ferricyanides P1; S1 except substances containing less than the equivalent of 0.1% w/w hydrogen cyanide (P1 only), and except in the case of a sale exempted by Section 4 of the Poisons Act 1972, it is not lawful to sell or supply calcium cyanide, potassium cyanide or sodium cyanide

Cycloheximide P2; S1; S5 listed sellers of poisons permitted to sell only if in preparations for use in forestry, and such sales are restricted to trade or business users

D

Demephion see Phosphorus compounds

Demeton-S-methyl see Phosphorus compounds

Demeton-S-methyl sulphone see Phosphorus compounds

Dialifos see Phosphorus compounds

Dichlorophenarsine hydrochloride P1; S1 except substances containing less than the equivalent of 0.0075% arsenic (P1 only)

Dichlorvos see Phosphorus compounds

Diethylamine acetarsol P1; S1 except substances containing less than the equivalent of 0.0075% arsenic (P1 only)

Diethylamine acetarsone P1; S1 except substances containing less than the equivalent of 0.0075% arsenic (P1 only)

Dinitrocresols (DNOC); their compounds with a metal or a base P2; S1 except winter washes containing not more than the equivalent of 5% dinitrocresols (P2 only); S5 listed sellers of poisons permitted to sell only if in preparations for use in agriculture, horticulture or forestry and except for the above mentioned winter washes, such sales are restricted to these trade or business users

Dinoseb, its compounds with a metal or a base P2; S1; S5 listed sellers of poisons permitted to sell only if in preparations for use in agriculture, horticulture or forestry and such sales are restricted to these trade or business users

Dinoterb, P2; S1; S5 listed sellers of poisons permitted to sell only if in preparations for use in agriculture, horticulture or forestry and such sales are restricted to these trade or business users

Dioxathion see Phosphorus compounds

Diphetarsone P1; S1 except substances containing less than the equivalent of 0.0075% arsenic (P1 only)

Drazoxolon; its salts P2; S1; S4 in treatments on seeds; S5 listed sellers of poisons permitted to sell only if in preparations for use in agriculture, horticulture or forestry and such sales are restricted to these trade or business users

Disulfoton see Phosphorus compounds

E

Endosulfan P2; S1; S5 listed sellers of poisons permitted to sell only if in preparations for use in agriculture, horticulture or forestry, and such sales are restricted to these trade or business users

Endothal, its salts P2; S1; S5 listed sellers of poisons permitted to sell only if in preparations for use in agriculture, horticulture or forestry, and such sales are restricted to these trade or business users

Endrin P2; S1; S5 listed sellers of poisons permitted to sell only if in preparations for use in agriculture, horticulture or forestry, and such sales are restricted to these trade or business users

F

Fentin, compounds of P2; S1; S5 listed sellers of poisons permitted to sell only if in preparations for use in agriculture, horticulture or forestry and such sales are restricted to these trade or business users

Ferric cacodylate P1; S1 except substances containing less than the equivalent of 0.0075% arsenic (P1 only)

Ferrous arsenate P1; S1 except substances containing less than the equivalent of 0.0075% arsenic (P1 only)

Fluoroacetic acid, its salts; fluoroacetamide P1; S1. Rule 12 prohibits sale or supply except in the cases mentioned in Section 1.4.2

Fonofos see Phosphorus compounds

Formaldehyde P2; S4 in substances containing less than 5%w/w formaldehyde, in photographic glazing or hardening solutions

Formic acid P2; S4 in substances containing less than 25% w/w formic acid

H

Hydrochloric acid P2; S4 in substances containing less than 10%w/w hydrochloric acid

Hydrofluoric acid P2

Hydrogen cyanide P1; S1 except substances containing less than 0.15%. w/w hydrogen cyanide (P1 only); S4 in preparations of wild cherry, in reagent kits supplied for medical or veterinary purposes composed of substances which contain less than the equivalent of 0.1% w/w hydrogen cyanide

4-Hydroxy-3-nitrophenyl-arsonic acid P1; S1 except substances containing less than the equivalent of 0.0075% arsenic (P1 only)

L

Lead acetates P1; S4 in substances containing less than the equivalent of 2.5% w/w of elemental lead (Pb)

Lead arsenates P2; S1 except substances containing less than the equivalent of 0.0075% arsenic (P2 only); S5 listed sellers of poisons permitted to sell only for use in agricultural, horticultural or forestal insecticides or fungicides, and such sales are restricted to these trade or business users

Lead arsenite P1; S1 except substances containing less than the equivalent of 0.0075% arsenic (P1 only)

Lead, compounds of, with acids from fixed oils P1; S1

M

Magnesium Phosphide P1; S1

Mecarbam see Phosphorus compounds

Melarsonyl potassium P1; S1 except substances containing less than the equivalent of 0.0075% arsenic (P1 only)

Melarsoprol P1; S1 except substances containing less than the equivalent of 0.0075% arsenic (P1 only)

Mephosfolan see Phosphorus compounds

Mercuric ammonium chloride P1

Mercuric chloride P2; S1 except substances containing less than 1% mercuric chloride (P2 only); S4 in batteries, in treatments on seeds or bulbs; S5 listed sellers of poisons permitted to sell only for use as agricultural, horticultural and forestal fungicides, seed and bulb treatments, insecticides, and such sales are restricted to these trade or business users

Mercuric cyanide P1; S1 except substances containing less than the equivalent of 0.1% w/w hydrogen cyanide (P1 only)

Mercuric cyanide oxides P1

Mercuric iodide P2; S1 except substances containing less than 2% mercuric iodide (P2 only); S4 in treatments on seeds or bulbs; S5 listed sellers of poisons permitted to sell only for use as agricultural, horticultural and forestal fungicides, seed and bulb treatments, and such sales are restricted to these trade or business users

Mercuric nitrates P1; S1 except substances containing less than the equivalent of 3% w/w mercury (P1 only)

Mercuric oxide, red P1

Mercuric oxide, yellow P1; S4 in canker and wound paints (for trees) containing not more than 3% w/w yellow mercuric oxide

Mercuric oxycyanide see Mercuric cyanide oxides

Mercuric sulphodyanide P1

Mercuric thiocyanate P1

Mercury (metal) not in the Poisons List

Mercury, ammoniated P1

Mercury biniodide see Mercuric iodide

Mercury, nitrates of P1; S1 except substances containing less than the equivalent of 3% w/w mercury (P1 only)

Mercury, oleated P1; S1 in aerosols and in substances containing the equivalent of 0.2% w/w mercury or more (otherwise P1 only)

Mercury, organic compounds of, which contain a methyl group directly linked to the mercury atom P1 (for all other organic compounds of mercury see next entry); S1 in aerosols and in substances containing the equivalent of 0.2% w/w mercury or more (otherwise P1 only); S4 in treatments on seeds or bulbs; S5 listed sellers of poisons permitted to sell only for use as agricultural, horticultural and forestal fungicides, seed and bulb treatments, and such sales are restricted to these trade or business users

Mercury, organic compounds of (except those which contain a methyl group directly linked to the mercury atom for these see previous entry) P2; S1 in aerosols and in substances containing the equivalent of 0.2% w/w mercury or more (otherwise P2 only); S4 in treatments on seeds or bulbs; S5 listed sellers of poisons permitted to sell only for use as agricultural, horticultural and forestal fungicides, seeds and bulb treatments and solutions containing not more than 5% w/v phenylmercuric acetate for use in swimming baths, and except for this last mentioned substance, such sales are restricted to trade or business users

Mercury, organic compounds in aerosols (whether P1 or P2) S1; S4 in treatments on seeds or bulbs; S5 (in the case of P2 aerosols only) listed sellers of poisons permitted to sell only for use as agricultural, horticultural and

forestal fungicides, seed and bulb treatments, and such sales are restricted to these trade or business users

Metallic oxalates see Oxalates, metallic

Methidathion see Phosphorus compounds

Methomyl P2; S1; S4 in solid substances containing not more than 1% w/w of methomyl; S5 listed sellers of poisons permitted to sell only if in preparations for use in agriculture, horticulture or forestry and such sales are restricted to these trade or business users

Mevinphos see phosphorus compounds

N

Neoarsphenamine P1; S1 except substances containing less than the equivalent of 0.0075% arsenic (P1 only)

Nicotine, its salts, its quaternary compounds P2; S1; S4 in tobacco, in cigarettes, the paper of a cigarette (excluding any part of that paper forming part of or surrounding a filter), where that paper in each cigarette does not have more than the equivalent of 10 milligrams of nicotine; in aerosol dispensers containing not more than 0.2% w/w nicotine; in other liquid preparations, and solid preparations with a soap base containing not more than 7.5% w/w nicotine (for Nicotine dusts see next entry)

Nicotine dusts P2; S1 except if present in agricultural and horticultural insecticides containing not more than 4% w/w nicotine; label "Poison" in red but no register entry needed

Nitric acid P2; S4 in substances containing less than 20% w/w nitric acid

Nitrobenzene P2; S4 in substances containing less than 0.1% nitrobenzene, in polishes; S5 listed sellers permitted to sell only for use as agricultural, horticultural and forestal insecticides, but such sales are not restricted to these trade or business users

O

Omethoate see Phosphorus compounds

Oxalates, metallic P2; S4 in laundry blue, polishes, cleaning powders or scouring products, containing the equivalent of not more than 10% oxalic acid dihydrate; S5 (except for potassium quadroxalate), listed sellers of poisons permitted to sell for use only as photographic solutions or materials, but such sales are not restricted to trade or business users

Oxalic acid P1; S4 in laundry blue, in polishes, in cleaning powders or scouring products, containing the equivalent of not more than 10% oxalic acid dihydrate

Oxamyl P2; S1; S4 in granular preparations; S5 listed sellers of poisons permitted to sell only if in preparations for use in agriculture, horticulture or forestry and such sales are restricted to these trade or business users

Oxophenarsine hydrochloride P1; S1 except substances containing less than the equivalent of 0.0075% arsenic (P1 only)

Oxophenarsine tartrate P1; S1 except substances containing less than the equivalent of 0.0075% arsenic (P1 only)

Oxydemeton-methyl see Phosphorus compounds

P

Paraquat, salts of P2; S1; S4 preparations in pellet form containing not more than 5% of salts of paraquat (calculated as paraquat ion); S5 listed sellers of poisons permitted to sell only if in preparations for use in agriculture, horticulture or forestry and such sales are restricted to these trade or business users

Parathion see Phosphorus compounds

Phenkapton see Phosphorus compounds

Phenols, substances containing 60% w/w phenols (or more) and compounds of phenol with a metal containing the equivalent of 60% w/w phenol (or more) P1 (for all other phenols see next entry)

Phenols, substances containing less than 60% w/w phenols and compounds of phenol with a metal containing the equivalent of less than 60% w/w phenols P2; S4 creosote obtained from coal tar, in liquid disinfectants and antiseptics containing less than 0.5% phenol and containing less than 5% of other phenols, motor fuel treatments not containing phenol and containing less than 2.5% of other phenols, in reagent kits supplied for medical or veterinary purposes, solid substances containing less than 60% of phenols, tar (coal or wood), crude or refined, in tar oil distillation fractions containing not more than 5% of phenols

Phenylmercuric acetate as for Phenylmercuric salts

Phenylmercuric borate P2; S1 in aerosols and in substances containing the equivalent of 0.2% w/w mercury or more (otherwise P2 only); S4 as for Phenylmercuric salts; S5 listed sellers of poisons permitted to sell only for use as agricultural, horticultural and forestal fungicides, seed and bulb treatments, and such sales are restricted to these trade or business users

Phenylmercuric nitrate P2; S1 in aerosols and in substances containing the equivalent of 0.2% w/w mercury or more (otherwise P2 only); S4 as for Phenylmercuric salts; S5 listed sellers of poisons permitted to sell only for use as agricultural, horticultural and forestal fungicides, seed and bulb treatments, and such sales are restricted to these trade or business users

Phenylmercuric salts P2; S1 in aerosols and in substances containing the equivalent of 0.2% w/w mercury or more (otherwise P2 only) S4 in antiseptic dressings on toothbrushes, in textiles containing not more than 0.01% phenylmercuric salts as a bacteriostat and fungicide; S5 listed sellers of poisons permitted to sell only for use as agricultural, horticultural and forestal fungicides, seed and bulb treatments and solutions containing not more than 5% w/v phenylmercuric acetate for use in swimming baths (when S1 restrictions apply), and except for this last mentioned substance, such sales are restricted to these trade or business users

Phorate see Phosphorus compounds

Phosphamidon see Phosphorus compounds

Phosphoric acid P2; S4 in substances containing phosphoric acid, not being descaling preparations containing more than 50% w/w orthophosphoric acid

Phosphorus compounds:
  Azinphos-methyl
  Demephion
  Demeton-S-methyl
  Demeton-S-methyl sulphone
  Dialifos
  Dioxathion
  Mecarbam
  Mephosfolan
  Methidathion
  Mevinphos
  Omethoate
  Phenkapton
  Phosphamidon
  Quinalphos
  Thiometon
  Vamidothion
P2; S1; S5 listed sellers of poisons permitted to sell only if in preparations for use in agriculture, horticulture or forestry such sales are restricted to these trade or business users
  Disulfoton
  Fonofos
  Parathion
  Phorate
  Thionazin
  Triazophos
P2; Sl; S4 in granular preparations; S5 listed sellers of poisons permitted to sell only if in preparations for use in agriculture, horticulture or forestry, and such sales are restricted to these trade or business users
  Chlorfenvinphos
P2; S1; S4 in treatments on seeds, in granular preparations; S5 listed sellers of poisons permitted to sell only if in preparations for use in agriculture, horticulture or forestry, and such sales are restricted to these trade or business users
  Dichlorvos
P2; S1; S4 in aerosol dispensers containing not more than 1% w/w dichlorvos, in materials impregnated with dichlorvos for slow release, in granular preparations, in ready for use liquid preparations containing not more than 1% w/v of dichlorvos; S5 listed sellers of poisons permitted to sell only if in preparations for use in agriculture, horticulture or forestry, and such sales are restricted to these trade or business users
  Oxydemeton-methyl
P2; S1; S4 in aerosol dispensers containing not more than 0.25% w/w oxydemeton-methyl; S5 listed sellers of poisons permitted to sell only if in preparations for use in agriculture, horticulture or forestry, and such

sales are restricted to these trade or business users
  Pirimiphos-ethyl
P2; S1; S4 in treatments on seeds; S5 listed sellers of poisons permitted to sell only if in preparations for use in agriculture, horticulture or forestry, and such sales are restricted to these trade or business users
Phosphorus, yellow P1
Pirimiphos-ethyl see Phosphorus compounds
Potassium arsenite* P1; S1 except substances containing less than the equivalent of 0.0075% arsenic (P1 only). Rule 12 prohibits sale or supply except in certain circumstances
Potassium cyanide* P1; S1 except substances containing less than the equivalent of 0.1% w/w hydrogen cyanide (P1 only), and except in the case of a sale exempted by Section 4 of the Poisons Act 1972 it is not lawful to sell or supply potassium cyanide
Potassium fluoride P2
Potassium hydroxide P2; S4 in substances containing the equivalent of less than 17% of total caustic alkalinity expressed as potassium hydroxide, in accumulators, in batteries
Potassium oxalate P2; S4 in laundry blue, polishes, cleaning powders or scouring products, containing the equivalent of not more than 10% oxalic acid dihydrate; S5 (except for potassium quadroxalate), listed sellers of poisons permitted to sell for use only as photographic solutions or materials, but such sales are not restricted to trade or business users
Potassium quadroxalate P2; S4 in laundry blue, polishes, cleaning powders or scouring products, containing the equivalent of not more than 10% oxalic acid dihydrate
Potassium tetroxalate see Oxalates, metallic

Q

Quinalphos see Phosphorus compounds

S

Sodium arsanilate P1; S1 except substances containing less than the equivalent of 0.0075% arsenic (P1 only)
Sodium arsenate P1; S1 except substances containing less than the

equivalent of 0.0075% arsenic (P1 only)
Sodium arsenite* P1; S1 except substances containing less than the equivalent of 0.0075% arsenic (P1 only). Rule 12 prohibits sale or supply except in certain circumstances
Sodium cacodylate P1; S1 except substances containing less than the equivalent of 0.0075% arsenic (P1 only)
Sodium cyanide* P1; S1 except substances containing less than the equivalent of 0.1% w/w hydrogen cyanide (P1 only), and except in the case of a sale exempted by Section 4 of the Poisons Act 1972 it is not lawful to sell or supply sodium cyanide
Sodium dimethylarsonate P1; S1 except substances containing less than the equivalent of 0.0075% arsenic (P1 only)
Sodium fluoride P2; S4 in substances containing less than 3% sodium fluoride as a preservative
Sodium glycarsamate P1; S1 except substances containing less than the equivalent of 0.0075% arsenic (P1 only)
Sodium glycollylarsanilate P1; S1 except substances containing less than the equivalent of 0.0075% arsenic (P1 only)
Sodium hydroxide P2; S4 in substances containing the equivalent of less than 12% of total caustic alkalinity expressed as sodium hydroxide
Sodium methylarsinate P1; S1 except substances containing less than the equivalent of 0.0075% arsenic (P1 only)
Sodium metharsinite P1; S1 except substances containing less than the equivalent of 0.0075% arsenic (P1 only)
Sodium nitrite P2; S4 in substances other than preparations containing more than 0.1% sodium nitrite for the destruction of rats or mice
Sodium oxalate P2; S4 in laundry blue, polishes, cleaning powders or scouring products, containing the equivalent of not more than 10% oxalic acid dihydrate; S5 (except for potassium quadroxalate), listed sellers of poisons permitted to sell for use only as photographic solutions of materials, but such sales are not restricted to trade or business users
Sodium silicofluoride P2; S4 in substances containing less than 3% sodium silicofluoride as a preservative

Sodium thioarsenate P1; S1 except substances containing less than the equivalent of 0.0075% arsenic (P1 only)

Strychnine; its salts and quaternary compounds P1; S1 except substances containing less than 0.2% strychnine (P1 only). Rule 12 prohibits sale or supply except in the cases mentioned in Section 1.4.2
Sulpharsobenzene P1; S1 except substances containing less than the equivalent of 0.0075% arsenic (P1 only)
Sulpharsphenamine P1; S1 except substances containing less than the equivalent of 0.0075% arsenic (P1 only)
Sulphuric acid P2; S4 in substances containing less than 15% w/w sulphuric acid, in accumulators, in batteries and sealed containers in which sulphuric acid is packed together with car batteries for use in those batteries; in fire extinguishers

T

Thallium*, salts of P1; S1. Rule 12 prohibits sale or supply except in certain circumstances
Thiofanox P2; S1; S4 in granular preparations; S5 listed sellers of poisons permitted to sell only if in preparations for use in agriculture, horticulture or forestry and such sales are restricted to these trade or business users
Thiometon see Phosphorus compounds
Thionazin see Phosphorus compounds
Triazophos see Phosphorus compounds

V

Vamidothion see Phosphorus compounds

Z

Zinc phosphide* P2; S1 except preparations used for the destruction of rats or mice; S5 listed sellers of poisons permitted to sell only if in preparations for the destruction of rats or mice, but such sales are not restricted to trade or business users. Rule 12 prohibits sale or supply except in certain circumstances

1.6 Chemicals

Chemicals in the UK are classified and labelled under the Chemicals (Hazard Information and Packaging for Supply) Regulations 2002 (also referred to here as CHIP) which came into effect on 24 July 2002. They implement the Dangerous Substances Directive (No 67/548/EEC) and Dangerous Preparations Directive (No 1999/45/EC) that are due to be replaced by the Classification, Labelling and Packaging of Substances and Mixtures (CLP) Regulation over a transitional period which adopts the Globally Harmonised System of Classification and Labelling of Chemicals (GHS) system in the EU.

The CHIP Regulations were amended by the Chemicals (Hazard Information and Packaging for Supply) Regulations 2009 (SI 2009/716) (CHIP4) which came into effect on 6 April 2009. These amendments do not introduce any new duties but consolidate all the amendments to CHIP3 since 2002. However, the existing classification and labelling system of chemicals has not changed.

CHIP4 ensures that UK law is consistent with the new EU Regulation during the transitional period and allows the CLP Regulation to be enforced. It enables suppliers to follow the CLP system as an alternative to CHIP during the transitional period. CHIP4 discontinues the Approved Supply List (ASL) referring instead to Table 3.2 of Annex VI of the CLP Regulation and repeals the requirement of CHIP (except for the enforcement of the CLP Regulation).

The requirements of CHIP and the supply of chemicals are mainly the same with a few changes (eg, advertising and safety data sheets). However suppliers can either use the CHIP or the CLP classification and labelling of chemicals during the transitional period.

Globally Harmonised System of Classification and Labelling of Chemicals (GHS)

The United Nations (UN) created the Globally Harmonised System of Classification and Labelling of Chemicals (GHS) which aims to have the same criteria for classifying chemicals worldwide according to their health, environmental, physical hazards, and hazard communication requirements for labelling and safety data sheets. The GHS is not legally binding, and each country has to introduce separate legislation to adopt it.

Classification, Labelling and Packaging of Substances and Mixtures (CLP) Regulation

The EU has introduced the Classification, Labelling and Packaging of Substances and Mixtures (CLP) Regulation ([EC] No 1272/2008) to adopt the GHS system in the EU. The CLP Regulation came into effect on 20 January 2009, subject to a transitional period, and is directly-acting in all Member States. This will replace the Dangerous Substances Directive, the Dangerous Preparations Directive and CHIP over a transitional period until 1 June 2015 when the Regulation will be fully in force

The transitional arrangements are:

Substances

20 January 2009 to 1 December 2010 Suppliers must classify substances according to CHIP, and may continue to label and package them according to regulations 6 to 11 of CHIP. However, they may as an alternative choose to classify, label and package substances according to CLP. In this case, they must in addition continue to classify under regulation 4 of CHIP, but the requirements on labelling and packaging in regulations 6 to 11 of CHIP no longer apply.

1 December 2010 to 1 June 2015 Suppliers must classify substances according to both CHIP and CLP. They must label and package according to CLP.

1 June 2015 onwards Suppliers must classify, label and package according to CLP.

Preparations

20 January 2009 to 1 June 2015 Suppliers must classify preparations according to CHIP, and may continue to label and package them according to regulations 6 to 11 of CHIP. However they may as an alternative choose to classify, label and package mixtures according to CLP. In this case, they must in addition continue to classify under regulation 4 of CHIP, but the requirements on labelling and packaging in regulations 6 to 11 of CHIP no longer apply.

1 June 2015 onwards Suppliers must classify, label and package according to CLP.

Chemicals (Hazard Information and Packaging for Supply) Regulations 2002 (CHIP)

CHIP does not apply to certain chemicals such as those that are intended for use as medicinal products, veterinary products, investigational medicinal products, Controlled Drugs, cosmetic products, substances or preparations which are in the form of waste to which the Waste Management Licensing Regulations 1994, the Special Waste Regulations 1996, the Hazardous Waste (Wales) Regulations 2005 or the Hazardous Waste (England and Wales) Regulations 2005 apply, food, animal feedingstuffs, radioactive substances or preparations, or medical devices. CHIP also does not apply to a substance or preparation which is a sample taken by an enforcement authority.

Because of the complex nature of CHIP, the information provided below is not comprehensive. Pharmacists involved in the supply, labelling or packaging of chemicals are advised to first consult the Health and Safety Executive (HSE) published guidance (*www.hse.gov.uk/chip/issues.htm*). For additional guidance, the HSE can be contacted on 0845 345 0055 (e-mail: *hse.infoline@connaught.plc.uk*).

The main objectives of CHIP are:
(a) the identification of harmful properties of chemicals (hazards) and the communication of this information to users by means of labels; and
(b) to cover hazards to health, safety and the environment, and use of chemicals both in the home and at work.

CHIP requires suppliers of dangerous substances and dangerous preparations to:
(a) identify the hazards (or dangers) of dangerous substances and dangerous preparations they supply (this process is called classification);
(b) give information about those hazards to the persons they supply - both on the label and methods of marking, with particular labelling requirements for certain preparations;

(c) package the chemicals safely, including child resistant fastenings, tactile warning devices and other consumer protection measures; and

(d) retain data for dangerous preparations (this will not apply on or after 1 June 2018).

These requirements are known as the supply requirements. The carriage or transportation of chemicals is not the same as supply. However, similar duties are placed on persons who transport chemicals by road or by rail.

1.6.1 Supply requirements

Classification of dangerous substances and dangerous preparations

The fundamental requirement of CHIP is to assess whether a particular chemical is hazardous (dangerous) or not. If it is, then it must be classified by precise identification of the hazard by assigning a category of danger (eg, "Toxic"), and a description of the hazard by allocation of a risk phrase (eg, "Harmful in contact with skin").

The main categories of danger can be subdivided into substances and preparations dangerous because of their:
- Physicochemical properties - explosive, oxidising, extremely flammable, highly flammable and flammable.
- Health effects - very toxic, toxic, harmful, corrosive, irritant, sensitising, carcinogenic, mutagenic, toxic for reproduction.
- Environmental effects.

CHIP makes it an offence to supply a dangerous chemical before it is classified. It is important that this process is carried out correctly as failure to do so could lead to errors being made in other requirements of CHIP (ie, labelling, SDS preparation and packaging). When chemicals are supplied to a pharmacy they should already have been properly classified by that supplier. If this is the case, the pharmacist could use this classification provided he is satisfied that it is correct and the competence of the supplier is known to him.

From 1 June 2015 all dangerous substances and dangerous preparations must be classified in accordance with the requirements of the CLP Regulation.

CHIP requires a supplier to exercise "all due diligence" in complying with its legal requirements. This means that if a pharmacist uses the classification assigned by a manufacturer or supplier higher up the supply chain, then he may wish to make appropriate enquiries about the classification to ensure accuracy. If suppliers are known to the pharmacist and there is confidence in their ability, only simple checks may be necessary. For example, using a common sense check, if an acid commonly known to cause burns has not been classified as being corrosive, enquiries should be made with the supplier or another person the pharmacist knows to be competent in this area.

CHIP makes suppliers of chemicals responsible for the classification of a chemical right down the supply chain and it must be remembered that pharmacists will be the final supplier.

Labelling

CHIP sets down requirements for the information which has to be provided to persons when they are supplied with dangerous substances and dangerous preparations on the labels.

Safety Data Sheet requirements are no longer a part of CHIP. CHIP4 refers to Annexe 31 of REACH, which signposts the provisions for SDSs.

For supplies to domestic users, the CHIP label will contain all the information required to be given under CHIP. There may be further specific labelling requirements determined by other regulations relating to other aspects of chemical supply such as transport and general product safety, etc. However, with regard to CHIP, chemicals obtained by a pharmacist in their original packs should be already labelled up to comply with CHIP. Where the chemicals are to be decanted from bulk into smaller packages appropriate for the contents, these packages must be correctly labelled in accordance with CHIP. In any case, as the supplier of the product the pharmacist will be responsible for the labelling, and it is advisable to make checks with all "due diligence". As a guide to the labelling requirements in relation to CHIP, *see* below. A common sense check would also be beneficial.

Labels and symbols must be clearly and indelibly marked, and securely fixed to the package with its entire surface in contact with it and the label itself must be placed so that it may be read horizontally when the package is set down. The colour and nature of the marking must be such that any symbol and the wording stand out clearly from the background and the wording must be of such size and spacing as to be easily read. The regulations also specify the minimum sizes of label depending on the quantity supplied (for quantities less than 3 litres, at least 52mm x 74mm, if possible) and where the label should be placed (on outer packaging as well as on the container).

CHIP specifies exactly what must appear on the label of a dangerous substance or dangerous preparation. This is partially dependent on whether it is a substance (usually a single chemical) or preparation (in general terms, a mixture of substances) being labelled. It is also dependent on how it has been classified under CHIP.

The particulars required for labelling in relation to a dangerous substance supplied in a package are:

(a) the name, full address and telephone number of a person in an EEA State who is responsible for supplying the substance, including the pharmacist, whether he be its manufacturer, importer or distributor;

(b) the name of the substance, being:

(i) where the substance appears in Table 3.2 of part 3 of Annex VI of the CLP Regulation, the name or one of the names listed therein for that substance; or

(ii) where the substance does not appear in Table 3.2 of part 3 of Annex VI of the CLP Regulation, an internationally recognised name; and

(c) the following particulars ascertained in accordance with Part I of Schedule 4, namely

(i) any indications of danger together with corresponding symbols;

(ii) the risk phrases, set out in full;

(iii) the safety phrases, set out in full; and

(iv) any EC number and, in the case of a substance which is listed in Table 3.2 of part 3 of Annex VI of the CLP Regulation, the words "EC label".

The particulars required for labelling in relation to a dangerous preparation supplied in a package are:

(a) the name, full address and telephone number of a person in an EEA State who is responsible for supplying the preparation, including the pharmacist, whether that person be its manufacturer, importer or distributor;

(b) the trade name or other designation of the preparation; and

(c) the following particulars ascertained in accordance with Part I of Schedule 4, namely

(i) identification of the constituents of the preparation which result in it being classified as a dangerous preparation,

(ii) any indications of danger together with corresponding symbols,

(iii) the risk phrases, set out in full,

(iv) the safety phrases, set out in full,

(v) in the case of a preparation intended for sale to the general public, the nominal quantity (nominal mass or nominal volume).

Indications such as "non-toxic", "non-harmful", "non-polluting", "ecological" or any other statement indicating that the dangerous substance or preparation is not dangerous or that is likely to lead to underestimation of the dangers of the dangerous substance or dangerous preparation must not appear on the package.

Where the package contains such small quantities of that substance or preparation that there is no foreseeable risk, under conditions of supply, use and disposal, arising from that hazardous property to persons handling that substance or preparation or to other persons, the packaging of a dangerous substance or dangerous preparation classified in one or more of the categories of danger harmful, extremely flammable, highly flammable, flammable, irritant or oxidising are not required to be labelled in respect of that hazardous property.

Where the package in which a dangerous substance is supplied does not contain more than 125 millilitres of that substance the risk phrases and safety phrases do not have to be shown if the dangerous substance is classified only in one or more of these categories of danger:

(a) highly flammable, flammable, oxidising or irritant; or

(b) harmful, provided the dangerous substance is not sold to the general public.

Where the package in which a dangerous preparation is supplied does not contain more than 125 millilitres of that preparation:

(a) the risk phrases and safety phrases do not have to be shown if the dangerous preparation is classified only in one or more of these categories of danger:

(i) irritant (except those assigned the risk phrase R41);

(ii) dangerous for the environment and assigned the N symbol;

(iii) oxidising; or

(iv) highly flammable; and

(b) the safety phrases need not be shown if the dangerous preparation is classified only in one or more of these categories of danger:

(i) flammable; or

(ii) dangerous for the environment and not assigned the N symbol.

Dangerous preparations to be supplied to the general public

The label on the packaging of dangerous preparations intended to be supplied to the general public must in addition to the relevant safety advice, bear the relevant safety phrase S1 (*Keep locked up*), S2 (*Keep out of reach of children*), S45 (*In case of accident or if you feel unwell seek medical advice immediately [show the label where possible]*) or S46 (*If swallowed, seek medical advice immediately and show the container or label*), in accordance with the approved classification and labelling guide. When the dangerous preparations are classified as very toxic, toxic or corrosive and where it is physically impossible to give the information on the package itself, packages containing such preparations must be accompanied by precise and easily understandable instructions for use including, where appropriate, instructions for the destruction of the empty package.

Pharmacists involved in preparing labels for dangerous substances and dangerous preparations should refer to CHIP and HSE guidance and also to Table 3.2 in Annex VI of the CLP Regulation.

Packaging

It is an offence to supply a dangerous chemical, unless it is in a suitable package. The packaging and fastenings should be strong and solid throughout to ensure that they will not loosen when subjected to the stresses and strains of normal handling. The container must not be adversely affected by the chemical or react with the chemical to form other dangerous chemicals. Where the package is fitted with a replaceable closure its integrity must remain with repeated use. Except where a special safety device has been fitted to make the receptacle closable, the package should be designed and constructed so that its contents cannot escape.

There is also a requirement for certain chemicals to be packaged with a child-resistant fastening (CRF), although they are not required if it can be shown that a child cannot gain access to the chemical without the help of a tool. CRFs must be used for chemicals which are sold to the public containing either:

(i) products classified as "toxic", "very toxic" or "corrosive";

(ii) methanol (3% or more by weight);

(iii) dichloromethane (1% or more by weight); or

(iv) substances which have been assigned the risk phrase (R65) in Table 3.2 of part 3 of Annex VI of the CLP Regulation, which states, "Harmful: may cause lung damage if swallowed" (except where the chemical is supplied in an aerosol dispenser or a container fitted with a sealed spray attachment);

(v) substances and preparations which are assigned the risk phrase R65 and are classified and labelled according to the approved classification and labelling guide, except where such a substance or preparation is supplied in an aerosol dispenser or a container fitted with a sealed spray attachment.

Chemicals sold to the public which are labelled "toxic", "very toxic", "corrosive", "harmful", "extremely flammable" or "highly flammable" must also have a tactile warning device (normally a small raised triangle) to alert the blind and partially sighted that they are handling a dangerous product. This does not apply to an aerosol dispenser which is classified and labelled only with the indication of danger "extremely flammable" or "highly flammable".

Pharmacists must check that packaging complies with the above before supplying chemicals to the public. It is important to remember the need for "due diligence" to be exercised and when there is a legal obligation to supply a SDS.

Where a substance or preparation has been classified, labelled and packaged in accordance with the CLP Regulation, the packaging or dangerous substances, dangerous preparations and certain other preparations, labelling and child resistant fastening, tactile warning devices and other consumer protection measures as detailed above do not apply to that substance (from 1 December 2010) or preparation (from 1 June 2015).

Advertising

The provisions for advertisements have been removed from CHIP and it is now the CLP Regulation which applies. The CLP Regulation requires all advertisements for a substance classified as hazardous to mention the hazard classes and hazard categories concerned. Any advertisement for a mixture classified as hazardous or covered by Article 25(6) which allows a member of the public to conclude a contract to purchase a dangerous chemical before they have seen the label relating to that chemical (eg, via mail order or the internet), must mention the type or types of hazard indicated on the label. The term "advertisement" does not include a price list and therefore this is unlikely to affect the majority of pharmacists.

Registration, Evaluation, Authorisation and restriction of Chemicals (REACH)

REACH is the European regulation on the Registration, Evaluation, Authorisation and restriction of Chemicals (REACH) Regulation ([EC] No 1907/2006), which came into effect on 1 June 2007. The regulations run in parallel to the European CLP regulations. They have direct legal impact within the EU, however, the enforcement is up to the individual Member State. The REACH Enforcement Regulations 2008 apply to the United Kingdom and provide for the enforcement of REACH.

REACH covers the registration, pre-registration, evaluation, authorisation, restrictions, classification and labelling and information provision of chemicals.

For further guidance pharmacists are advised to contact *www.hse.gov.uk/reach* or *ukreachca@hse.gsi.gov.uk*

Substances of Very High Concern (SVHC)

REACH contains a list of substances of very high concern, the registration and use of which is subject to further restrictions including authorisation and the provision of information. SVHCs are substances which are classified as:
- carcinogenic, mutagenic or toxic for reproduction (CMR) category 1 or 2;
- persistent, bio-accumulative and toxic (PBT;
- very persistent and very bio-accumulative (vPvB)
- substances not classified as above but where there is scientific evidence of probable serious effects to human health or the environment.

Substances meeting the above criteria may be placed on the Candidate List (published by ECHA) and the Annex XIV List. It is possible that some substances that meet the criteria will not appear on either list.

Pharmacists supplying any substance should check with the HSE whether it is a SVHC and for further guidance refer to *www.hse.gov.uk/reach/svhc.pdf*

Safety data sheets for substances and preparations (SDS)

The rules relating to Safety Data Sheets (SDS) are now to be found in the REACH regulations. They were previously covered in the CHIP regulations.

The supplier of a substance or a preparation must provide the recipient with a SDS compiled in accordance with Annex 2 where the substance or preparation is:
- classified;
- a PBT or vPvB;
- a SVHC or on the Candidate list; or
- hazardous as it contains at least one substance in an individual concentration less than or equal to: 1% by weight for non-gaseous preparations; 0.2% by volume for gaseous

preparations; or less than or equal to: 0.1% by weight for non-gaseous preparations which is a PBT or vPvB in accordance with specified criteria; or
- there are workplace exposure criteria.

A SDS does not need to be provided where dangerous substances or preparations are sold to the general public where sufficient information is given to enable the user to take measures which are necessary for the protection of health and safety and the environment, unless requested by a downstream user or distributor.

The headings under which information must be provided are listed below together with a general description of the information which may be found under the heading. These descriptions are not all encompassing. For further information contact the HSE.

(1) *Identification of the substance/preparation and company/undertaking* The name of the substance/preparation should be identical to the name used on the label. It should indicate the intended or recommended uses of the substance/preparation. The name, full address, telephone number and email address of the competent person responsible for the SDS. Where this person is not in the Member State where the substance or preparation is placed on the market, the full address and telephone number for the person responsible in that member state. An emergency telephone number of the company and/or relevant advisory body should be added if access to advice in the event of an emergency is not available on the number already given and specify if the phone number is available only during office hours.

(2) *Hazards identification* The classification of the substance or preparation under the classification rules should be stated here. The most important hazards of the substance or preparation to man and the environment should be stated.

(3) *Composition/information on ingredients* Sufficient information must be given to enable the recipient to readily identify the hazards of the components of the preparation. The hazards of the preparation itself are listed in (2).

(4) *First aid measures* The information should state whether immediate medical attention or professional assistance by a doctor is needed or advisable. The information should be brief and easy to understand by the victim, bystanders and first aiders. Subheadings should be given for different routes of exposure, eg, skin and eye contact, inhalation or ingestion. If immediate medical attention or if a specific form of treatment is required, that should be stated.

(5) *Fire fighting measures* Suitable extinguishing media should be stated, together with details of extinguishing media which are not safe to be used, and details of special protective equipment for fire fighters. Exposure hazards arising from the substance or preparation, combustion products and resulting gases should be stated.

(6) *Accidental release measures* Information should be provided on personal precautions, eg,"removal of ignition sources", "provision for sufficient ventilation/respiratory protection", environmental precautions, eg, "keep away from drains, surface and ground water and soil", and methods of cleaning up, eg,"use of absorbent material" "sand". Consideration should also be given to using statements such as "Never use with..." or "Neutralise with...."

(7) *Handling and storage* This information relates to the protection of human health, safety and the environment and assist the employer in implementing suitable working procedures and organizational measures. Precautions necessary for safe handling,

such as measures to prevent dust generation, fire, etc, and conditions for storage, eg, ventilation, temperature, light and humidity should also be stated. For end products designed for specific use(s), recommendations must refer to the identified use, with reference to industry/sector specific approved guidance.

(8) *Exposure control and personal protection* This should include the full range of precautionary measures to be taken during use to minimise worker and environmental exposure. It should specify where necessary the type of equipment to afford suitable protection, eg respiratory, eye, skin and hand protection.

(9) *Physical and chemical properties* The following information should be provided: Appearance, eg, white solid; odour, if perceptible a brief description; pH; boiling point/melting range; flash point; flammability (solid, gas); explosive properties; oxidising properties; vapour pressure; relative density; solubility (water or fat); partition coefficient; viscosity; vapour density; evaporation rate; other important safety parameters of the product.

(10) *Stability and reactivity* State the stability of the substance or preparation and the possibility of hazardous reactions occurring under certain conditions of use and also if released into the environment, ie, conditions to avoid (temperature, pressure, shock, etc); materials to avoid (water, air, etc); hazardous materials produced in dangerous amounts on decomposition., addressing specifically the need for and the presence of stabilizers; the possibility of a hazardous exothermic reaction; safety significance, if any, of a change in physical appearance of the substance or preparation, hazardous decomposition products, if any, formed upon contact with water;and the possibility of degradation to unstable products.

(11) *Toxicological information* Provide a concise but complete and comprehensive description of the toxicological effects resulting from contact with the substance or preparation. Known delayed and immediate and chronic effects from short and long term exposure should be stated. Information on different routes of exposure and a description of the symptoms related to the physical, chemical and toxicological characteristics should be given.

(12) *Ecological information* An assessment should be given of the possible effects on the environment in relation to such factors as ecotoxicity, mobility, persistence and degradability, bioaccumulative potential, results of a persistent, bioaccumulative and toxic assessment (PBT) and any other adverse effects.

(13) *Disposal considerations* Information should be provided on the dangers associated with disposal. Safety and appropriate methods of disposal should be given together with references to appropriate legislation.

(14) *Transport information* Details of special precautions relating to transport or conveyance, either within or outside premises.

(15) *Regulatory information* The health, safety and environmental information on the label required by CHIP should be given. Reference to the Control of Substances Hazardous to Health Regulations 2002, as amended (COSHH), may also be made.

(16) *Other information* Advice on other information which may be of importance for health and safety of the user and for the protection of the environment, eg, training advice, recommended restrictions on use, further information, ie, written references and /or technical contact point, sources of key data used to compile the safety data sheet. A list of the relevant R-phrases referred to under headings (2) and (3) above, the full text of which must be written out in full, must appear under this heading on the SDS. A revised SDS should clearly indicate the information which has been added, deleted or revised (unless this has been indicated elsewhere).

Pharmacists may be able to use the SDSs provided by their supplier, who is responsible for the accuracy of the SDS. The pharmacist may wish to make the following "due diligence" checks: that
(i) all the safety headings (as detailed above) are present;
(ii) the SDS is comparable with those for similar products;
(iii) the sections dealing with safe use/storage, etc, are adequate for the intended applications of the pharmacy's customers; and
(iv) the SDS covers foreseeable eventualities.

Substances restricted to professional users

Certain substances specified in Annex XVII of REACH, in addition to the classification, packaging and labelling requirements of dangerous substances and preparations must contain the safety labelling phrase, legible and indelibly marked, 'Restricted to professional users'. The substances to which this restriction applies are those classified as "carcinogenic", "mutagenic", or "toxic to reproduction" and are listed as categories 1 or 2. (These products are not normally sold through pharmacies to the general public.)

A SDS and any updated version should be provided free of charge on paper or electronically, and be dated, in an official language of the Member State where the substance or preparation is placed on the market. The suppliers must update the SDS as soon as new information on risks and hazards becomes available or there are changes to the authorisation or restrictions imposed. The new, dated version of the information, identified as "Revision: (date)", including the registration number, must be supplied to all persons who have received the substance or preparation within the preceding 12 months. For this reason it would be wise to keep a record of sales of such products.

Pharmacists are advised to check the HSE website for further details on Safety Data Sheets: *www.hse.gov.uk/reach/ resources/reachsds.pdf*

Chloroform and certain other halogenated hydrocarbons

Chloroform and certain other halogenated hydrocarbons (including carbon tetrachloride) are listed in Annex XVII of REACH, with specific restrictions on their use (and also in Schedule 2 COSHH). Chloroform and carbon tetrachloride must not be used in concentrations equal to or greater than 0.1% by weight, in substances and preparations placed on the market, for sale to the general public, and/or in diffusive applications such as in surface cleaning and cleaning of fabrics. In addition to the classification, packaging and labelling requirements of dangerous substances and preparations the packaging of such substances and preparations containing them in concentrations equal to or greater than 0.1% must be legible and indelibly marked with: "For use in industrial installations only". This does not however apply to medicinal, veterinary products or cosmetic products as defined in the Directives.

1.7 Denatured alcohol

Denatured alcohol is alcohol that has been made unsuitable for drinking by the addition of denaturants.

Law affecting denatured alcohol

In England and Wales Section 77 of the Alcoholic Liquor Duties Act 1979 gives HM Revenue and Customs the power to make regulations laying down requirements for the manufacture, supply and use of denatured alcohol. Section 78 of the Act prescribes penalties for offences in connection with denatured alcohol. The requirements are set out in the Denatured Alcohol Regulations 2005 (SI 2005/1524) which revoked the Methylated Spirits Regulations 1987 and The Iso-Propyl Alcohol Regulations 1927 and further implements Articles 27 (1)(a) and (b) of Council Directive 92/83/EEC.

In Scotland The Deregulated Methylated Spirits (Sale by Retail) (Scotland) Order 1998 removed some requirements of the Methylated Spirits (Sale by Retail)(Scotland)Act 1937.

NB: On 1 September 2009 the Licensing (Scotland) Act 2005 will revoke the Methylated Spirits (Sale by Retail) (Scotland) Act 1937 and Section 26 of the Revenue Act 1889. The Denatured Alcohol Regulations 2005 also apply in Scotland. Therefore, the Denatured Alcohol Regulations 2005 cover the whole of the United Kingdom.

1.7.1 Type of denatured alcohol

There are three approved classes of denatured alcohol in the UK: completely denatured alcohol; industrial denatured alcohol; and trade specific denatured alcohol, although most pharmacists will deal only with the first two.

(a) Completely denatured alcohol (CDA) (Formerly known as Mineralised Methylated Spirits - MMS)

Completely denatured alcohol is the most heavily denatured alcohol. CDA is suitable for heating, lighting, cleaning and general domestic use. Pharmacists can obtain CDA from wholesalers in any quantity.
· CDA is a mixture of 90 parts by volume of alcohol, 9.5 parts by volume of wood naphtha or a substitute for wood naphtha and 0.5 parts by volume of crude pyridine, to each 1000 litres of the mixture of which is added 3.75 litres mineral naphtha (petroleum oil) and 1.5g of synthetic organic dyestuff (methyl violet). A full list of formulations of CDA used in EU Member States can be found in HM Customs and Excise Notice 473 (July 2005), available from HM Revenue and Customs National Advice Service (0845 010 9000).

(b) Industrial denatured alcohol (IDA) (Formerly known as Industrial Methylated Spirits - IMS)

Industrial denatured alcohol is the grade of denatured alcohol designed for industrial use. IDA is usually approved for use in industrial, scientific and external medical applications. A full list of authorised uses can be found in HM Customs and Excise Notice 473 (July 2005). To use IDA in a way not on the approved list, the National Registration Unit should be contacted with the details of the proposed use. They may approve its use as an alternative.

IDA consists of 95 parts by volume of alcohol and 5 parts by volume of wood naphtha, or a substitute for wood naphtha. Where a substitute for wood naphtha is used, the volume mixed with every 95 parts of alcohol may be less than 5 parts depending on: (i) the proportion of the marker in the resulting mixture, and (ii) the resulting mixture contains the other substances that the Commissioners approved when they approved the substitute for wood naphtha in the proportions that they specify.

Denatured alcohol that is not CDA, which has been made in another Member State, in accordance with a CDA formulation of that Member State and has been incorporated into a product that is not for human consumption, must be accepted in the UK free of duty.

(c) Trade specific denatured alcohol (TSDA) (includes Denatured Ethanol B - DEB)

Trade specific denatured alcohol formulations are types of denatured alcohol approved to meet specific trade needs. TSDA can only be obtained by persons specifically authorised by HM Revenue and Customs to receive them. TSDA can only be used in certain formulations for specific approved purposes. For example, the TDSA formulation for the former Denatured Ethanol B (DEB) - Tertiary Butyl Alcohol 0.1% vol and Denatonium benzoate added to the resulting mixture in the proportion of 10 micrograms per millilitre; is approved for use in the manufacture of skin preparations (perfumes, toiletries, cosmetics and external medical applications such as medicated creams and ointments), printing ink and as a biocide reagent.

There is a list of formulations of, and uses for, TSDA, which have been approved by the Commissioners of HM Revenue and Customs. This list can be found in HM Customs and Excise Notice 473 (July 2005). To use a TSDA in a way that is not on the approved list, the National Registration Unit should be contacted with the details of the proposed use. They may approve its use as an alternative.

To use a new formulation of TSDA, the National Registration Unit should be contacted in writing with the following details:
(i) the proposed TSDA formulation;
(ii) the use; and
(iii) the reason why CDA, IDA and the approved TSDA formulations would be unsuitable for the intended use.

1.7.2 Application for authority to receive IDA or TSDA

Pharmacists must be authorised by HM Revenue and Customs to receive IDA or TDSA (except where this is contained in a ready prepared medicinal product containing the denatured alcohol). In order to obtain authority to receive IDA or TSDA, an application has to be made to HM Revenue and Customs National Registration Unit (NRU). The application form can be found at the back of HM Customs and Excise Notice 473 (July, 2005) (see Figure 1.2). If approved, the Commissioners may authorise a person in writing to receive IDA or TSDA, stating what they are entitled to receive, what it can be used for, and the conditions that must be observed (see 1.7.4 below). The authority and conditions can be changed or

Application for authorisation to receive and use IDA or TSDA

Application for Authority to receive Industrial Denatured Alcohol/Trade Specific Denatured Alcohol*

Part A *I/We (name of company, partnership, proprietor, as appropriate) apply for authority to receive IDA/TSDA* formulation(s)
....
....
....

for use at (address of premises):
....
....
....

Type of business/activity...
VAT Registration Number...

Part B The *IDA/TSDA is to be used for the following purpose(s):
....
....

Part C (only for requests to use TSDA for a use not previously approved)
CDA/IDA is unsuitable because
....
....

Part D *My/Our estimated annual requirement is:
*Industrial Denatured Alcohol.......................................litres
*Trade Specific Denatured Alcohol..............................litres
Signature...
Full name...
Status...
(proprietor, partner, director, company secretary etc.)
Date...
Telephone Number...
Fax Number..
E-mail address..

*Delete as necessary

Figure 1.2. Application for authorisation to receive and use IDA or TSDA

revoked by HM Revenue and Customs at any time, but authorised users must comply with any conditions or restrictions imposed by the Commissioners.

IDA and TSDA may be supplied to persons specifically authorised by HM Revenue and Customs to receive it. Users must furnish the pharmacist (the supplier) with a copy of their authorisation before they may receive IDA or TSDA. These statements are valid indefinitely, but the supplier must notify HM Revenue and Customs of any changes to its use or formulation. Medical and veterinary practitioners do not need to be authorised to obtain IDA from an authorised pharmacist against a written order or prescription.

1.7.3 Supply of denatured alcohol by authorised users

Authorised users may supply denatured alcohol or articles containing denatured alcohol as follows:

CDA

England and Wales There are no restrictions on the quantity of CDA that can be supplied. There are also no conditions on its use.
Scotland No more than four gallons of CDA may be sold to any person unless it is for resale. It is an offence to knowingly sell CDA or surgical spirits to a person aged under 14, otherwise

than on a prescription. The restriction on the sale of CDA between the hours of 10pm on Saturday and 8am on the following Monday applies in Scotland only. This restriction also applies to the supply on a prescription and on a written request.

NB: From 1 September 2009, the restrictions in Scotland will no longer apply, and the sale will be the same as for England and Wales.

CDA may be received free of duty if the denatured alcohol made in a Member State is in accordance with a formulation of that Member State, or it is made as near as possible in accordance with the UK CDA formulation or a CDA formulation of another Member State. The acceptability of the formulation should be checked with the National Advice Service (See C& E Notice 473 July 2005). CDA may be imported directly to your premises from a Member State if the CDA is denatured in accordance with a CDA formulation of a Member State, otherwise it has to be consigned to an excise warehouse with the relevant approval to hold such goods.

IDA and TSDA

IDA and TSDA can only be supplied to other producers or distributors who are authorised by HM Revenue and Customs as users. The pharmacist must hold a copy of that user's authorisation to receive and use IDA/TSDA and must not supply it for any other use. The authorisation may cover any number of consignments of IDA or TSDA supplied. Supply of IDA or TSDA must not be made without holding a copy of the user's authorisation or for a use that is not included in the user's authorisation.

An authorised user may supply IDA/TSDA in quantities of less than 20 litres at any one time to another authorised user provided the supplier's authority does not specifically restrict this.

Only licensed, or authorised producers or distributors are permitted to supply denatured alcohol in quantities of greater than 20 litres (wholesale quantities).

Supply of IDA by a pharmacist

Users must furnish the pharmacist (supplier) with a copy of the authorisation before they may receive IDA.

When a pharmacist supplies IDA for "medical use" on a prescription or order of a medical or veterinary practitioner, a copy of the person's authorisation to receive and use denatured alcohol is not needed. Where the IDA is not intended for medical use, it can only be supplied in the quantity and for the purpose stated in the authoirsation from HM Revenue and Customs. An "order" is a request to be supplied with a specific quantity of denatured alcohol. There is no set format for an order, but should include the quantity and class of denatured alcohol required.

The definitions for the above section are:
"Pharmacist" has the meaning given in section 132(1) of the Medicines Act 1968;
"Medical or veterinary practitioner" means a person entitled by law to provide medical or veterinary services in the United Kingdom (HM Revenue and Customs have confirmed that this does include a dentist, nurse and chiropodist);
"Medical use" means any medical, veterinary, surgical or dental purpose other than administration internally.

Isle of Man

IDA/TSDA can be supplied to users in the Isle of Man who are authorised to receive that IDA/TSDA in accordance with the laws of the Isle of Man. The user in the Isle of Man must supply the pharmacist with a written statement showing:
(i) the date the user was authorised to receive the denatured alcohol of the formulation requested;
(ii) the intended use(s) for that denatured alcohol;
(iii) any conditions or restrictions imposed by his authorisation to receive denatured alcohol; and
(iv) the uses to which he is entitled to put the received denatured alcohol.

Do I need to "make entry" of premises?

If stocks of denatured alcohol are held by the pharmacist, an entry of the premises will need to be made before beginning to hold denatured alcohol (unless the premises are approved as an excise warehouse). To do this, Form EX 103 for a sole trader or partnership, or Form EX 103A for an incorporated company, should be completed.

Each continuation sheet to the EX 103(A) must be signed and dated. To obtain copies of these forms or help in completing them, the HM Revenue and Customs National Advice Service should be contacted.

1.7.4 Conditions of use of IDA and TSDA

The authority to receive denatured alcohol states what is authorised to be received, what it can be used for and the conditions that must be observed. The authority will be reviewed from time to time and the conditions may be varied or the authorisation revoked. The user must notify the National Registration Unit of any changes and may not receive any further supplies of IDA or TSDA until the National Registration Unit has been notified.

The main conditions are:
(a) *Storage* All stocks of IDA and TSDA must be kept under lock and key and under the pharmacist's control or that of a responsible person appointed by him.
(b) *Use* IDA and TSDA can be used only as set out in the letter of authority and all conditions must be complied with.
(c) *Supply* Suppliers can only distribute the formulations of denatured alcohol that are approved in the UK. For supply, the following must be kept for inspection by the local HM Revenue and Customs officer:
(i) written statements from authorised users;
(ii) written signed orders from medical practitioners.
These records are not required for a supply made against a prescription.
(d) *Closing or transfer of business* If the business is discontinued while holding stocks of denatured alcohol, the authority to hold stocks of denatured alcohol is revoked, and the National Advice Service should be contacted to arrange how the stocks must be disposed of and within what time period. Once all stocks are disposed of, the National Registration Unit must be contacted to cancel the licence or the authority. If the discontinuation of the business is caused by the death of a producer or distributor or other person, their personal representative must contact the National Advice Service.

Records

Authorised persons must keep and preserve records relating to their use of denatured alcohol as specified by the Commissioners, and must also comply with any conditions or restrictions imposed by them.

On receipt of IDA or TSDA the following must be kept:
- a record of the amount of denatured alcohol received; and
- one copy of the supplier's dispatch document signed as a receipt and returned to the supplier, and the other copy retained on the premises for records. These will need to be shown to the HM Revenue and Customs officer when the premises are visited.

Distribution

For a pharmacist to be considered a distributor, the following criteria would need to be met:
(a) holds an excise licence for the purpose of Section 75 of the Act;
(b) does not denature alcohol at any premises on which denatured alcohol is kept;
(c) deals or intends to deal wholesale in denatured alcohol.

Only the denatured alcohols which are detailed on the licence may be distributed. To apply for a licence the application form L5 should be sent to the National Registration Unit with a letter stating which denatured alcohol will be distributed. In the "specified trade" section on the licence application, "distributor" must be entered. The licence may cover more than one set of premises and any proposed changes must be notified to the NRU. If stocks of denatured alcohol are held, an authorisation from HM Revenue and Customs, as a user in order to receive denatured alcohol from producers and other distributors, would be required.

An entry of premises must be made where stocks of denatured alcohol are held, and this must be done before holding the stock. An entry of premises is not required if stocks of denatured alcohol are not held. Denatured alcohol can be sold without holding stock, but the distributor would have to be licensed in the same way as a distributor holding stock.

A pharmacist may hold stocks of denatured alcohol up to the level for which they are authorised.

Users with multi-premises businesses (eg, retail chains, etc) may apply to be authorised to distribute IDA/TSDA to premises, eg, branches, under their control. A multisite application form must be used for authorisation to receive and use IDA or TSDA (see Customs and Excise Notice 473 July 2005).

Specific record keeping requirements for producers/distributors

Under the Denatured Alcohol Regulations 2005, there is a requirement to keep records which show the following information:
(i) purchases of materials used in the production of denatured alcohol;
(ii) imports of denatured alcohol, including details of the country of origin;
(iii) the class of denatured alcohol held in containers, that is whether it is CDA, IDA or TSDA;
(iv) quantities of alcohols, denaturants, markers, dyes and denatured alcohol held and used on your premises;

(v) the results of stocktakes and action taken to investigate deficiencies and surpluses identified by those stocktakes;
(vi) exports and sales of denatured alcohol;
(vii) copy authorisations received in support of orders for denatured alcohols.

Specific record keeping requirements for users

Under the Denatured Alcohol Regulations 2005, there is a requirement to keep records which show the following information:
(i) purchases of IDA or TSDA;
(ii) imports of IDA or TSDA, including details of the country of origin;
(iii) the class of denatured alcohol held in containers, where IDA or TSDA;
(iv) quantities of IDA or TSDA held and used on the premises;
(v) the results of stocktakes and action taken to investigate deficiencies and surpluses identified by those stocktakes;
(vi) sales of IDA or TSDA to other authorised users;
(vii) copy authorisations received in support of orders for IDA or TSDA.

HM Revenue and Customs will visit from time to time to inspect the premises and examine any denatured alcohol on the premises.

Pharmacists may be liable to penalties, required to repay the duty on the alcohol lost in any unauthorised processes and supplies and could have their authorisation withdrawn, if there are unexplained losses of denatured alcohol where:
(a) as a distributor supplies have been made to users without receiving a copy of the authorisations, or
(b) supplies have been made to persons who are not authorised users, or
(c) as a user the denatured alcohol has not been used in accordance with its authorised use.

Some EU countries may require a certificate of denaturing for cosmetics or toiletries which are exported to them. The National Advice Service should be contacted for more details.

Surplus/deficiency in stocks of denatured alcohol as a distributor

Any surplus or deficiency would have to be investigated and the reasons recorded for the deficiency/surplus in the business records and the National Advice Service notified in writing. For any surplus the records would have to be amended to reflect the quantities of alcohols actually in stock.

Surplus/deficiency in stocks of denatured alcohol as a user

Any surplus or deficiency would have to be investigated and the reasons recorded for the deficiency/surplus in the business records and the National Advice Service notified in writing. If the denatured alcohol cannot be accounted for and has been supplied to an unauthorised user, or for an unauthorised purpose, a demand may be issued to pay the duty on the alcohol in the missing amount.

Contacts

For further information on the Denatured Alcohol Regulations 2005 please contact HM Revenue and Customs National Advice Service Helpline (tel 0845 010 9000; for information in Welsh 0845 010 0300; www.hmrc.gov.uk).

HM Revenue and Customs, National Advice Service - Written Enquiries Section, Alexander House, Victoria Avenue, Southend, Essex SS99 1BD
National Advice Service - email service:
enquiries.estn@hmrc.gsi.gov.uk

HM Revenue and Customs, National Registration Unit, Portcullis House, 21 India Street, Glasgow G2 4PZ
e-mail: enquiries.sco@hmrc.gsi.gov.uk

Isopropyl alcohol

Isopropyl alcohol 70% (which is isopropyl alcohol diluted down with water) is not a denatured alcohol and is not covered by the Denatured Alcohol Regulations 2005. Therefore, there is no requirement to be authorised by HM Revenue and Customs to receive or supply isopropyl alcohol 70%.

Ether (Ethyl ether)

Ether does not come under the Denatured Alcohol Regulations 2005; it is classed as a Chemical (see Section 1.6) except when it is licensed as a medicinal product.

Duty Free Spirits (DFS)

Duty free spirits cannot be used for general cleaning and other purposes. Duty free spirits are not permitted to be used for making for sale: any product which contains spirits (other than, subject to special conditions, ethyl esters and ethyl ethers); or use any beverage, foodstuff, flavouring essence, perfumery or cosmetic preparation.

There is no definitive list of allowable medicinal uses of DFS. The HMRC would consider each case on its merits, however the general medical applications and uses for which DFS will be allowed include:

- for the production of recognised medical products, drugs and pharmaceuticals (whether or not the final product contains spirits) including veterinary products, including DFS to be used in the manufacture of any product (including herbal or homoeopathic) which has a Medicines and Healthcare products Regulatory Agency (MHRA) product licence;
- herbal or homoeopathic remedies which do not have an MHRA licence. They must be recognised, by Customs and Excise as having medicinal properties;
- the manufacture of intermediate products used exclusively for the production of medical products (as above);
- for use in hospitals, and, where applicable, dental and veterinary surgeries for specific uses:

DFS can be used in the manufacture of any product prescribed by a doctor to be made up by a pharmacist. This includes "specials" which may be made up on behalf of a pharmacist and which may not have an MHRA product licence.

A pharmacist would have to apply for authorisation to obtain or use duty free spirits. Further details can be obtained from HMRC Notice 47 (January 2002, amended 2004) "Duty free spirits: use in manufacture or for medical or scientific purposes."

The application for authority to receive duty free spirits (Form EX 240) is available from HMRC National Advice Service and should also be returned there.

1.8 Medicines for veterinary use

Section 1.8 covers the following:

Prescriptions (1.8.1)
Prescribing cascade (1.8.2)
Records (1.8.3)
Labelling (1.8.4)
Wholesale dealing (1.8.5)
Sheep dips (1.8.6)
MFS prescriptions (1.8.7)
Medicated animal feedingstuffs (1.8.8)
Advertising (1.8.9)
Small Animal Exemption Scheme (SAES) (1.8.10)
Suspected adverse reactions (1.8.11)

A veterinary medicinal product (VMP) is defined in the Veterinary Medicines Regulations 2008 as any substance or combination of substances presented as having properties for treating or preventing disease in animals, or any substance or combination of substances that may be used in, or administered to, animals with a view either to restoring, correcting or modifying physiological functions by exerting a pharmacological, immunological or metabolic action, or to making a medical diagnosis.

The Veterinary Medicines Regulations 2008 which came into force on 1 October 2008 revoked the Veterinary Medicines Regulations 2007. The Veterinary Medicines Regulations replaced the Medicines Act as far as veterinary legislation is concerned. The classes of VMPs include:
1. Prescription-only medicines - veterinarian (POM-V)
2. Prescription-only medicines - veterinarian, pharmacist, suitably qualified person (POM-VPS)
3. Non-food animal - veterinarian, pharmacist, suitably qualified person (NFA-VPS)
4. Authorised veterinary medicine - general sales list (AVM-GSL).

See table, p92, for further information on the different classes of VMPs.

Pharmacists may only supply VMPs classified as a POM-V, POM-VPS or NFA-VPS from registered pharmacy premises and from 1 April 2009 from premises registered as being premises from which a veterinary surgeon supplies VMPs, or, in the case of VMPs classified as POM-VPS or NFA-VPS from premises which are registered under Schedule 3, paragraph 14 of the Regulations

The Veterinary Medicines Regulations 2009 are expected to come into force on 1 October 2009. After this date, pharmacists are advised to consult the Royal Pharmaceutical Society's website, *www.rpsgb.org*, for up-to-date guidance on the sale and supply of veterinary medicinal products.

1.8.1 Prescriptions

A POM-V or POM-VPS may only be supplied by retail in accordance with a prescription (*see* table, p92, for guidance on who may prescribe VMPs authorised as either POM-V or POM-VPS). The prescription may be oral (eg, if the pharmacist prescribing a POM-VPS medicine also supplies it) or written (eg, where a veterinary surgeon issues a prescription to be

separately dispensed by a pharmacist). Where a VMP is not supplied by the person who has prescribed it, the prescription must be written.

A written prescription must include the following particulars:
(a) the name, address and telephone number of the person prescribing the product;
(b) the qualifications enabling the person to prescribe the product;
(c) the name and address of the owner or keeper;
(d) the identification (including the species) of the animal or group of animals to be treated;
(e) the premises at which the animals are kept if different from that of the owner/keeper;
(f) the date of the prescription;
(g) the signature or other authentication of the prescriber (NB: "other authentication" is not acceptable for a CD);
(h) the name and amount of the product prescribed;
(i) the dosage and administration instructions (NB: the VMD have advised that a dosage of "as directed" is not acceptable);
(j) any necessary warnings;
(k) the withdrawal period if relevant;
(l) if it is prescribed under the cascade, a statement to that effect.

A prescription for any medicine, other than a Schedule 1-4 Controlled Drug, is valid for six months or shorter if specified by the prescriber. In the case of a repeatable prescription it must specify the number of times the VMP may be supplied.

Controlled Drug prescriptions

Where the VMP prescribed is also a Schedule 2 or 3 Controlled Drug (CD) (except temazepam), the prescription must also include the following:

(a) the address of the prescriber which must be in the UK;
(b) the form of the preparation;
(c) the strength of the preparation (when more than one strength of the preparation is available);
(d) the total quantity (in both words and figures) of the preparation to be supplied. This must be in dosage units;
(e) a declaration written on it that the CD is prescribed for an animal or herd under the veterinary surgeon's or veterinary practitioner's care;
(f) the name and address of the person to whom the CD is to be delivered;
(g) a CD to be dispensed in daily instalments must contain a direction specifying the amount of the instalment which may be supplied and the intervals to be observed when supplying.

The requirement to use standardised prescription forms when prescribing Schedule 2 and 3 CDs does not apply to veterinary prescriptions. Similarly, there is currently no requirement for veterinary prescriptions for Controlled Drugs or copies of such prescriptions to be submitted to the relevant NHS agency.

A written prescription for a Schedule 1-4 CD is valid for 28 days. A repeat of a Schedule 2 or 3 CD is not acceptable.

Classification of veterinary medicinal products

Legal category	Retail supply and record keeping	Restrictions on supply

POM-V (POM-veterinarian)	May be supplied by a veterinary surgeon or pharmacist in accordance with a prescription from a veterinary surgeon. Records must be kept of all supplies for a period of at least five years (*see* Section 1.8.3)	A pharmacist supplying a POM-V under a written prescription:
		- may only supply the product specified in that prescription
		- must take all reasonable steps to be satisfied that the prescription has been written and signed by a person entitled to prescribe the product; and
		- must take all reasonable steps to ensure that it is supplied to the person named in the prescription.
		- must be present when it is handed over, unless the pharmacist:
		  • authorises each transaction individually before the product is supplied; and
		  • is satisfied that the person handing it over is competent to do so.
		- may only supply the product from registered pharmacy premises, or from 1 April 2009 from premises registered under the Regulations as being premises from which a veterinary surgeon supplies VMPs.

POM-VPS	May be supplied by a veterinary surgeon, pharmacist or suitably qualified person[2] in accordance with a prescription from one of those persons. Records must be kept of all supplies for a period of at least five years (*see* Section 1.8.3)	A pharmacist supplying a POM-VPS under a written prescription:
		- may only supply the product specified in that prescription
		- must take all reasonable steps to be satisfied that the prescription has been written and signed by a person entitled to prescribe the product; and
		- must take all reasonable steps to ensure that it is supplied to the person named in the prescription.
		
		A pharmacist supplying a POM-VPS:
		- must be present when it is handed over, unless the pharmacist:
		  • authorises each transaction individually before the product is supplied; and
		  • is satisfied that the person handing it over is competent to do so.
		- may only supply the product from registered pharmacy premises, or from 1 April 2009 from premises registered under the Regulations as being premises from which a veterinary surgeon supplies VMPs, or from premises which are registered under Schedule 3, Paragraph 14 of the Veterinary Medicines Regulations 2008.
		
		A pharmacist prescribing a POM-VPS must:
		- always advise on the safe administration of the product
		- advise as necessary on any warnings or contraindications on the label/package leaflet
		- be satisfied that the person using it is competent, and intends to use it for an authorised use
		- not prescribe more than the minimum amount required for the treatment; unless the product supplied is in a container specified in the marketing authorisation; the manufacturer does not supply that VMP in a smaller container; and he is not a person authorised to break open the package before supply (NB: A pharmacist may break open any package other than the immediate packaging of injectable products).

NFA-VPS (Non food-producing animal-veterinarian, pharmacist and suitably qualified person[1])	May be supplied by veterinary surgeon, pharmacist or suitably qualified person[2]. It is a good practice requirement to keep records of NFA-VPS medicines received or supplied	A pharmacist supplying a NFA-VPS must:
		- always advise on the safe administration of the product
		- advise as necessary on any warnings or contraindications on the label/package leaflet
		- be satisfied that the person using it is competent, and intends to use it for an authorised use
		- not supply more than the minimum amount required for the treatment; unless the product supplied is in a container; and he is not a person authorised to break open the package before supply (NB: A pharmacist may break open any package other than the immediate packaging of injectable products)
		- be present when it is handed over, unless the pharmacist:
		  • authorises each transaction individually before the product is supplied; and
		  • is satisfied that the person handing it over is competent to do so.
		- may only supply the product from registered pharmacy premises, or from 1 April 2009 from premises registered under the Regulations as being premises from which a veterinary surgeon supplies VMPs, or from premises which are registered under Schedule 3, Paragraph 14 of the Veterinary Medicines Regulations 2008.

AVM-GSL (Authorised veterinary medicine-GSL)	There are no restrictions on supply	No additional restrictions

[1] Suitably qualified person who must be registered with Animal Medicines Training Regulatory Agency (AMTRA)
[2] In accordance with paragraph 14 of the Regulations

1.8.2 Prescribing cascade

The Veterinary Medicines Regulations 2008 make it an offence to place on the market (which includes sale or supply by wholesale or retail) or to administer (or cause or permit to be administered) any medicinal product unless it is an authorised veterinary medicinal product.

Where no authorised veterinary medicinal product exists in the UK for a condition, the veterinary surgeon responsible for the animal may treat the animal concerned by invoking the "cascade", as follows:

(a) A veterinary medicinal product authorised in the UK for use in another animal species or for another condition in the same species (off-label use);
(b) If no product as described in (a) exists, either;
(i) a human medicinal product authorised in the UK, or
(ii) a veterinary medicinal product not authorised in the UK but authorised in another member State for use with any animal species (in the case of a food-producing animal, it must be a food-producing species); or
(c) If no product as described in (b) is suitable, a veterinary medicinal product prepared extemporaneously (i.e. made up at the time of need) by a registered pharmacist, a veterinary surgeon or the holder of an appropriate manufacturer's licence in accordance with a veterinary prescription.
(NB: Pharmacists who are asked to provide medicines, eg, against a prescription, for animal treatment under the circumstances used in (a), (b) or (c) above should ensure that the veterinary surgeon has prescribed that product specifying that it is to be used under the "cascade".)

The supply and administration of medicines under the "cascade" is permitted only if it is in accordance with a prescription issued by a veterinary surgeon under whose care the animal has been placed.

Under the Regulations, it is an offence to supply an authorised human medicinal product for administration to an animal, otherwise than in accordance with a prescription from a veterinary surgeon. The prescription must specifically state that the medicinal product is for administration under the cascade, either by that veterinary surgeon or under his direction and responsibility. This includes authorised human GSL or P medicines. Pharmacists must not supply human GSL or P medicines over the counter if they are intended for animal administration, even where oral authorisation from a veterinary surgeon has been given.

1.8.3 Records

Pharmacists must keep records of the receipt and supply of POM-V and POM-VPS products. They must keep all documents relating to the transaction. All documents and records must be retained for at least five years. The information retained must include:

(a) the date;
(b) the name of the VMP;
(c) the batch number (NB: in the case of a VMP for a non-food-producing animal, the batch number need only be recorded either on the date that batch is received or on the date that the VMP from that batch is first supplied);
(d) the quantity received or supplied;

(e) the name and address of the supplier or recipient; and
(f) if there is a written prescription, the name and address of the person who wrote the prescription and a copy of the prescription.

If the document relating to the transaction (for example, the prescription) does not include all of this information, the pharmacist must make a record of the missing information as soon as is reasonably practicable following the transaction.

Audit

It is a legal requirement for a detailed audit to be carried out at least once a year by every person who is entitled to supply a VMP on prescription. All incoming and outgoing VMPs must be reconciled with products currently held in stock, with any discrepancies being recorded.

The VMD has stated that the legal requirement to audit VMPs applies to products licensed as POM-V and POM-VPS. It would be good practice to audit stocks of NFA-VPS, however this is not mandatory. There is no requirement to audit stocks of AVM-GSL.

Proof of purchase

The keeper of a food-producing animal must keep proof of purchase of all veterinary medicinal products acquired for the animal (or, if they were not bought, documentary evidence of how they were acquired). An itemised EPOS till receipt or handwritten receipt would constitute proof of purchase.

1.8.4 Labelling

The label of a veterinary medicine supplied against a prescription for administration under the cascade should contain the following information:

- the name and address of the pharmacy, veterinary surgery or approved premises supplying the VMP;
- the name of the veterinary surgeon who prescribed it;
- the name and address of the animal owner;
- the identification (including the species) of the animal or group of animals;
- the date of supply;
- the expiry date of the product, if applicable;
- the name or description of the product which should at least include the name and quantity of active ingredients;
- dosage and administration instructions;
- any special storage precautions;
- any necessary warnings for the user, target species, administration or disposal of the product;
- the withdrawal period, if relevant; and
- the words "Keep out of the reach of children" and "For animal treatment only".

Manufacturers' labelling

The following are labelling and leaflet requirements for manufacturers.

All labels and package leaflets of authorised veterinary medicinal products must be in English and may contain in legible characters "UK authorised veterinary medicinal product" or other wording as specified in the marketing authorisation to indicate that the product is authorised in the UK. The labels and package leaflets may contain other languages provided that all the information is identical in all the languages.

Where it is reasonably practicable, the following information must be present on the immediate packaging, in legible characters:

(1)

(a) the name, strength and pharmaceutical form of the veterinary medicinal product;

(b) the name and strength of each active substance, and of any excipient if this is required under the summary of product characteristics;

(c) the route of administration (if not immediately apparent);

(d) the batch number;

(e) the expiry date;

(f) the words "For Animal Treatment Only" and if appropriate "To be supplied only on a veterinary prescription";

(g) the contents by weight, volume or number of dose units;

(h) the marketing authorisation number;

(i) the name and address of the marketing authorisation holder or, if there is a distributor authorised in the marketing authorisation, that distributor;

(j) a suitably labelled space to record discard date (if relevant);

(k) the target species;

(l) the distribution category;

(m) the words "Keep out of reach of children";

(n) storage instructions;

(o) the in-use shelf-life (if appropriate);

(p) for food-producing species, the withdrawal period for each species or animal product concerned;

(q) any warning specified in the marketing authorisation;

(r) disposal advice;

(s) full indications;

(t) dosage instructions;

(u) contraindications;

(v) further information required in the marketing authorisation;

(w) if the product is one that is requires a dose to be specified for the animal being treated, a space for this.

Where all of this information is present on the immediate packaging there is no need for a package leaflet or any outer packaging. Where it is not reasonably practicable to have all of the above information on the immediate packaging, then the immediate packaging must at least have the following:

(2)

(a) the name of the veterinary medicinal product, including its strength and pharmaceutical form;

(b) the name and proportion of each active substance, and of any excipient if knowledge of this excipient is needed for safety reasons;

(c) the route of administration (if not immediately apparent);

(d) the batch number;

(e) the expiry date;

(f) the words "For Animal Treatment Only" and if appropriate "To be supplied only on a veterinary prescription";

(g) the words "Keep the container in the outer carton".

The outer package must also contain as much as possible of the information set out above in list (2), but where this is not reasonably practicable, a package leaflet must be supplied with the product.

The package leaflet must relate solely to the VMP with which it is included, and be approved in the marketing authorisation for that product.

The package leaflet must be written in plain English.

The leaflet must contain the information set out above in list (1), except for the batch number and the expiry date, and include the name of both the marketing authorisation holder and, if different, the name of the distributor named in the marketing authorisation.

If there is a package leaflet, the immediate packaging and the outer packaging must both refer the user to it.

1.8.5 Wholesale dealing

There are specific restrictions on wholesale dealing. However, there is provision for a person lawfully conducting a retail pharmacy business to wholesale to another retailer (eg, a veterinary practitioner) provided that in any one year the amount supplied does not exceed five per cent in terms of value of turnover of the retail pharmacy business (see Section 1.2.4 for requirements for that must be followed when a retail pharmacy business wholesales medicines).

The holder of a wholesale dealer's authorisation must record, as soon as is reasonably practicable after each incoming or outgoing transaction (including disposal), the following:

(a) the date and nature of the transaction;

(b) the name of the VMP;

(c) the manufacturer's batch number;

(d) the expiry date;

(e) the quantity; and

(f) the name and address of the supplier or recipient.

The records retained in respect of wholesale dealing must be kept for at least three years.

1.8.6 Sheep dips

The supply must be to a person (or a person acting on that person's behalf) who holds a Certificate of Competence in the Safe Use of Sheep Dips showing that Parts 1 and 2 or units 1 and 2 of the assessment referred to in the Certificate have been satisfactorily completed and issued by:

(a) in England, Wales, and Northern Ireland by the National Proficiency Tests Council, or by NPTC Part of the City & Guilds Group; or

(b) in Scotland, by one of those organisations or the Scottish Skills Testing Service.

The supplier must make a record of the certificate number as soon as is reasonably practicable and keep it for three years.

If the active ingredient of the VMP is an organophosphorus compound, the supplier must give the buyer:

(a) a double sided laminate notice. (NB: This is not necessary where the notice has been provided to the buyer within the previous twelve months and the supplier knows or has reasonable cause to believe that the buyer still has it available for use.)

The notice must meet the following specifications.

The notice must be at least A4 size with a laminated cover and must tell the user of the sheep dip:
(i) to read and act in accordance with the label, including instructions on measuring and diluting concentrate;
(ii) that sheep dip is absorbed through the skin;
(iii) always to wear the recommended protective clothing, including gloves, and have spare protective clothing available;
(iv) always to wash protective clothing before taking it off; and
(v) to direct any questions to the supplier or manufacturer.
The notice must contain a diagram showing recommended protective clothing.
(b) two pairs of gloves as specified in the above notice or providing demonstrably superior protection to the user against exposure to the sheep dip.

1.8.7 Medicated feedingstuffs prescriptions (MFS)

The supply of a feedingstuff containing a VMP can only be supplied in accordance with a written prescription. The prescription must include:

(a) the name and address of the person prescribing the product;
(b) the qualifications enabling the person to prescribe the product;
(c) the name and address of the keeper of the animal(s) to be treated;
(d) the species of animal, identification and number of animals;
(e) the premises at which the animals are kept if different from the address of the keeper;
(f) the date of the prescription;
(g) the signature or other authentication of the person prescribing the product (NB: "other authentication" is not acceptable for a CD);
(h) the name and amount of the product prescribed;
(i) the dosage and administration instructions (NB: the VMD have advised that a dosage of "as directed" is not acceptable);
(j) any necessary warnings;
(k) the withdrawal period;
(l) the manufacturer or distributor of the feedingstuffs (who must be approved for the purpose);
(m) if the validity exceeds one month, a statement that not more than 31 days supply may be provided at any time;
(n) the name, type and quantity of feedingstuffs to be used;
(o) the inclusion rate of the veterinary medicinal product and the resulting inclusion rate of the active substance;
(p) any special instructions;
(q) the percentage of the prescribed feedingstuffs to be added to the daily ration; and
(r) if it is prescribed under the cascade, a statement to that effect.

A prescription for a feedingstuff is valid for three months or shorter if specified on the prescription, and should be sufficient for only one course of treatment. Where a prescription is for longer than one month, the supplier cannot provide more than one month's supply at a time.

The person supplying the feedingstuff must keep the prescription for five years.

1.8.8 Medicated animal feedingstuffs

Pharmacists who wish to supply VMPs or specified feed additives for incorporation into feedingstuffs or premixtures/feedingstuffs containing such products should consult the Animal Medicines Inspectorate (AMI) of the VMD for advice (see contact details below).

For further information regarding medicated/specified feed additives or products, contact the AMI:

Animal Medicines Inspectorate
Veterinary Medicines Directorate
Stoneleigh Park
Warwickshire CV8 2LZ
Tel: 024 7684 9260
Fax: 024 7684 9261
e-mail: *amienquiries@vmd.defra.gsi.gov.uk*

1.8.9 Advertising

A VMP may be advertised provided that the advertisement is not misleading, and does not make a medicinal claim that is not in the SPC. There are additional requirements for advertisements for VMPs which are only available on prescription, POM-V and POM-VPS.

A POM-V cannot be advertised except as a price list, or where the advertisement is aimed at veterinary surgeons, pharmacists, veterinary nurses, or professional keepers of animals.

A POM-VPS cannot be advertised except as a price list, or where the advertisement is aimed at veterinary surgeons, pharmacists, professional keepers of animals, owners or keepers of horses, other veterinary healthcare professionals (includes veterinary nurses) and suitably qualified persons.

It is an offence to advertise a VMP that contains psychotropic drugs or narcotics, except where this is aimed at a veterinary surgeon or a pharmacist. It is also an offence to advertise an authorised human medicinal product for administration to animals. This includes sending a price list of or including authorised human medicinal products to a veterinary surgeon or veterinary practice, except in certain circumstances.

1.8.10 Small Animal Exemption Scheme (SAES)

There is an exemption in the Regulations in relation to VMPs intended solely for the following animals: aquarium fish; cage birds; ferrets; homing pigeons; rabbits; small rodents; and terrarium animals, where the animal is kept exclusively as a pet. This exemption allows those VMPs, intended solely for these animals and which comply with the requirements of Schedule 6 of the Regulations to be placed on the market, imported or administered without a marketing authorisation. For further information on the SAES contact the VMD.

1.8.11 Suspected adverse reactions

The Suspected Adverse Reaction Surveillance Scheme (SARSS) is a national surveillance scheme run by the Veterinary Medicines Directorate (VMD). The scheme aims to record and monitor reports of suspected adverse reactions to veterinary medicines and human medicines in both animals (any species) and humans. A human SAR may occur in a person administering a veterinary medicinal product, or a person exposed to a recently treated animal. The scheme also records lack of efficacy, adverse environmental effects, and suspected residues in milk and meat.

Suspected adverse reactions in animals or humans should be reported on Form MLA 252A to:

Department for Environment, Food and Rural Affairs (Defra), Veterinary Medicines Directorate, FREEPOST KT 4503, Woodham Lane New Haw, Addlestone, Surrey KT15 3BR

Forms are available on request from the VMD (tel 01932 338427; fax 01932 336618) and from the VMD website, *www.vmd.gov.uk*. Tear-out copies are included in the *The Veterinary Formulary* and *NOAH Compendium of Data Sheets for Animal Medicines*.

1.9: Alphabetical list of medicines for veterinary use

This list of medicines for veterinary use brings together zootechnical feed additives (ZFA) and veterinary medicines. Where INNs differ from BANs, these are indicated in square brackets. For current lists of prescription only medicines-veterinarian (POM-V), prescription only medicines-veterinarian, pharmacist, suitably qualified person (POM-VPS), non-food animal medicine-veterinarian, pharmacist, suitably qualified person (NFA-VPS), authorised veterinary medicine-general sale list (AVM-GSL), small animal exemption scheme (SAES), see the Veterinary Medicines Directorate (VMD) website, *www.vmd.gov.uk*. The Royal Pharmaceutical Society's Legal and Ethical Advisory Service welcomes, in writing, details of any errors or omissions.

A

Abbotsbury Insecticidal shampoo AVM-GSL
Acetarsol: for Poisons Act 1972 restrictions see poisons section
ACP preparations POM-V
Action Actodine New Formulation AVM-GSL
Action Actodip and Spray RTU AVM-GSL
Action Actodip Supreme RTU AVM-GSL
Action Super teat dip 1:3 AVM-GSL
Action Super teat dip 15 AVM-GSL
Activyl tablets POM-V
Actodine Pink teat dip RTU AVM-GSL
Actodip Supreme Concentrate AVM-GSL
Adequan preparations POM-V
Adocam oral suspension POM-V
Adrenocaine injection POM-VPS
Advantage preparations POM-V
Advantix preparations POM-V
Advasure POM-V
Advocate preparations POM-V
Advocin preparations POM-V
Aeroclens aerosol AVM-GSL
Aftopur preparations POM-V
Aivlosin preparations POM-V
Alamycin preparations POM-V
Albacert POM-VPS
Albazole 2.5% SC POM-VPS
Albencare POM-VPS
Albenil preparations POM-VPS
Albensure preparations POM-VPS
Albex preparations POM-VPS
Alcide Uddergold Platinum teat dip AVM-GSL

Alfamed spot on for Small, medium, Very Large Dogs NFA-VPS
Alfamed spot on for Large Dogs POM-V
Alfamed spray POM-V
Alfaxan injection POM-V
Alizin injection POM-V
Allverm preparations POM-VPS
Alphaject 1200 vaccine POM-VPS
Alphaject 2-2 vaccine POM-V
Alphaject 4000 vaccine POM-VPS
Alstomec preparations POM-VPS
Altresyn oral solution POM-V
Aludex solution POM-V
Amfipen preparations POM-V
Amoxicure POM-V
Amoxinsol preparations POM-V
Amoxival tablets POM-V
Amoxycare preparations POM-V
Amoxycillin [Amoxicillin] tablets POM-V
Amoxygen preparations POM-V
Amoxypen preparations POM-V
Amoxyvet preparations POM-V
Ampibrittin injection POM-V
Ampicaps capsules POM-V
Ampicare preparations POM-V
Ampicillin vet capsules POM-V
Ampitab preparations POM-V
AMX concentrate for solution for Fish Treatment POM-V
Anarthron injection POM-V
Animal Welfare Insecticidal shampoo for Dogs AVM-GSL
Animalintex AVM-GSL
Animalintex Hoof Treatment AVM-GSL
Animec preparations POM-VPS
Animedazon spray POM-V

Animeloxam oral suspension POM-V
Anipyrl tablets POM-V
Anivit B12 injection POM-VPS
Anivit 4BC injection POM-VPS
Antirobe capsules POM-V
Antisedan injection POM-V
Antiseptic Teat ointment AVM-GSL
Apiguard gel AVM-GSL
Apistan AVM-GSL
Appertex tablets AVM-GSL
Apralan preparations POM-V
Aquarium Bactocide SAES
Aquarium Diseasolve SAES
Aquarium Ichcide SAES
Aquatet POM-V
AquaVac ERM vaccines POM-VPS
AquaVac FNM Plus vaccine POM-V
AquaVac Furovac 5 vaccine POM-V
AquaVac RELERA POM-V
AquaVac Vibrio vaccines POM-V
Aqupharm preparations POM-V
Armitage Felt Flea collar Twin Pack AVM-GSL
Armitage Pet Care Felt Flea collar AVM-GSL
Armitage Pet Care Flea and Tick drops AVM-GSL
Armitage Pet Care Flea shampoo for Dogs AVM-GSL
Armitage Pet Care Flea spray for Cats/Dogs AVM-GSL
Armitage Pet Care Insecticidal Flea shampoo + conditioner AVM-GSL
Armitage Pet Care Protect Flea collar for Cats AVM-GSL
Armitage Pet Care Protect Flea and Tick collar for Dogs AVM-GSL

Armitage Pet Care Single Dose Wormer for Dogs AVM-GSL
Arquel V granules POM-V
Arsanilic acid: for Poisons Act 1972 restrictions see poisons section
Artervac vaccine POM-V
Atipam injection POM-V
Atopica capsules POM-V
Atrocare injection POM-V
Aureomycin preparations POM-V
Auriplak ear tag POM-VPS
Auriplak Fly and Scab dip POM-VPS
Aurizon ear drops POM-V
Aurofac preparations POM-V
Aurogran preparations POM-V
Auroto ear drops POM-V
Autoworm preparations POM-VPS
Avatec 15% CC (Game Birds) POM-V
Avatec 150G premix ZFA
Avian Tuberculin PPD POM-V
Avicas tablets AVM-GSL
Avinew vaccine POM-V
AviPro vaccines POM-V

B

Banacep vet tablets POM-V
Barricade 5% EC liquid concentrate POM-VPS
Battle's Ketosis drench AVM-GSL
Baycox preparations POM-V
Bayer Dog Wormer tablets NFA-VPS
Baymec pour on POM-VPS
Bayopal NFA-VPS
Baytril preparations POM-V
Bayvarol strips AVM-GSL
BCK granules AVM-GSL

KEY TO ANNOTATIONS

CD: A substance controlled by the Misuse of Drugs Act 1971 to which the principal restrictions of the Misuse of Drugs Regulations 2001 apply

CD Lic: A substance controlled by the Misuse of Drugs Act to which the restrictions of the Regulations apply and, in addition, the production, possession and supply of which is limited in the public interest to purposes of research or other special purposes. A Home Office licence is required for such purposes

CD No Register: A substance controlled by the Misuse of Drugs Act to which the restrictions of the Regulations apply except that no entry in the Controlled Drugs Register is required and invoices must be retained for two years

CD Anab: A substance controlled by the Misuse of Drugs Act to which the restrictions of the Regulations apply but with the following relaxation: no restriction on possession and labelling requirements (except those under the Veterinary Medicines Regulations 2008), prescription requirements, except for the validity of a prescription being limited to 28 days, do not apply, except those falling under the controls of the Veterinary Medicines Regulations 2008, records need not be kept by retailers, destruction requirements apply only to importers/exporters and manufacturers, there are no safe custody requirements

CD Benz : A substance controlled by the Misuse of Drugs Act to which the restrictions of the Regulations apply but with the following relaxation: no restriction on import and export, possession and labelling requirements (except those under the Veterinary Medicines Regulations 2008), prescription requirements, except for the validity of a prescription being limited to 28 days, do not apply, except those falling under the controls of the Veterinary Medicines Regulations 2008, records need not be kept by retailers, destruction requirents apply

only to importers, exporters and manufacturers, there are no safe custody requirements

CD Inv: A substance controlled by the Misuse of Drugs Act but which is exempt from all restrictions under the Regulations except that the invoice or a copy of it must be kept for two years

POM-V: A substance that may be sold or supplied to the public by a veterinary surgeon or pharmacist but only in accordance with a veterinary surgeon's prescription as described in the Veterinary Medicines Regulations 2008

POM-VPS: A substance that may be prescribed and supplied by a veterinary surgeon, pharmacist or suitably qualified person as described in the Veterinary Medicines Regulations 2008

NFA-VPS: A substance for a non-food producing animal that may supplied by a veterinary surgeon, pharmacist or suitably qualified person as described in the Veterinary Medicines Regulations 2008

AVM-GSL: A substance to which there are no restrictions on the retail supply

SAES: a substance for use in certain animals kept exclusively as pets under the Small Animal Exemption Scheme as described in the Veterinary Medicines Regulations 2008

ZFA: Zootechnical feed additive incorporated in feed as indicated in the relevant Annex entry of Directive 1831/2003/EC

Beaphar Cat Flea collar Twin Pack AVM-GSL
Beaphar Cat Flea powder/ spray AVM-GSL
Beaphar Dog Flea and Tick drops AVM-GSL
Beaphar Dog Flea powder/ shampoo/ spray AVM-GSL
Beaphar Ear drops AVM-GSL
Beaphar Flea and Tick collar for Dogs AVM-GSL
Beaphar Flea collar for Cats AVM-GSL
Beaphar Flea spray AVM-GSL
Beaphar Soft Cat Flea collar AVM-GSL
Benazecare tablets POM-V
Betamox preparations POM-V
Betsolan preparations POM-V
Big Dog Wormer tablets NFA-VPS
Bilosin injection POM-V
Bimamast MC POM-V
Bimamix POM-V
Bimectin preparations POM-VPS
Bimotrim Co injection POM-V
Bimoxyl preparations POM-V
Binixin injection POM-V
BioTech's Anti-Flea and Anti-Tick drops for Dogs AVM-GSL
BioTech's Flea and Tick drops for Dogs AVM-GSL
BioTech's Flea shampoo for Dogs AVM-GSL
Biozine AVM-GSL
Birnagen Forte AS POM-V
Birp AVM-GSL
Bisolvon preparations POM-V
Blackleg vaccine POM-VPS
Bloat Guard drench POM-VPS
Bloat Guard premix POM-V
Blockade AVM-GSL
Blu-Gard AVM-GSL
Blu-Gard teat spray AVM-GSL

Bob Martin 2 in 1 Dewormer tablets for Cats AVM-GSL
Bob Martin All-In-One Dewormer tablets for Dogs AVM-GSL
Bob Martin Antiflatulence tablets AVM-GSL
Bob Martin Coat Conditioning Flea and Tick shampoo for Dogs AVM-GSL
Bob Martin Dewormer tablets for Dogs AVM-GSL
Bob Martin Diarrhoea tablets AVM-GSL
Bob Martin Dog spot on AVM-GSL
Bob Martin Double Action spot on for Cats/Dogs AVM-GSL
Bob Martin Dual Dewormer for Cats/Dogs AVM-GSL
Bob Martin Easy to Use Dewormer granules for Cats/Dogs AVM-GSL
Bob Martin Flash Cat Reflective collar AVM-GSL
Bob Martin Flea and Tick collar for Dogs AVM-GSL
Bob Martin Flea and Tick collar Plus Coat Conditioner AVM-GSL
Bob Martin Flea and Tick spot on AVM-GSL
Bob Martin Flea collar for Cats AVM-GSL
Bob Martin Flea Killing Mousse Plus for Cats AVM-GSL
Bob Martin Flea powder for Cats and Dogs AVM-GSL
Bob Martin Flea shampoo for Dogs AVM-GSL
Bob Martin Flea spray for Dogs AVM-GSL
Bob Martin Flea tablets AVM-GSL
Bob Martin Laxative tablets AVM-GSL
Bob Martin Multi-purpose Flea spray AVM-GSL
Bob Martin Natural Flea Killing spray for Dogs AVM-GSL
Bob Martin Natural Flea shampoo for Dogs AVM-GSL
Bob Martin Permethrin Dog spot on AVM-GSL

Bob Martin Permethrin Reflective Flea collar AVM-GSL
Bob Martin Pump Action Flea spray for Cats and Dogs AVM-GSL
Bob Martin Silent Flea spray for Cats AVM-GSL
Bob Martin Spot on Dewormer AVM-GSL
Bob Martin Velvet Flea collar Twin Pack AVM-GSL
Bob Martin Vetcare Flea collar for Cats AVM-GSL
Bob Martin Vetcare spot-on for Cats/Dogs AVM-GSL
Bolfo Flea spray AVM-GSL
Borgal preparations POM-V
Bovaclox preparations POM-V
Bovex preparations POM-VPS
Bovidec vaccine POM-V
Bovidip preparations AVM-GSL
Bovilis vaccines POM-V
Bovine Tuberculin PPD POM-V
Bovivac S vaccine POM-V
Bravoxin injection POM-VPS
Bronchi-Shield vaccine POM-V
BTVPUR Alsap 8 POM-V
Buprecare injection CD No Register POM-V
Bupregesic preparations POM-V
Buprenodale injection POM-V
Bursamune in Ovo vaccine POM-V
Buscopan preparations POM-V
Busol injection POM-V
Butox Swish POM-VPS

C

C Dip AVM-GSL
Calcibor preparations POM-VPS
Calciject preparations POM-VPS
Calcium borogluconate 40% POM-VPS
Calcium borogluconate 40% CM POM-VPS
Calcium borogluconate 20% MPD POM-VPS
Calicide POM-V
Calicivac POM-V
Calmivet preparations POM-V
Canac Dog Flea and Tick collar AVM-GSL
Canac Easy Worming granules for Cats/Dogs AVM-GSL
Canac One Dose Worming tablets for Dogs AVM-GSL
Canac Soft Flea collar for Cats AVM-GSL
Canaural ear drops POM-V
Canidryl tablets AVM-GSL
Canine Parafluvac POM-V
Caninsulin injection POM-V
Canovel Catovel Insecticidal powder AVM-GSL
Canovel Flea collar for Dogs AVM-GSL
Canovel Flea drops AVM-GSL
Canovel Insecticidal and Conditioning shampoo AVM-GSL
Canovel Insecticidal Conditioning collar for Dogs AVM-GSL
Canovel Insecticidal Flea and Tick shampoo and conditioner AVM-GSL
Canovel Long Acting Flea and Tick spray AVM-GSL
Canovel Palatable Wormer tablets AVM-GSL
Capstar tablets AVM-GSL
Carprieve tablets POM-V
Carprodyl tablets POM-V
Carprogesic tablets POM-V
Cartrophen Vet injection POM-V
Casofend POM-VPS
Catovel Insecticidal Conditioning collar for Cats AVM-GSL
Catovel Palatable Wormer tablets AVM-GSL
Cefadale tablets POM-V
Cefalexin tablets POM-V

Cefaseptin preparations POM-V
Cefa-Tabs POM-V
Cepesedan POM-V
Cephacare tablets POM-V
Cephaguard preparations POM-V
Cephorum tablets POM-V
Ceporex preparations POM-V
Cepravin preparations POM-V
Cerenia preparations POM-V
Cevac vaccines POM-V
Cevaxel injection POM-V
Chanamast DC intramammary preparation POM-V
Chanaverm preparations POM-VPS
Chanazine preparations POM-V
Chanazole SC solution POM-VPS
Chanoprim preparations POM-V
Chlorhexidine teat dip/spray AVM-GSL
Chlorsol 50 POM-V
Chorulon CD Anab POM-V
Chronogest POM-V
CIDR vaginal delivery system for Cattle POM-V
Circovac vaccine POM-V
Clamoxyl preparations POM-V
Clavaseptin tablets POM-V
Clavucill tablets POM-V
Clik pour on POM-VPS
Clinacin tablets POM-V
Clinacox ZFA
Clinagel Vet POM-V
Clindacyl tablets POM-V
Clinidip L Concentrate AVM-GSL
Clinidip Superconcentrate AVM-GSL
Clomicalm tablets POM-V
Closamectin injection POM-VPS
Closiver injection POM-VPS
CM + D injection POM-VPS
Cobactan preparations POM-V
Coliscour POM-V
Colisorb vaccine POM-VPS
Colombo Morenicol Alparex SAES
Colombo Morenicol FMC-50 SAES
Colombovac vaccines POM-VPS
Colombovac PMV/Pox vaccine POM-VPS
Colvasone injection POM-V
Combiclav preparations POM-V
Combimox preparations POM-V
Combinex preparations POM-VPS
Combisyn preparations POM-V
Combivit injection POM-VPS
Comforion Vet injection POM-V
Compagel POM-V
Companazone 25 tablets POM-V
Convenia injection POM-V
Coopers Ectoforce sheep dip POM-VPS
Coopers Fly Repellent Plus for horses AVM-GSL
Coopers Head to Tail Veterinary Flea powder AVM-GSL
Coopers Head to Tail Veterinary Flea shampoo AVM-GSL
Coopers Spot On Insecticide POM-VPS
Copasure 24G capsules AVM-GSL
Copinox preparations AVM-GSL
Copper sulphate MA 02987/4005 POM-V
Copprite preparations POM-VPS
Coprin injection POM-V
Cortavance spray POM-V
Corvental-D capsules POM-V
Cosecure bolus POM-VPS
Cosumix Plus POM-V
Co-Trimazine tablets POM-V
Cotrimoxgen tablets POM-V
Countdown 1:4 AVM-GSL
Countdown Extra AVM-GSL
Countdown He teat dip AVM-GSL
Countrywide Farmers Concentrated Iodine teat dip/spray AVM-GSL
Countrywide Farmers Ready to Use Iodine teat dip/spray AVM-GSL
Countrywide Farmers Ready to Use Iodine teatsoft dip/spray AVM-GSL
Covexin 7 vaccine POM-VPS
Covexin 8 vaccine POM-VPS
Covexin 10 vaccine POM-V

Coxi Plus oral powder POM-V
Coxicure POM-VPS
Coxidin premix ZFA
CPF Dairyclene Iodine RTU AVM-GSL
Crestar POM-V
Cronyxin injection POM-V
Crovect preparations POM-VPS
Cryomarex Rispens vaccine POM-VPS
Crystapen 5 Mega for injection (Veterinary) POM-V
Curazole preparations POM-VPS
Cyclio spot on preparations AVM-GSL
Cyclix preparations POM-V
Cyclo spray POM-V
Cycloprost POM-V
Cyclosol LA injection POM-V
Cycostat 66G premix ZFA
Cydectin preparations POM-VPS
Cyfac HS granular POM-V
Cygro 1% premix ZFA
Cylap vaccine POM-V
CynoVAX vaccines POM-V
CZV Avian Tuberculin PPD POM-V

D

Dairyclene Chlorhexidine RTU teat dip and spray AVM-GSL
Dairyclene Iodine Concentrate teat dip and spray AVM-GSL
Dairyclene Iodine RTU teat dip and spray AVM-GSL
Dales Glucose 40% w/v injection POM-VPS
Dalmazin POM-V
Dalocain POM-VPS
Dalophylline gel POM-VPS
Damiana and Kola tablets AVM-GSL
Danilon Equidos oral granules POM-V
Decazole Forte drench POM-VPS
Deccox preparations POM-V
Dectomax preparations POM-VPS
Defencare shampoo AVM-GSL
Defendog AVM-GSL
Delvosteron injection POM-V
Denagard preparations POM-V
Denex tablets AVM-GSL
Deosan Flyaway POM-VPS
Deosan Iodip Concentrate AVM-GSL
Deosan Summer Teatcare Plus AVM-GSL
Deosan Super Ex-Cel AVM-GSL
Deosan Super Iodip AVM-GSL
Deosan Teatcare Plus AVM-GSL
Deosan Thixodip AVM-GSL
Deosect spray POM-VPS
Depidex preparations POM-VPS
Depocillin injection POM-V
Depo-Medrone V injection POM-V
Deposel injection POM-V
Derasect Flea drops AVM-GSL
Dermisol preparations POM-VPS
Dermobion Clear POM-V
Dermobion Green POM-V
Dermoline Louse powder AVM-GSL
Dermoline Insecticidal shampoo for Horses AVM-GSL
Dermoline Sweet Itch lotion AVM-GSL
Detogesic injection POM-V
Devomycin preparations POM-V
Dexadreson injection POM-V
Dexafort injection POM-V
Dexamedium injection POM-V
Dexdomitor injection POM-V
Dextrose 40% POM-VPS
Diaproof K AVM-GSL
Dichlorophen tablets BP AVM-GSL
Dicural preparations POM-V
Dilumarex POM-V
Diluvac Forte POM-V
Dimazon preparations POM-V
Dinalgen preparations POM-V
Dipal Concentrate AVM-GSL
Divamectin pour on POM-VPS
Dog Wormer tablets NFA-VPS
Dolagis tablets POM-V
Dolethal injection CD No Register POM-V

Dolorex injection POM-V
Dolpac tablets POM-V
Domidine injection POM-V
Domitor injection POM-V
Domosedan injection POM-V
Dopram-V drops POM-VPS
Dopram-V injection POM-V
Dorbene Vet injection POM-V
Dormilan injection POM-V
Dosalid preparations POM-V
Downland Antiseptic aerosol AVM-GSL
Downland Calcium Borogluconate 20%
    PMD POM-VPS
Downland Calcium Borogluconate 40%
    CM POM-VPS
Downland Fluke and Worm drench
    POM-VPS
Downland Levamisole injection POM-
    VPS
Doxirobe gel POM-V
Doxyseptin preparations POM-V
Draxxin injection POM-V
Droncit injection POM-V
Droncit pills AVM-GSL
Droncit spot on AVM-GSL
Droncit tablets AVM-GSL
Drontal preparations NFA-VPS
Dual Action Worming tablets for
    Cats/Dogs AVM-GSL
Dufulvin preparations POM-V
Dunlop's 20 CM POM-VPS
Dunlop's 20 PMD POM-VPS
Dunlop's 40 CB POM-VPS
Dunlop's 40 CM POM-VPS
Dunlop's 4BC Vitamin injection POM-
    VPS
Dunlop's Water for injection POM-V
Duofast POM-V
Duowin POM-V
Duphacillin injection POM-V
Duphacort Q injection POM-V
Duphacycline preparations POM-V
Duphafral Extravite injection POM-VPS
Duphafral Multivitamin 9 injection
    POM-VPS
Duphalyte solution POM-V
Duphamox preparations POM-V
Duphapen preparations POM-V
Duphapen + Strep injection POM-V
Duphatrim preparations POM-V
Duramune vaccines POM-V
Durateston injection CD Anab POM-V
Duvaxyn vaccines POM-V
Dynaclav injection POM-V
Dysect preparations POM-VPS
Dystosel injection POM-V

E

Eazi-Breed CIDR POM-V
Ecomec 1% injection POM-VPS
Ecomectin preparations POM-VPS
Econor preparations POM-V
Ecotel 2.5% oral drench POM-VPS
Efficur injection POM-V
Effipro spot on NFA-VPS
Effipro spray POM-V
Effydral solution AVM-GSL
Elancoban G200 ZFA
Elderberry tablets AVM-GSL
Embotape oral paste POM-VPS
Emprasan Lanolin teat dip concentrate
    AVM-GSL
Emprasan Sovereign AVM-GSL
Emprasan Super Concentrated teat dip
    AVM-GSL
Enacard tablets POM-V
Endofluke 10 POM-VPS
Endospec preparations POM-VPS
Endoworm POM-VPS
Energaid AVM-GSL
Engemycin preparations POM-V
Enovex preparations POM-VPS
Enroxil preparations POM-V
Enterisol Ileitis vaccine POM-V
Enurace 50 tablets POM-V
Enviracor vaccine POM-V
Enzaprost injection POM-V

Enzex Injection for Cattle POM-VPS
Enzovax vaccine POM-V
Epiphen preparations CD No Register
    POM-V
Eprinex pour on POM-VPS
Equest preparations POM-VPS
EquibactinVet POM-V
Equifulvin granules POM-V
Equilis vaccines POM-V
Equimax oral paste POM-VPS
Equimidine injection POM-V
Equinixin granules POM-V
Equioxx POM-VPS
Equip vaccines POM-V
Equipalazone preparations POM-V
Equitape paste POM-VPS
Equitrim preparations POM-V
Eqvalan preparations POM-VPS
Eraquell oral paste POM-VPS
Ermogen vaccine POM-VPS
Erysorb Plus vaccine POM-VPS
Erythrocin preparations POM-V
Eryvac vaccine POM-VPS
Estroplan injection POM-V
Estrumate injection POM-V
Eurican vaccines POM-V
Euthatal solution CD No Register POM-
    V
Excenel preparations POM-V
Excis solution POM-V
Exelpet Wormer for Cats/Dogs AVM-GSL
Exhelm suspension POM-VPS
Exodus POM-VPS
Exspot Insecticide for Dogs AVM-GSL

F

Farmcare Concentrated teat dip AVM-
    GSL
Farmcare RTU teat dip AVM-GSL
Fasimec Duo POM-VPS
Fasinex preparations POM-VPS
FCB Teatcare 1:3 Conc. AVM-GSL
Feligen RCP vaccine POM-V
Felimazole tablets POM-V
Feline 3 POM-V
Felocell CVR vaccine POM-V
Fenflor injection POM-V
Fenzol 5% solution POM-VPS
Fertagyl injection POM-V
Fevaxyn vaccines POM-V
Finadyne preparations POM-V
Fiproline spot on NFA-VPS
Fiproline spray POM-V
Fitergol tablets POM-V
Flea collar from Bob Martin (Cat) AVM-
    GSL
Flea spot on preparations POM-V
Flectron Fly tags POM-VPS
Fleegard preparations POM-V
Flexicam POM-V
Florocol premix POM-V
Florvetol injection POM-V
Flubenol preparations POM-VPS; but if
    Flubenol Easy preparations AVM-GSL
Flubenvet premix POM-VPS
Flukiver suspension POM-VPS
Flunixin preparations POM-V
Flypor solution POM-VPS
Folltropin POM-V
Footrot aerosol AVM-GSL
Footvax vaccine POM-VPS
Forgastrin AVM-GSL
Forketos AVM-GSL
Fortekor tablets POM-V
Forthyron tablets POM-V
Fostim injection CD Anab POM-V
Foston injection POM-V
Four Paws Magic Coat Dog Flea sham-
    poo AVM-GSL
Framomycin injection POM-V
Freedom Cat collar AVM-GSL
Friends Dog Flea spray AVM-GSL
Friskies Cat Flea collar AVM-GSL
Friskies Flea & Tick collar for Dogs AVM-
    GSL
Friskies Pro Control Flea and Tick collar
    AVM-GSL

Friskies Pro Control Flea and Tick spray
    AVM-GSL
Friskies Pro Control Flea collar for Cats
    AVM-GSL
Friskies Pro Control Flea foam for Cats
    AVM-GSL
Frontline Combo spot on preparations
    POM-V
Frontline spot on NFA-VPS
Frontline spray POM-V
Frusecare tablets POM-V
Frusedale 40 tablets POM-V
Frusemide [Furosemide] tablets BP POM-
    V
Fuciderm gel POM-V
Fucithalmic Vet POM-V
Fumidil B AVM-GSL
Furexel preparations POM-VPS
Furogen 2 vaccine POM-V

G

Gabbrostim injection POM-V
GAC ear drops POM-V
Galastop solution POM-V
Galaxy vaccines POM-V
Gallimune vaccines POM-V
Gallivac vaccines POM-V
Garlic and Fenugreek tablets AVM-GSL
Garlic tablets AVM-GSL
Gastric tablets AVM-GSL
Gastrogard oral paste POM-V
Gelofusine Veterinary POM-V
Genestran injection POM-V
Genitrix Anti-flatulence tablets AVM-
    GSL
Genitrix Diarrhoea tablets AVM-GSL
Genus teat dip and spray concentrate
    AVM-GSL
Genus teat dip and spray solution RTU
    AVM-GSL
Gleptosil injection POM-VPS
Gletvax 6 vaccine POM-VPS
Glucose 40% w/v injection POM-VPS
Gold Glycodip AVM-GSL
Gold teat dip concentrate AVM-GSL
Golden-Hoof AVM-GSL
Golden-Hoof Plus AVM-GSL
Golden-Mane AVM-GSL
Golden-Udder AVM-GSL
Goldfish Start Up Pack SAES
Gonazon POM-V
Granofen Wormer for Cats and Dogs
    NFA-VPS
Granofen Wormer for Pigs POM-VPS
Greenleaf tablets AVM-GSL
Grisol-V preparations POM-V

H

Haemaccel infusion solution
    (Veterinary) POM-V
Haemo 15 injection POM-V
Halocur solution POM-V
Halothane-Vet POM-V
Hamra Blue AVM-GSL
Hapadex preparations POM-VPS
Harkers Pigeon Coccidiosis Treatment
    AVM-GSL
Hartz Control Pet Care System Flea
    shampoo for Dogs AVM-GSL
Hartz Control Pet Care System Flea col-
    lar for Cats AVM-GSL
Hartz Control Pet Care System Longlife
    Flea collar for Cats/Dogs AVM-GSL
Hartz Control Pet Care System One Spot
    Flea and Tick Remedy AVM-GSL
Hartz Health Measures Rid Worm for
    Dogs AVM-GSL
Hartz Rid Flea collar for Dogs AVM-GSL
HatchPak Avinew POM-V
HatchPak Avinew IB120 POM-V
HatchPak IB120 POM-V
Hartz Rid Flea powder for Cats/Dogs
    AVM-GSL
Hemovet dressings AVM-GSL
Hemovet swabs AVM-GSL
Heptavac vaccines POM-VPS

Hexamine and sodium acid phosphate
    tablets POM-V
Hexasol LA POM-V
Hexiprotect WS AVM-GSL
Hexodip AVM-GSL
Hexodip Extra AVM-GSL
Hi-Craft Insecticidal Dog shampoo
    AVM-GSL
Hi-Craft Flea & Tick collar for Dogs
    AVM-GSL
Hi-Craft Flea collar for Cats AVM-GSL
High Emollient AVM-GSL
High Emollient Ready to Use teat dip or
    spray AVM-GSL
Hiprabovis Pneumos POM-V
Hipracox Broilers POM-V
Hipragumboro GM97 POM-V
Hornex Calf Dehorning paste POM-VPS
Hy-50 Vet injection POM-V
Hyalovet 20 injection POM-V
Hydrocortisone and Neomycin
    Veterinary cream POM-V
HydroDoxx POM-V
Hydrogen cyanide: for Poisons Act 1972
    restrictions see poisons section
Hydrolect HE AVM-GSL
Hylartil Vet injection POM-V
Hyonate injection POM-V
Hyoresp vaccine POM-V
Hypercard 10 tablets POM-V
Hyperdrug Veterinary Flea and Tick
    drops AVM-GSL
Hypermune preparations POM-V
Hypnorm CD POM-V
Hypurin Vet preparations POM-V

I

Ibaflin preparations POM-V
Ibraxion Emulsion for Injection POM-V
Imaverol POM-VPS
Imizol injection POM-V
Imposil POM-VPS
Imuresp RP vaccine POM-V
Incurin tablets POM-V
Ingelvac vaccines POM-V
Insuvet preparations POM-V
Intra-Epicaine injection POM-V
Intrac vaccine POM-V
Intradine injection POM-V
Intraval sodium injection POM-V
Intravit 12 injection POM-VPS
Intubeaze spray POM-V
Iodactiv AVM-GSL
Iodine Glycerine teat dip RTU AVM-GSL
Iodine Teat Dip Spray Concentrate
    AVM-GSL
Iodine Teat Dip Spray RTU AVM-GSL
Iodypro AVM-GSL
Ioprotect WS AVM-GSL
Iosan preparations AVM-GSL
Isoba POM-V
Isocare POM-V
Isofane POM-V
IsoFlo POM-V
IsoFlo Vet POM-V
Isoflurane Vet POM-V
Isolec POM-V
Isovet POM-V
Isoxetol POM-V
Itrafungol oral solution POM-V
Ivermectin Virbac 18.7 mg/g oral paste
    POM-VPS
Ivertin Cattle POM-V
Ivomec preparations POM-VPS

J

Johnes Disease vaccine living POM-V
Johnson's 4fleas Cat collar AVM-GSL
Johnson's 4fleas powder for Cats and
    Dogs AVM-GSL
Johnson's 4fleas Protector spot-on for
    Cats/Dogs AVM-GSL
Johnson's 4fleas shampoo for Dogs
    AVM-GSL
Johnson's 4fleas 11.4 mg, 57 mg tablets
    for Cats and Dogs AVM-GSL

Johnson's Anti-Mite & Insect spray AVM-GSL

Johnson's Anti-Pest Insect spray AVM-GSL

Johnson's Anti-Scratch powder AVM-GSL

Johnson's Antiseptic Wound powder AVM-GSL

Johnson's Cat Flea powder AVM-GSL

Johnson's Cat Flea pump spray AVM-GSL

Johnson's Cat Flea spray AVM-GSL

Johnson's Diarrhoea tablets AVM-GSL

Johnson's Dog Flea powder AVM-GSL

Johnson's Dog Flea pump spray AVM-GSL

Johnson's Dog Flea shampoo AVM-GSL

Johnson's Dog Flea spray AVM-GSL

Johnson's ear drops AVM-GSL

Johnson's Easy Roundwormer for Kittens/Puppies AVM-GSL

Johnson's Easy Tapewormer for Cats/Dogs AVM-GSL

Johnson's Easy Wormer granules for Cats/Dogs AVM-GSL

Johnson's Extra Guard Flea and Tick shampoo with Permethrin AVM-GSL

Johnson's Extra Guard Flea and Tick spray with Permethrin AVM-GSL

Johnson's Felt Cat Flea collar AVM-GSL

Johnson's Flavoured Tapeworm tablets AVM-GSL

Johnson's Flea & Tick drops AVM-GSL

Johnson's Flea collar for Dogs AVM-GSL

Johnson's Flea Guard collar for Cats AVM-GSL

Johnson's Flea Guard Waterproof Flea and Tick collar for Dogs AVM-GSL

Johnson's Insecticidal Flea and Tick drops AVM-GSL

Johnson's Kil-Pest Insect powder AVM-GSL

Johnson's Kitten/Cat Easy Worm syrup AVM-GSL

Johnson's One Dose Easy Wormer for Dogs AVM-GSL

Johnson's Palatable Roundworm tablets AVM-GSL

Johnson's Pigeon Insect powder AVM-GSL

Johnson's Pigeon Insect spray AVM-GSL

Johnson's Puppy Easy Worm syrup AVM-GSL

Johnson's Puppy Flea powder AVM-GSL

Johnson's Rid-Mite Insect powder AVM-GSL

Johnson's Scaly lotion AVM-GSL

Johnson's Twin-Wormer for Cats/Dogs AVM-GSL

Juramate injection POM-V

K

K dip AVM-GSL

K L One Minute poultice AVM-GSL

Kaobiotic tablets POM-V

Kaogel VP suspension AVM-GSL

Kaolin poultice AVM-GSL

Karidox oral solution POM-V

Katavac vaccines POM-V

Kavak vaccines POM-V

Kelp Seaweed tablets AVM-GSL

Kenostart teat dip AVM-GSL

Ketaset injection CD Benz POM-V

Ketofen preparations POM-V

Ketol AVM-GSL

KetoProPig POM-V

Ketosaid AVM-GSL

Kidney tablets AVM-GSL

Killitch AVM-GSL

King British Bacteria Control SAES

King British Disease Clear SAES

King British Fin Rot & Fungus Control SAES

King British Methylene Blue SAES

King British Original Formula WS3 White Spot Terminator SAES

King British Pond Fish Treatment SAES

King British Professional Fin Rot & Fungus Control SAES

King British Professional Original Formula WS3 White Spot Terminator SAES

King British Professional Pond Fish Treatment SAES

King British Professional Ulcer & Open Wound Treatment SAES

King British Professional White Spot Control SAES

King British Revitaliser Tonic SAES

King British Ulcer & Open Wound Treatment SAES

King British Velvet Control SAES

King British White Spot Control SAES

Kitzyme Flearid Dual Action Insecticidal spray AVM-GSL

Kitzyme Flearid Insecticidal spray AVM-GSL

Kitzyme Granule Wormer for Cats AVM-GSL

Kitzyme Insecticidal Flea powder AVM-GSL

Kitzyme Insecticidal powder AVM-GSL

Kitzyme Veterinary Antiseptic ointment AVM-GSL

Kitzyme Veterinary Antiseptic powder AVM-GSL

Kitzyme Veterinary Combined Wormer AVM-GSL

Kitzyme Veterinary ear drops AVM-GSL

Kitzyme Veterinary Tapewormer AVM-GSL

Kloxerate preparations POM-V

KoiCare Acriflavin SAES

KoiCare B-D-S Fluke Treatment SAES

KoiCare Ex-5 SAES

KoiCare F-M-G SAES

KoiCare Formaldehyde SAES

KoiCare Koi Calm SAES

KoiCare Malachite SAES

KoiCare Permanganate dip SAES

L

Lactaclox intramammary preparation POM-V

Lactatrim MC intramammary preparation POM-V

Lactovac vaccine POM-V

Ladoxyn preparations POM-V

Lambivac vaccine POM-VPS

Lanodip preparations AVM-GSL

Lapinject VHD vaccine POM-V

Lapizole SAES

Large Animal Immobilon CD POM-V

Large Animal Revivon POM-V

Laurabolin injections CD Anab POM-V

Lectade preparations AVM-GSL

Lenticillin injection POM-V

Leptavoid-H vaccine POM-V

Lethobarb CD No Register POM-V

Leucogen vaccine POM-V

Leukocell 2 vaccine POM-V

Levacide preparations POM-VPS

Levacur preparations POM-VPS

Levadren POM-VPS

Levafas preparations POM-VPS

Levasure 7.5% POM-VPS

Levazole 7.5% POM-VPS

Leventa POM-V

Levitape POM-VPS

Leyodip Concentrate teat dip and udderwash AVM-GSL

Leyodip RTU teat dip and teat spray AVM-GSL

Lice Killing shampoo AVM-GSL

Life-Aid preparations AVM-GSL

Lignadrin injection POM-VPS

Lignocaine and adrenaline injection POM-VPS

Lignol injection NFA-VPS

Lincocin preparations POM-V

Lincoject POM-V

Lincomix POM-V

Linco-Spectin preparations POM-V

Liquid Fungus Care SAES

Liquid Lectade AVM-GSL

Liquid Life-Aid AVM-GSL

Locaine 2% injection POM-VPS

Locatim oral solution POM-V

Locovetic injection POM-V

Lopatol tablets AVM-GSL

Louping Ill vaccine POM-VPS

Louse powder AVM-GSL

Lutalyse injection POM-V

Luteosyl injection POM-V

Luxspray 50V teat dip/spray AVM-GSL

M

Magnesium sulphate injection BP(Vet) 25% w/v POM-VPS

Magniject POM-VPS

Malaseb shampoo POM-V

Malted Kelp tablets AVM-GSL

Mamyzin injection POM-V

Marbocyl preparations POM-V

Masocare preparations AVM-GSL

Masodine preparations AVM-GSL

Masodip preparations AVM-GSL

Mastex AVM-GSL

Mastiplan LC intramammary preparation POM-V

Maxiban G160 ZFA

Maximec Horse oral paste POM-VPS

Mebadown preparations POM-VPS

Medesedan injection POM-V

Medetor injection POM-V

Medicinal Oxygen POM-V

Medrone V tablets POM-V

Meflosyl injection POM-V

Megacal-M POM-VPS

Megodine preparations AVM-GSL

Megorex AVM-GSL

Melafix preparations SAES

Meloxidyl POM-V

Meloxivet POM-V

Mesalin injection POM-V

Metacam preparations POM-V

Metricure POM-V

Micotil injection POM-V

Milbemax tablets POM-V

Milk-Line Teat Plus teat dip and spray AVM-GSL

Millophyline-V preparations POM-V

Mixed Vegetable tablets AVM-GSL

Monteban G100 ZFA

Monzaldon injection POM-V

M+PAC vaccine POM-V

MS222 POM-VPS

Multiject IMM POM-V

Multivitamin injection (MA 02000/4131) POM-VPS

Multiworm tablets for Cats NFA-VPS

MV Chlorhexidine RTU teat dip and spray AVM-GSL

MV Iodine RTU teat dip and spray AVM-GSL

Mycophyt POM-VPS

Mycozole spray SAES

Mydiavac vaccine POM-V

Myolaxin 15% POM-V

Mypravac suis POM-V

Mysoline Veterinary tablets POM-V

N

Nafpenzal preparations POM-V

Nandoral tablets CD Anab POM-V

Nandrolin injections CD Anab POM-V

Narketan 10 injection CD Benz POM-V

Natura Insecticidal collars AVM-GSL

Natural Herb tablets AVM-GSL

Navilox oral powder POM-V

Naxcel injection POM-V

Nelio tablets POM-V

Nemovac vaccine POM-V

Neobiotic preparations POM-V

Neocolipor vaccine POM-V

Neomycin Premix (MA 04188/4026) POM-V

Neopen injection POM-V

Nerve tablets AVM-GSL

Nilverm preparations POM-VPS

Nilzan preparations POM-VPS

Nisamox preparations POM-V

Nitroscanate tablets AVM-GSL

Nobilis AE 1143 vaccine POM-VPS

Nobilis CAV-P4 vaccine POM-V

Nobilis diluent CA POM-VPS

Nobilis diluent Oculonasal POM-V

Nobilis Duck Plague vaccine POM-VPS

Nobilis E coli inac vaccine POM-V

Nobilis EDS vaccine POM-VPS

Nobilis Gumboro 228E vaccine POM-V

Nobilis Gumboro D78 vaccine POM-V

Nobilis IB 4-91 vaccine POM-V

Nobilis IB+G+ND vaccine POM-VPS

Nobilis IB H-120 vaccine POM-VPS

Nobilis IB-Ma5 vaccine POM-VPS

Nobilis IB Multi+ND+EDS vaccine POM-V

Nobilis IB+ND+EDS vaccine POM-VPS

Nobilis Influenza vaccine POM-V

Nobilis Influenza H5N2 vaccine POM-V

Nobilis Influenza H5N6 vaccine POM-V

Nobilis Influenza H7N1 vaccine POM-V

Nobilis Ma5 + Clone 30 vaccine POM-VPS

Nobilis Marek THV lyo vaccine POM-VPS

Nobilis Marexine CA126 vaccine POM-VPS

Nobilis MG 6/85 vaccine POM-V

Nobilis ND C2 vaccine POM-V

Nobilis ND Clone 30 Live vaccine POM-VPS

Nobilis ND Hitchner vaccine POM-VPS

Nobilis Newcavac vaccine POM-VPS

Nobilis ORT inac vaccine POM-V

Nobilis Paramyxo P201 vaccine POM-VPS

Nobilis Pasteurella Erysipelas vaccine POM-VPS

Nobilis Reo ERS inac POM-V

Nobilis Reo inac vaccine POM-V

Nobilis Reo+IB+G+ND vaccine POM-V

Nobilis Rhino CV vaccine POM-V

Nobilis Rismavac vaccine POM-VPS

Nobilis Rismavac + CA126 vaccine POM-VPS

Nobilis RT+IB Multi+G+ND vaccine POM-V

Nobilis RT+IB Multi+ND+EDS vaccine POM-V

Nobilis Salenvac vaccine POM-V

Nobilis Salenvac T vaccine POM-V

Nobilis Tri-OR inac vaccine POM-V

Nobilis TRT inac vaccine POM-V

Nobilis TRT live vaccine POM-V

Nobilis TRT+ND vaccine POM-V

Nobivac Bb for Cats vaccine POM-V

Nobivac DH vaccine POM-V

Nobivac DHP vaccine POM-V

Nobivac DHPPi vaccine POM-V

Nobivac Ducat vaccine POM-V

Nobivac Ducat-Chlam vaccine POM-V

Nobivac FeLV vaccine POM-V

Nobivac Forcat vaccine POM-V

Nobivac KC vaccine POM-V

Nobivac Lepto 2 vaccine POM-V

Nobivac Myxo vaccine POM-V

Nobivac Parvo-C vaccine POM-V

Nobivac Pi vaccine POM-V

Nobivac Pigeon Pox vaccine POM-VPS

Nobivac Piro vaccine POM-V

Nobivac PPi vaccine POM-V

Nobivac Rabies vaccine POM-V

Nobivac solvent for vaccines POM-V

Nobivac Tricat vaccine POM-V

Nobivac Tricat Trio vaccine POM-V

Norbet tablets POM-V

Norcal preparations POM-VPS

Norixin injection POM-V

Norobrittin POM-V

Norocarp preparations POM-V

Norocillin preparations POM-V

Noroclav preparations POM-V

Noroclox preparations POM-V

Norodine preparations POM-V

Norodyl preparations POM-V

Norofas injection POM-VPS
Norofol injection POM-V
Norofulvin preparations POM-V
Noromectin preparations POM-VPS
Noroprost injection POM-V
Norotyl LA injection POM-V
Norvax Compact PD vaccine POM-V
Norworm AVM-GSL
Novem preparations POM-V
Nuflor preparations POM-V

O

Occrycetin preparations POM-V
Octacillin WSP POM-V
Oestradiol benzoate [Estradiol benzoate] 5mg injection POM-V
Opticlox eye ointment POM-V
Opticorten tablets POM-V
Optimmune eye ointment POM-V
Oralject preparations POM-V
Oramec preparations POM-VPS
Orandrone tablets CD Anab POM-V
Orbax preparations POM-V
Orbenin preparations POM-V
Orbeseal paste POM-V
Ornicure powder POM-V
Original Extra Tail preparations AVM-GSL
Orojet preparations POM-V
Osmonds Gold Fleece sheep dip POM-VPS
Otello Insecticidal collars for Cats/Dogs AVM-GSL
Oterna ear drops POM-V
Otodex Insecticidal Shampoo for Dogs AVM-GSL
Otodex Skin cream AVM-GSL
Otodex Veterinary ear drops AVM-GSL
Otomax ear drops POM-V
Ovagen POM-V
Ovarelin injection POM-V
Ovarid tablets POM-V
Ovidown preparations POM-VPS
Ovipast Plus vaccine POM-VPS
Ovispec S&C preparations POM-VPS
Ovitelmin preparations POM-VPS
Ovitrol Cat collar AVM-GSL
Ovitrol Dog collar POM-V
Ovivac vaccines POM-VPS
Ovuplant implant POM-V
Oxfencare preparations POM-VPS
Oxycare preparations POM-V
Oxycomplex NS injection POM-V
Oxyglobin POM-V
Oxytetrin preparations POM-V
Oxytocin-S injection POM-V

P

Pabac vaccine POM-VPS
Panacur preparations POM-VPS; but if (a) Panacur 2.5%, 10% Small Animal oral suspension, Panacur granules, Panacur Favourites, Panacur 18.75% oral paste NFA-VPS; (b) Panacur capsules AVM-GSL; (c) Panacur Rabbit 18.75% oral paste SAES
Pangram 5% injection POM-V
Panolog ointment POM-V
Panomec preparations POM-VPS
Paracide preparations POM-VPS
Paracox vaccines POM-V
Parafend preparations POM-VPS
Paramectin preparations POM-VPS
Parasitex Insecticidal collar AVM-GSL
Paratect Flex Bolus POM-VPS
Pardale-V tablets NFA-VPS
Parvovax POM-V
Pastobov vaccine POM-V
Pathocef intramammary suspension POM-V
Paxcutol shampoo POM-V
Pedigree Care Anti Flea shampoo AVM-GSL
Pedigree Care Flea and Tick collar AVM-GSL
Pedigree Care Flea spray AVM-GSL

Pedigree Care Single Dose Worming tablets AVM-GSL
Pedigree Care Wormer for Dogs AVM-GSL
Pen & Strep injection POM-V
Penacare injection POM-V
Penbenocillin injection POM-V
Penillin preparations POM-V
Pentobarbital Solution 20% for Euthanasia CD No Register POM-V
Pentoject injection CD No Register POM-V
PEP 2% powder POM-V
Peridale preparations AVM-GSL
Perlutex tablets POM-V
Permethrin 2% spray for Dogs AVM-GSL
Pestroy 3 months Cat Flea collar AVM-GSL
Pet Mail Insecticidal shampoo AVM-GSL
Pet Rescue Flea spray AVM-GSL
Pet Rescue Worming powder for Cats/Dogs AVM-GSL
Pet Rescue Worming tablets for Dogs AVM-GSL
Pet Star Cat Flea collar AVM-GSL
Pet Star Dog Flea and Tick collar AVM-GSL
Petacol Insecticidal shampoo AVM-GSL
Pethidine injection CD POM-V
Petsulin preparations POM-V
Pfizer Scour Formula AVM-GSL
Pfizer Scour Formula Extra AVM-GSL
Pfizer Twin Lamb Formula AVM-GSL
PG 600 injection POM-V
Pharmaq Ivermectin spot on drops SAES
Pharmasin oral solution POM-V
Phenoxypen POM-V
Phenycare tablets POM-V
Phenylbutazone tablets POM-V
Phosphorus Supplement injection POM-V
Pigzin premix POM-V
Pimafix SAES
Piperazine citrate tablets AVM-GSL
Pirsue intramammary solution POM-V
Planate injection POM-V
Planipart CD Anab POM-V
Plerion tablets NFA-VPS
PLT tablets POM-V
Pluset POM-V
PMSG-Intervet CD Anab POM-V
Pond Aid All You Need Health SAES
Pond Aid Bacterad SAES
Pond Aid Eradick SAES
Pond Care Melafix SAES
Pond Care Pimafix SAES
Pond Care Stress Coat SAES
Porcilis AR-T vaccine POM-VPS
Porcilis AR-T DF vaccine POM-V
Porcilis Begonia DF vaccine POM-V
Porcilis Begonia IDAL vaccine POM-V
Porcilis Coli 6C POM-VPS
Porcilis Ery vaccine POM-VPS
Porcilis Ery + Parvo vaccine POM-V
Porcilis Glässer vaccine POM-V
Porcilis M Hyo vaccine POM-V
Porcilis Pesti vaccine POM-V
Porcilis Porcol 5 vaccine POM-VPS
Porcilis Porcoli vaccines POM-V
Porcilis Porcoli Diluvac Forte POM-VPS
Porcilis PRRS vaccine POM-V
Porcovac Plus vaccine POM-VPS
Posatex ear drops POM-V
Potencil POM-V
Poulvac AE vaccine POM-VPS
Poulvac Bursa Plus vaccine POM-V
Poulvac Bursine 2 vaccine POM-V
Poulvac Flufend i-AIH5N3RG vaccine POM-V
Poulvac Flufend i-AIH5N9 vaccine POM-V
Poulvac Hitchner B1 vaccine POM-VPS
Poulvac IB H120 vaccine POM-VPS
Poulvac IB Primer vaccine POM-V
Poulvac IBMM vaccine POM-VPS
Poulvac IBMM + ARK vaccine POM-V
Poulvac i-IB,ND,EDS,IBD,SHS vaccine POM-V

Poulvac ILT vaccine POM-VPS
Poulvac iSE vaccine POM-V
Poulvac Marek CVI vaccine POM-VPS
Poulvac Marek CVI + HVT vaccine POM-VPS
Poulvac MD-Vac lyophilised vaccine POM-VPS
Poulvac MD-Vac (Frozen-Wet) vaccine POM-VPS
Poulvac NDW vaccine POM-VPS
Poulvac Pabac vaccine POM-VPS
Poulvac SHS vaccine POM-V
Poulvac TRT vaccine POM-V
Pracetam premix POM-V
Prac-Tic spot on POM-V
Prednicare tablets POM-V
Prednidale tablets POM-V
Prednisolone tablets BP (Vet) POM-V
Pregsure BVD vaccine POM-V
Premadex preparations POM-VPS
Prevac vaccines POM-V
Prevender preparations AVM-GSL
Preventef Insecticidal collar for Dogs AVM-GSL
Previcox tablets POM-V
Prid intrauterine device POM-V
Prilactone tablets POM-V
Prilben POM-V
Prilenal preparations POM-V
Prilium preparations POM-V
Primex SC POM-VPS
Proactive teat dip and spray AVM-GSL
Procare preparations POM-V
Procyon Dog vaccines POM-V
Pro-dynam powder POM-V
Profender preparations POM-V
Program injection POM-V
Program Plus tablets POM-V
Program oral suspension for Cats AVM-GSL
Program tablets for Dogs AVM-GSL
Progressis vaccine POM-V
Promeris spot on POM-V
Promone-E injection POM-V
Propalin syrup POM-V
Prophalin POM-V
Propisderm AVM-GSL
PropoFlip POM-V
PropoFlo POM-V
PropoFlo Vet POM-V
Prosolvin injection POM-V
Prostapar injection POM-V
Prostavet injection POM-V
Protech vaccines POM-V
Protect spot Flea and Tick drops for Dogs AVM-GSL
Protection 300 Insecticidal collar AVM-GSL
ProteqFlu vaccines POM-V
Protocon Gold AVM-GSL
Provid 44% paste POM-VPS
Provita Protect for Newborn Calves POM-VPS
Pruban 0.1% cream POM-V
Pulmodox oral paste POM-V
Pulmotil preparations POM-V
Pulsaflox oral solution POM-V
Purevax vaccines POM-V
Pyceze POM-V
Pyratape P Horse Wormer POM-VPS
Pyriproxyfen premix POM-V
Pyroflam injection POM-V

Q

Quadrisol preparations POM-V
Qualimec preparations POM-VPS
Qualminthic preparations POM-VPS
Quantum vaccines POM-V
QuarterMate AVM-GSL
Quazitel 2.5% suspension POM-VPS

R

Rabguard POM-V
Rabigen SAG2 oral suspension POM-V
Rabisin vaccine POM-V

Radiol Insecticidal Soapless shampoo with Conditioner AVM-GSL
Rapidex pour on POM-VPS
Rapidexon injection POM-V
Rapinovet injection POM-V
Raspberry Leaf tablets AVM-GSL
Ready to Use teat dip and teat spray AVM-GSL
Readymix Gold teat dip or spray AVM-GSL
Readymix teat dip or spray AVM-GSL
Rearguard solution POM-V
Receptal injection POM-V
Regulin implant POM-VPS
Regumate preparations POM-V
Release injection POM-V
Renegade pour on POM-VPS
Reprocine injection POM-V
Reproval injection POM-V
Resflor injection POM-V
Resprixin injection POM-V
Resugel POM-VPS
Retarbolin CD Anab POM-V
Revertor injection POM-V
Revivon (Large Animal) POM-V
Rheumocam POM-V
Rhubarb tablets AVM-GSL
Ridect pour on POM-VPS
Rilexine tablets POM-V
Rimadyl preparations POM-V
Rimifin tablets POM-V
Ripercol preparations POM-VPS
Rispoval vaccines POM-V
Robust dip POM-VPS
Romidys injection POM-V
Rompun preparations POM-V
Ronaxan tablets POM-V
Rotavec vaccines POM-V
RTU teat dip or spray AVM-GSL
Ruby Paragard Veterinary Insecticidal spray AVM-GSL
Ruby Teatguard AVM-GSL
Ruby Veterinary ear drops AVM-GSL
Rumbul Magnesium bullets POM-VPS
Rumbul Rumen Bullet Cattle POM-VPS
Rumbul Rumen Bullet Sheep POM-VPS
Rumetrace Ezymin Cobalt pellets AVM-GSL
Rupinal POM-V
Rycoben preparations POM-VPS

S

Sacox 120 ZFA
Salinomax 120G premix ZFA
Salmosan POM-V
Saniphor spray AVM-GSL
Sapphire preparations AVM-GSL
Savlon Veterinary Antiseptic Concentrate AVM-GSL
Scabivax vaccines POM-V
Scalibor collar POM-V
Scordex injection POM-VPS
Scourproof solution AVM-GSL
Scullcap and Valerian tablets AVM-GSL
Seaweed tablets AVM-GSL
Sebolyse shampoo POM-V
Sectine pour on AVM-GSL
Sedalin preparations POM-V
Sedator injection POM-V
Sedaxylan injection POM-V
Sededorm injection POM-V
Sedivet injection POM-V
Selectan injection POM-V
Seleen shampoo AVM-GSL
Selgian tablets POM-V
Sensospray teat dip and spray AVM-GSL
Sentinel Spectrum preparations POM-V
Sergeants Flea collar for Cats/Dogs AVM-GSL
Sergeants Pet Patrol AVM-GSL
Seven Seas Kitzyme Flea Rid Reflective Flea collar AVM-GSL
Seven Seas Vetzyme Flea Rid Reflective Flea collar AVM-GSL
Sevoflo POM-V
Shake AVM-GSL
Sheptaclox DC POM-V

Sherley's Easy Treat Wormer AVM-GSL
Sherley's Easy Treat Worming cream AVM-GSL
Sherley's Felt Flea collar AVM-GSL
Sherley's Flea and Tick collar for Dogs AVM-GSL
Sherley's Flea collar for Cats AVM-GSL
Sherley's Flea spray AVM-GSL
Sherley's Insecticidal Dog shampoo AVM-GSL
Sherley's Multiwormer for Cats/Dogs AVM-GSL
Sherley's One Dose Wormer for Dogs AVM-GSL
Sherley's Permethrin Flea powder AVM-GSL
Sherley's Rheumatine Tablets for Adult Dogs AVM-GSL
Sherley's Worming cream AVM-GSL
Sherley's Worming granules for Cats/Dogs AVM-GSL
Sherley's Worming syrup AVM-GSL
Sherley's Worming tablets for Cats/Dogs AVM-GSL
Shotaflor injection POM-V
Silkidip AVM-GSL
Slentrol POM-V
Slice premix POM-V
Skin Cure AVM-GSL
Sodium calciumedetate POM-V
Solacyl POM-V
Soldoxin POM-V
Soloxine tablets POM-V
Solubenol POM-VPS
Soludox POM-V
Solu-Medrone V injection POM-V
Somulose injection CD POM-V
Spartakon tablets AVM-GSL
Spartrix tablets AVM-GSL
Spectam preparations POM-V
Spirovac vaccine POM-V
Spunhill Gold AVM-GSL
Sputolosin powder POM-V
Stabox preparations POM-V
Star Iodocare Concentrate AVM-GSL
Star Ready-Dip AVM-GSL
Star Teat-ex AVM-GSL
Stegantox preparations POM-V
Stellamune vaccines POM-V
Stenoral premix ZFA
Sterile water for injections BP POM-V
SteroVet POM-V
Stomorgyl preparations POM-V
Streptacare injection POM-V
Streptopen preparations POM-V
Stresnil injection POM-V
Stress Coat SAES
Strinacin II tablets POM-V
Stronghold preparations POM-V
Strongid Caramel POM-VPS
Strongid P preparations POM-VPS
Strongid paste for Dogs NFA-VPS
Sulfatrim preparations POM-V
Sulphur Colecton preparations AVM-GSL
Sumex pour on POM-VPS
Summer C dip AVM-GSL
Summer Teatguard AVM-GSL
Supaverm oral suspension POM-VPS
Super Concentrate teat dip or spray AVM-GSL
Super Gold dip AVM-GSL
Super Ov POM-V
Super Ruby dip AVM-GSL
Super Zinc AVM-GSL
Supercal preparations POM-VPS
Supercare Four AVM-GSL
Supercare Summer Tg AVM-GSL
Supercare Three teat dip Concentrate AVM-GSL
Supercare Two Iodine teat dip Ready to Use AVM-GSL
Superteat AVM-GSL
Suprelorin implant POM-V
Suredip preparations AVM-GSL
Surolan POM-V
Suvaxyn Aujeszky 783+O/W vaccine POM-V

Suvaxyn E Coli P4 vaccine POM-VPS
Suvaxyn Ery vaccine POM-V
Suvaxyn M. hyo vaccine POM-V
Suvaxyn M. hyo-Parasuis vaccine POM-V
Suvaxyn MH One POM-V
Suvaxyn Parvo vaccine POM-V
Suvaxyn Parvo/e vaccine POM-V
Suvaxyn Parvo ST POM-V
Suvaxyn Respifend POM-V
Swaycop injection POM-VPS
Switch AVM-GSL
Synermast Lactating Cow Intramammary suspension POM-V
Synulox preparations POM-V
Synutrim preparations POM-V
Systamex preparations POM-VPS

T

Tapewormer tablets for Cats/Dogs AVM-GSL
Tardak injection POM-V
1:3 Teat dip/spray and udder wash AVM-GSL
Tecvax Pasteurella vaccine POM-V
Telmin preparations POM-VPS
Telzenac injection POM-V
Tensolvet gel POM-VPS
Terramycin preparations POM-V
Terrexine POM-V
Tetanus Antitoxin Behring POM-V
Tetanus Toxoid Concentrated POM-V
Tetcin preparations POM-V
Tetra Delta preparations POM-V
TetraMedica ContraSpot SAES
TetraMedica FungiStop SAES
TetraMedica General Tonic SAES
TetraMedica Gold Med SAES
Tetramin preparations POM-V
TetraPond MediFin SAES
Tetraseptin preparations POM-V
Tetroxy LA injection POM-V
Tetsol 800 POM-V
Therios tablets POM-V
Thiovet preparations POM-V
Thyroxyl tablets POM-V
Tiacil Ophthalmic solution POM-V
Tiamvet POM-V
Tildren POM-V
Tilmovet preparations POM-V
Tirade spray POM-VPS
Tivafol injection POM-V
Tolfedine preparations POM-V
Tolfine injection POM-V
Top Drop preparations POM-V
Torbugesic injection POM-V
Torbutrol tablets POM-V
Torvac vaccines POM-V
Toxovax vaccine POM-V
Tracherine vaccine POM-V
Tramazole 2.5% drench POM-VPS
Trempex AVM-GSL
Tri Lyte Plus AVM-GSL
Tribex preparations POM-VPS
Tribovax-T vaccine POM-VPS
Tribrissen preparations POM-V
Triclacert preparations POM-VPS
Triclafas drench POM-VPS
Trimacare preparations POM-V
Trimediazine preparations POM-V
Trimedoxine preparations POM-V
Trinacol injection POM-V
Trioxyl LA injection POM-V
Trivacton 6 vaccine POM-VPS
Trodax 34% injection POM-VPS
Tropical Fish Start Up Pack SAES
Troscan preparations AVM-GSL
True Dip Pink teat dip and teat spray AVM-GSL
True Dip RTU teat dip and spray AVM-GSL
Tryplase capsules AVM-GSL
TUR 3 vaccine POM-V
Twin Pack Two Collars Bob Martin Flea and Tick for Dogs AVM-GSL
Twinox preparations POM-V

3TX 1:3 Concentrate for teat dip and spray AVM-GSL
Tylan preparations POM-V
Tyluvet-20 injection POM-V

U

Ubro Red Dry Cow POM-V
Ubro Yellow Milking Cow POM-V
Ubrolexin POM-V
Udder Guard AVM-GSL
Ultrapen LA injection POM-V
Uniferon injection POM-VPS
Uniprim preparations POM-V
Unisolve POM-VPS
Urilin syrup POM-V
Utocyl pessaries POM-V

V

Valbazen preparations POM-VPS
Vanguard vaccines POM-V
Vasotop tablets POM-V
Vaxxitek HVT + IBD vaccine POM-V
Vecoxan suspension POM-VPS
Vectin preparations POM-VPS
Ventipulmin preparations CD Anab POM-V
Venture 321 AVM-GSL
Venture Io-care AVM-GSL
Venture Satinex AVM-GSL
Veramix Sheep Sponge POM-V
Vetalar V injection CD Benz POM-V
Vetergesic injection CD No Register POM-V
Veterinary Antiseptic spray AVM-GSL
Veterinary Wound powder AVM-GSL
Vetflurane POM-V
Vetical 40+M POM-VPS
Veticop injection POM-VPS
Vetivex preparations POM-V
VetKem collar AVM-GSL
VetKem Dog spray POM-V
Vetmedin preparations POM-V
Vetmulin preparations POM-V
Vetodale cream POM-V
Vetodex skin cream AVM-GSL
Vetofol injection POM-V
Vetoryl preparations POM-V
Vetrazin pour on POM-VPS
Vetremox preparations POM-V
Vetrimoxin preparations POM-V
Vetzyme Antiseptic ointment/ powder AVM-GSL
Vetzyme Cat Wormer AVM-GSL
Vetzyme Combined Wormer AVM-GSL
Vetzyme Flearid Dual Action Insecticidal spray AVM-GSL
Vetzyme Flearid Insecticidal spray AVM-GSL
Vetzyme Flearid shampoo for Dogs AVM-GSL
Vetzyme Granule Wormer for Dogs AVM-GSL
Vetzyme Insecticidal Flea powder AVM-GSL
Vetzyme JDS Insecticidal shampoo AVM-GSL
Vetzyme Kitzyme Ear drops AVM-GSL
Vetzyme One Dose Wormer for Dogs AVM-GSL
Vetzyme Pet Antiseptic AVM-GSL
Vetzyme Skin cream AVM-GSL
Vetzyme Veterinary Antiseptic lotion/ ointment/ powder AVM-GSL
Vetzyme Veterinary Combined wormer AVM-GSL
Vetzyme Veterinary ear drops AVM-GSL
Vetzyme Veterinary skin cream AVM-GSL
Vetzyme Veterinary Tapewormer tablets AVM-GSL
Vidalta tablets POM-V
Virbac Ivermectin & Praziquantel oral gel for Horses POM-VPS
Virbac Prevender AVM-GSL
Virbacef injection POM-V
Virbagen preparations POM-V

Virbagest oral solution POM-V
Virbamec preparations POM-VPS
Virbaxyl preparations POM-V
Vitamin B1 injection POM-V
Vitbee preparations POM-VPS
Vitenium injection POM-V
Vitesel POM-V
Vivitonin preparations POM-V
Voren injections POM-V

W

Walpole's Buffer solution POM-V
Water for injection POM-V
Whiskas Care Flea collar/ spray AVM-GSL
Whiskas Care Worming tablets AVM-GSL
Whiskas Wormer for Cats AVM-GSL
White Spot Cure SAES
Wilko Cat Felt Flea collar AVM-GSL
Wilko Cat Flea powder AVM-GSL
Wilko Cat Flea spray AVM-GSL
Wilko Dog Flea drops AVM-GSL
Wilko Dog Flea powder AVM-GSL
Wilko Dog Flea spray AVM-GSL
Wilko Dual Action Worming tablets for Cats AVM-GSL
Wilko Insecticidal Dog shampoo AVM-GSL
Wilko Long Lasting Flea and Tick collar for Dogs AVM-GSL
Wilko Long Lasting Flea collar for Cats AVM-GSL
Wilko Silent Action Cat/Dog Flea spray AVM-GSL
Wilko Single Dose Wormer for Dogs AVM-GSL
Wilko Vinyl Cat Flea collar AVM-GSL
Wilko Vinyl Dog Flea and Tick collar AVM-GSL
Wilko White Spot Control SAES
Willcain injection POM-VPS
Willows Dry Cow Xtra POM-V
Worm tablets for Cats/Dogs NFA-VPS
Wormazole NFA-VPS
Wynnstay 1:3 Concentrated Iodophor teat dip/spray AVM-GSL
Wynnstay RTU Iodophor teat dip/spray AVM-GSL

X

Xeden tablets POM-V
Xenex Ultra spot on SAES
Xeno preparations SAES
Xylacare 2% injection POM-V
Xylapan injection POM-V
Xylazine 2% POM-V

Y

Yarvitan POM-V
Ypozane POM-V

Z

Zactran POM-V
Zanil Fluke drench POM-VPS
Zermasect preparations POM-VPS
Zermex preparations POM-VPS
Zerofen preparations POM-VPS; but if Zerofen 22% granules (small animals) AVM-GSL
Zincoped solution AVM-GSL
Zincotec Zinc Oxide POM-V
Zitac Vet tablets POM-V
Zodiac Five Month Flea collar for Cats/Dogs AVM-GSL
Zodiac Flea and Tick for Dogs AVM-GSL
Zodiac Pet spray AVM-GSL
Zodiac Single Dose Wormer 100 AVM-GSL
Zodiac Single Dose Wormer 500 AVM-GSL
Zodiac Twelve Month Flea collar for Cats AVM-GSL
Zolan tablets POM-V
Zubrin preparations POM-V
Zulvac 8 vaccines POM-V

2: Code of Ethics and Professional Standards and Guidance

2.1 Code of Ethics for Pharmacists and Pharmacy Technicians

About this document

Registration as a pharmacist or pharmacy technician carries obligations as well as privileges. It requires you to:

- develop and use your professional knowledge and skills for the benefit of those who seek your professional services,
- maintain good professional relationships with others, and
- act in a way that promotes confidence and trust in the pharmacy professions.

The Code of Ethics sets out the principles that you must follow as a pharmacist or pharmacy technician. The Code is the Society's core guidance on the conduct, practice and professional performance expected of you. It is designed to meet our obligations under The Pharmacists and Pharmacy Technicians Order 2007 and other relevant legislation. The principles of the Code are intended to guide and support the work you do and the decisions you make. They also inform the general public of the standards of behaviour that can be expected from the pharmacy professions. The Code underpins all other standards and guidance we issue. We will review the Code in the light of changes within the professions or health-care environment.

The Code is founded on seven principles which express the values central to the identity of the pharmacy professions. The seven principles and their supporting explanations encapsulate what it means to be a registered pharmacist or pharmacy technician. Making these principles part of your professional life will maintain patient safety and public confidence in the professions.

As well as the Code of Ethics, we have produced supporting standards and guidance documents that expand on aspects of the Code, or provide more detailed guidance on specific areas of pharmacy practice. You can download these documents and more copies of the Code from our website at *www.rpsgb.org*, or you can telephone us on 020 7735 9141.

Status of the Code of Ethics

The principles of the Code of Ethics are mandatory. As a registered pharmacist or pharmacy technician your professional and personal conduct will be judged against the Code. You must abide by its principles irrespective of the job you do. Disreputable behaviour, even if it is not directly connected to your professional practice, or failure to comply with the principles identified in the Code could put your registration at risk. The Society's fitness to practise committees will take account of the Code in considering cases that come before them but are not limited solely to the matters mentioned in it. They will consider the circumstances of an individual case when deciding whether or not action should follow.

The seven principles

As a pharmacist or pharmacy technician you must:

1. Make the care of patients your first concern
2. Exercise your professional judgement in the interests of patients and the public
3. Show respect for others
4. Encourage patients to participate in decisions about their care
5. Develop your professional knowledge and competence
6. Be honest and trustworthy
7. Take responsibility for your working practices

Applying the principles

Pharmacists have overall responsibility for the provision of pharmaceutical services. Pharmacy technicians undertake work to support, develop or provide these services. Every registered pharmacy professional is responsible for their own actions.

It is your responsibility as a pharmacist or pharmacy technician to apply the principles of the Code of Ethics to your daily work, whether or not you routinely treat or care for patients. You must be able to show that you are aware of the Code and have followed the principles it lays down.

You are professionally accountable for your practice. This means that you are answerable for your acts and omissions, regardless of advice or directions from your manager or another professional. You are expected to use your professional judgement in the light of the principles of the Code and must be prepared to justify your actions if asked to do so.

Users of pharmaceutical services include patients, customers and clients. The Code uses the term patient(s) to encompass any individuals or groups who access or are affected by your professional pharmacy services or advice. If you offer veterinary pharmacy services, the term patient also extends to the animals you provide services for.

The work of pharmacists and pharmacy technicians takes many different forms and accordingly not all of the principles will be applicable to every situation you find yourself in. The seven principles are of equal importance. Each principle is supported by a series of statements that explain the types of action and behaviour expected of you when applying the principles in practice. These are not exhaustive. In meeting the principles of the Code you are expected to comply with other accepted standards and take account of guidance issued by the Society or other relevant organisations.

From time to time you may be faced with conflicting professional obligations or legal requirements. In these circumstances you must consider fully the options available to you, evaluate the risks and benefits associated with possible courses of action and determine what is most appropriate in the interests of patients and the public.

1. Make the care of patients your first concern

The care, well-being and safety of patients are at the centre of everyday professional practice. They must be your primary and continuing concern when practising, irrespective of your field of work. Even if you do not have direct contact with patients your actions or behaviour can still impact on their care or safety. You must:

1.1 Provide a proper standard of practice and care to those for whom you provide professional services.
1.2 Take steps to safeguard the well-being of patients, particularly children and other vulnerable individuals.
1.3 Promote the health of patients.
1.4 Seek all relevant information required to assess an individual's needs and provide appropriate treatment and care. Where necessary, refer patients to other health or social care professionals or other relevant organisations.
1.5 Seek to ensure safe and timely access to medicines and take steps to be satisfied of the clinical appropriateness of medicines supplied to individual patients.
1.6 Encourage the effective use of medicines and be satisfied that patients, or those who care for them, know how to use their medicines.
1.7 Be satisfied as to the integrity and quality of products to be supplied to patients.
1.8 Maintain timely, accurate and adequate records and include all relevant information in a clear and legible form.

1.9 Ensure you have access to the facilities, equipment and materials necessary to provide services to professionally accepted standards.
1.10 Undertake regular reviews, audits and risk assessments to improve the quality of services and minimise risks to patient and public safety.

2. Exercise your professional judgement in the interests of patients and the public

The need to balance the requirements of individuals with society as a whole and manage competing priorities and obligations is a feature of professional life. Guidelines, targets and financial constraints need to be taken into account, but they must not be allowed to compromise your ability to make an informed professional judgement on what is appropriate for patients in specific situations. When acting in your professional capacity you must:

2.1 Consider and act in the best interests of individual patients and the public.
2.2 Make sure that your professional judgement is not impaired by personal or commercial interests, incentives, targets or similar measures.
2.3 Make best use of the resources available to you.
2.4 Be prepared to challenge the judgement of colleagues and other health or social care professionals if you have reason to believe that their decisions could compromise the safety or care of others.
2.5 Conduct research and development with integrity and obtain any necessary permissions from the appropriate regulatory authorities.
2.6 In an emergency take appropriate action to provide care and reduce risks to patients and the public, taking into account your competence and other options for assistance or care available.

3. Show respect for others

Demonstrating respect for the dignity, views and rights of others is fundamental in forming and maintaining professionally appropriate relationships with patients, their carers, colleagues and other individuals with whom you come into contact with. In your professional practice you must:

3.1 Recognise diversity and respect the cultural differences, values and beliefs of others.
3.2 Treat others politely and considerately.
3.3 Make sure your views about a person's lifestyle, beliefs, race, gender, age, sexuality, disability or other perceived status do not prejudice their treatment or care.
3.4 Ensure that if your religious or moral beliefs prevent you from providing a particular professional service, the relevant persons or authorities are informed of this and patients are referred to alternative providers for the service they require.
3.5 Respect and protect the dignity and privacy of others. Take all reasonable steps to prevent accidental disclosure or unauthorised access to confidential information and ensure that you do not disclose confidential information without consent, apart from where permitted to do so by the law or in exceptional circumstances.

3.6 Obtain consent for the professional services, treatment or care you provide and the patient information you use.

3.7 Use information obtained in the course of professional practice only for the purposes for which it was given or where otherwise lawful.

3.8 Take all reasonable steps to ensure appropriate levels of privacy for patient consultations.

3.9 Maintain proper professional boundaries in the relationships you have with patients and other individuals that you come into contact with during the course of your professional practice, taking special care when dealing with vulnerable individuals.

4. Encourage patients to participate in decisions about their care

Patients have a right to be involved in decisions about their treatment and care. They should be encouraged to work in partnership with you and other members of the professional team to manage their healthcare needs. Successful partnership working requires effective communication and an ability to identify the individual needs of patients. Where patients are not legally capable of making decisions about their care you must seek the authority of persons who are empowered to make decisions on their behalf. You must:

4.1 When possible, work in partnership with patients, their carers and other healthcare professionals to manage the patient's treatment and care. Explain the options available and help individuals to make informed decisions about whether they wish to use particular services or treatment options.

4.2 Listen to patients and their carers and endeavour to communicate effectively with them. Ensure that, whenever possible, reasonable steps are taken to meet the particular communication needs of the patient.

4.3 Take all reasonable steps to share information that patients or their carers want or need in a way that they can understand, and make sure that the information you provide is impartial, relevant and up to date.

4.4 Subject to paragraph 3.5, ensure that information is shared appropriately with other health and social care professionals involved in the care of the patient.

4.5 Respect a patient's right to refuse to receive treatment, care or other professional services.

4.6 Consider and whenever possible take steps to address factors that may prevent or deter individuals from obtaining or taking their treatment.

4.7 Ensure that when a patient is not legally competent, any treatment or care you provide is in accordance with the appropriate legal requirements.

5. Develop your professional knowledge and competence

At all stages of your professional working life you must ensure that your knowledge, skills and performance are of a high quality, up to date and relevant to your field of practice. You must:

5.1 Maintain and improve the quality of your work by keeping your knowledge and skills up to date, evidence-based and relevant to your role and responsibilities.

5.2 Apply your knowledge and skills appropriately to your professional responsibilities.

5.3 Recognise the limits of your professional competence; practise only in those areas in which you are competent to do so and refer to others where necessary.

5.4 Undertake and maintain up-to-date evidence of continuing professional development relevant to your field of practice.

5.5 Respond constructively to the outcomes of assessments, appraisals and reviews of your professional performance and undertake further training where necessary.

5.6 Practise only if you are fit and competent to do so. Promptly declare to the Society, your employer and other relevant authorities any circumstances that may call into question your fitness to practise or bring the pharmacy professions into disrepute, including ill health that impairs your ability to practise, criminal convictions and findings by other regulatory bodies or organisations.

6. Be honest and trustworthy

Patients, colleagues and the public at large place their trust in you as a pharmacy professional. You must behave in a way that justifies this trust and maintains the reputation of your profession. You must:

6.1 Uphold public trust and confidence in your profession by acting with honesty and integrity.

6.2 Ensure you do not abuse your professional position or exploit the vulnerability or lack of knowledge of others.

6.3 Avoid conflicts of interest and declare any personal or professional interests to those who may be affected. Do not ask for or accept gifts, inducements, hospitality or referrals that may affect, or be perceived to affect, your professional judgement.

6.4 Be accurate and impartial when teaching others and when providing or publishing information to ensure that you do not mislead others or make claims that cannot be justified.

6.5 Adhere to accepted standards of personal and professional conduct.

6.6 Comply with legal requirements, mandatory professional standards and accepted best practice guidance.

6.7 Honour commitments, agreements and arrangements for the provision of professional services.

6.8 Respond honestly, openly and courteously to complaints and criticism.

7. Take responsibility for your working practices

Team working is a key feature of everyday professional practice and requires respect, co-operation and communication with colleagues from your own and other professions. When working as part of a team you remain accountable for your own decisions, behaviour and any work done under your supervision. You must:

7.1 Communicate and work effectively with colleagues from your own and other professions and ensure that both you and those you employ or supervise have sufficient language competence to do this.

7.2 Contribute to the development, education and training of colleagues and students, sharing relevant knowledge, skills and expertise.

7.3 Take responsibility for all work done by you or under your supervision. Ensure that individuals to whom you delegate tasks are competent and fit to practise and have undertaken, or are in the process of undertaking, the training required for their duties.

7.4 Be satisfied that appropriate standard operating procedures exist and are adhered to, and that clear lines of accountability and verifiable audit trails are in place.

7.5 Ensure that you are able to comply with your legal and professional obligations and that your workload or working conditions do not compromise patient care or public safety.

7.6 Make sure that your actions do not prevent others from complying with their legal and professional obligations, or present a risk to patient care or public safety.

7.7 Ensure that all professional activities undertaken by you, or under your control, are covered by appropriate professional indemnity arrangements.

7.8 Be satisfied that there is an effective complaints procedure where you work and follow it at all times.

7.9 Raise concerns if policies, systems, working conditions, or the actions, professional performance or health of others may compromise patient care or public safety. Take appropriate action if something goes wrong or if others report concerns to you.

7.10 Co-operate with investigations into your or another healthcare professional's fitness to practise and abide by undertakings you give or any restrictions placed on your practice.

Guidance that supports the Code of Ethics

Supporting standards and guidance documents that expand on aspects of the Code, or provide more detailed guidance on specific areas of pharmacy practice are available below and on the Society's website at _www.rpsgb.org_. You can also telephone us on 020 7735 9141 or e-mail us at _enquiries@rpsgb.org_.

Other sources of advice

For further advice on the Code, or other professional or legal obligations, contact our legal and ethical advisory service on 020 7572 2308; or e-mail _leadvice@rpsgb.org_.

2.2 Professional Standards and Guidance Documents

The Code of Ethics for Pharmacists and Pharmacy Technicians is supported by the following nine Professional Standards and Guidance Documents:

- Professional Standards for **Pharmacists and Pharmacy Technicians in Positions of Authority** (_see_ p106) (Amended version, effective from 1 October 2009, available on the RPSGB website _www.rpsgb.org_)
- Professional Standards and Guidance for **Patient Consent** (_see_ p110)
- Professional Standards and Guidance for **Patient Confidentiality** (_see_ p114)
- Professional Standards and Guidance for the **Sale and Supply of Medicines** (_see_ p117)
- Professional Standards and Guidance for **Advertising Medicines and Professional Services** (_see_ p122)
- Professional Standards and Guidance for **Internet Pharmacy Services** (_see_ p123)
- Professional Standards and Guidance for **Pharmacist Prescribers** (_see_ p126)
- Professional Standards and Guidance for **Continuing Professional Development** (_see_ p133)
- Professional Standards and Guidance for **Responsible Pharmacists** (Effective from 1 October 2009) (_see_ p134)

Status of these documents Principle 6.6 of the Code of Ethics states that you must comply with legal requirements, mandatory professional standards and accepted best practice guidance. These documents contain:

- Mandatory professional standards (indicated by the word 'must') for all registered pharmacists and pharmacy technicians; and
- Guidance on good practice (indicated by the word 'should') which you should follow in all normal circumstances.

If a complaint is made against you the Society's fitness to practise committees will take account of the requirements of the Code of Ethics and underpinning documents including these documents. You will be expected to justify any decision to act outside their terms.

Other sources of Society advice Further information or advice on the professional or legal obligations of the pharmacy profession can be obtained by contacting the Society's Legal and Ethical Advisory Service on 020 7572 2308, or e-mail _leadvice@rpsgb.org_.

Professional Standards for Pharmacists and Pharmacy Technicians in Positions of Authority

About this document

The Code of Ethics sets out seven principles of ethical practice that you must follow as a pharmacist or pharmacy technician. It is your responsibility to apply the principles to your daily work, using your judgement in the light of the principles.

The Code of Ethics says that you must **'Take responsibility for your working practices'** and sets out what you are expected to do when applying this principle in practice.

This document expands on the principles of the Code of Ethics to set out your professional responsibilities if you are in a position of authority. It is designed to meet the Society's obligations under the Pharmacists and Pharmacy Technicians Order 2007 and other relevant legislation.

The term 'position of authority' encompasses the wide range of managerial responsibilities pharmacists and pharmacy technicians undertake, including managing a pharmacy, pharmacy team or department, being a superintendent pharmacist or pharmacy owner, or managing services in a hospital, trust or other field of practice such as industry or academia. The standards in this document are intended to apply to all practice settings. As pharmacists and pharmacy technicians take on management responsibilities to varying degrees, the ability to put into effect parts of this document will depend on the authority your position gives you and the area of practice in which you work.

If you have overall responsibility for the provision of pharmacy services within your organisation (for example, if you own a registered pharmacy premises, are a superintendent pharmacist, or are a chief pharmacist), you must ensure that all the standards set out in this document are met. Where you have delegated the day-to-day implementation of any of the standards you retain overall responsibility for ensuring that the standards are met.

If you are a pharmacist or pharmacy technician with other management responsibilities, for example, if you assume responsibility for the day-to-day running of a department or pharmacy premises, or if you have management responsibilities for a group of pharmacies or staff within your organisation, you must ensure that the standards in this document are met wherever it is your responsibility and within your power to do so. Where it is not, you must raise awareness of any problems with those who are in a position to make change.

This document does not detail legislative requirements, but when in a position of authority you must comply with the legislative and contractual requirements, such as NHS terms of service, relevant to your management responsibilities.

1. Accepting positions of authority

Standards
You must accept work only where you have the skills and competence for the tasks to be performed. When taking on any position of authority you must:

1.1 establish the scope of your role and responsibilities and clarify any ambiguities or uncertainties about where your responsibilities lie.
1.2 have the necessary knowledge, skills and experience, including sufficient language competence, to undertake the role.
1.3 be able to comply with your legal and professional obligations and manage effectively the activities you are responsible for.
1.4 keep up to date with and observe the laws, statutory codes and professional obligations relevant to your particular responsibilities.
1.5 declare to the relevant person or authority any interests that could be perceived to influence your judgement in financial or commercial dealings which impact on patient care or public safety.

2. Policies and procedures

Standards
You must ensure that all legal and professional requirements are observed in relation to the pharmaceutical aspects of the business or professional services you manage. It is essential that appropriate policies and procedures are established, maintained and reviewed. Policies and procedures must be made readily available to relevant staff. There must be clarity on areas of responsibility and clear lines of accountability must exist.

If you are a pharmacy owner, superintendent pharmacist or pharmacy manager in a hospital, trust, or other field of practice you have overall responsibility for setting out the standards and policies for the provision of pharmacy services by your organisation. If you are a pharmacist or pharmacy technician with management responsibilities for the day-to-day running of one or more departments or pharmacy premises, you must ensure that policies and procedures are appropriate for the particular department or premises you are responsible for.

You must, as appropriate to your particular management responsibilities, ensure that:

2.1 policies and standard operating procedures to ensure the safe and effective provision of pharmacy services in accordance with relevant legal and professional requirements are in place, maintained and regularly reviewed.
2.2 clear lines of accountability exist and a retrievable audit trail of the health professional taking responsibility for the provision of each pharmacy service is maintained.
2.3 appropriate policies for the number and required experience levels of staff for the business or department(s) you manage are in place and are made known to relevant staff.
2.4 suitable arrangements are in place when members of staff are off duty and effective handover procedures are followed.
2.5 there are systems to identify and manage risks to patients, the public and those you employ. There must be procedures to deal with incidents that pose a threat to patient, public or employee safety and to review practices in light of such incidents.
2.6 procedures are in place to record errors or near miss incidents, notify the person responsible, and review procedures as appropriate.
2.7 procedures respect and protect confidential information about patients and employees in accordance with current legislation, relevant codes of practice and professional guidelines.
2.8 systems are in place to ensure that the supplier and the quality of any medicines, devices and pharmaceutical ingredients obtained are reputable.
2.9 appropriate security measures are in place to protect stocks of medicinal products, devices, and pharmaceutical ingredients, especially those which may be at particular risk of theft or abuse.
2.10 any advertising and promotional activity you authorise for professional services or medicinal products complies with appropriate advertising codes of practice, professional guidance and the law.

3. Pharmacy premises and facilities

Standards
The pharmacy premises, department or facilities you manage must enable safe systems of work and be appropriate to the professional services being provided. You must ensure that:

3.1 the pharmacy premises, department or facilities you are responsible for do not bring the pharmacy profession into disrepute.
3.2 all relevant statutory requirements and regulations are complied with.

3.3 any part of the premises from which professional services are provided is readily identifiable and well maintained.

3.4 medicines, pharmaceutical ingredients, devices and other stock at the pharmacy premises or facilities are stored under conditions appropriate to the nature and stability of the product concerned.

4. Responsibilities to those you employ, manage or lead

Standards

You must make sure that those you employ, manage or lead, including temporary staff and locums, are not prevented or hindered from performing their professional and legal duties. You must ensure that:

4.1 the views, beliefs and rights of those you employ, manage or lead are respected and protected.

4.2 financial or other targets do not compromise the professional services you and your staff provide.

4.3 those you employ, manage or lead:
- are aware of and are able to comply with their professional and legal responsibilities;
- are able to exercise their professional judgement in the best interest of patients and the public;
- understand their individual roles and responsibilities, including the activities and decisions which have and have not been delegated to them;
- are provided with the information necessary to enable them to perform their duties safely and effectively;
- are not required to undertake tasks that they are not competent and trained, or being trained, to do;
- have appropriate supervision, either through close personal supervision (trainee staff, for example) or, where legislation permits and the staff are appropriately trained and qualified, through a managed system with clear reporting structures.

4.4 working conditions and practices are lawful and resources, facilities and equipment enable staff to provide services to professionally accepted standards.

4.5 staff are able and encouraged to take appropriate rest breaks. When agreeing working hours and rest breaks with employees you must take into account legislative requirements, individual requirements for breaks and the needs of patients.

5. Employing others

Standards

Individuals who are employed or engaged to provide pharmacy services, including temporary staff and locums, must be suitable for the role given to them. If you employ or engage pharmacists, pharmacy technicians or other pharmacy staff (including trainees and students), or if you have overall responsibility for their employment within your organisation, you must be satisfied that:

5.1 appropriate checks are carried out before employment commences and that adverse findings do not make employing or engaging the individual untenable. Depending on the remit and responsibilities of the role this may include inquiries about previous criminal convictions, verification of professional registration status and checks on any conditions or limitations on practice.

5.2 the individual to be employed has or will undertake appropriate training to attain the skills, knowledge and competency, including sufficient language competence for their role.

5.3 reliable references are sought and provided.

5.4 the requirements of the Code of Ethics are taken into account when making decisions relating to the conduct of pharmacists, pharmacy technicians, pre-registration trainees or student pharmacy technicians.

5.5 the Society is informed if there is concern that the professional competence or fitness to practise of a pharmacist, pharmacy technician, pre-registration trainee or student pharmacy technician may compromise patient care or public safety.

5.6 there is co-operation with investigations or inquiries into the fitness to practise of anyone you employ and the impact of any findings and decisions on the employee's role and responsibilities are taken into account.

6. Training and development

Standards

Pharmacists, pharmacy technicians and other staff must have the appropriate knowledge, skills and competence for the roles they undertake and must be provided with training and development opportunities to strengthen and improve these. Where you employ, manage or lead others you must ensure that:

6.1 individuals have access to the training they need and undertake any accredited training requirements relevant to their duties in a timely manner.

6.2 you take steps to satisfy yourself that the pharmacists and pharmacy technicians you employ, manage or lead are aware of their obligation to undertake continuing professional development relevant to their professional duties, and are supported to meet this requirement.

6.3 staff who seek assistance because they do not feel able to carry out their professional work are reasonably and effectively supported.

6.4 the progress and performance of staff, particularly trainees, is regularly reviewed with honest and constructive feedback.

6.5 when training pre-registration trainees or student pharmacy technicians:
- the trainee is fit to practise throughout their training contract,
- the training meets the development needs of the trainee and provides the necessary range of experiences of professional practice,
- the trainee is appropriately supervised and monitored by their pre-registration tutor or supervisor and their performance is honestly and impartially evaluated,
- training is provided in approved premises and the Society is notified when such training is being provided.

7. Enabling others to raise concerns

Standards

It is important that those you employ, manage or lead, including temporary staff and locums, are able to raise concerns about risks to patients or the public. Appropriate systems need to be in place to deal with these concerns. You must make sure that:

7.1 there is an appropriate and effective mechanism for staff to raise concerns about risks to patients or the public, including concerns about inadequate resources, policies and procedures, or problems with the health, behaviour or professional performance of others.

7.2 staff have ready access to information on how to raise concerns, and who they should be raised with.

7.3 staff who raise genuine concerns are appropriately supported and protected.

7.4 systems are in place to investigate concerns promptly, fully and fairly, and appropriate records are maintained of any investigations and action taken.

7.5 concerns which cannot be addressed at a local level are referred to senior management and/or the appropriate authority, such as a regulatory body.

Further information and advice on raising concerns can be found in the Society's guidance document 'Raising concerns-guidance for pharmacists and registered pharmacy technicians' (www.rpsgb.org).

8. Handling complaints

Standards

All complaints about individuals, activities or services under your managerial control must be dealt with in an appropriate and professional manner. Where applicable, NHS complaints procedures must be followed. If you are in a position of authority you must be satisfied that:

8.1 an effective complaints handling procedure exists to deal with all complaints promptly, constructively and honestly.

8.2 those you employ, manage or lead, including temporary staff and locums, are familiar with the complaints procedure.

8.3 complainants receive a timely and constructive response and are informed about the way in which the complaints process will proceed.

8.4 anyone being investigated is treated fairly and individuals who are being asked to account for their conduct are made fully aware of the allegations made against them.

8.5 appropriate records are maintained of any complaints received and the action taken.

9. Indemnity arrangements

Standards

All pharmacists and pharmacy technicians have a responsibility to ensure that their professional activities are covered by adequate professional indemnity arrangements. Where you employ or engage pharmacists, pharmacy technicians or other staff you must ensure that:

9.1 all professional activities undertaken by you or under your control are covered by adequate professional indemnity cover.

9.2 those you employ or engage are aware of the extent of the professional indemnity cover provided to them.

10. Superintendent pharmacists and pharmacists responsible for a registered pharmacy premises

Superintendent pharmacists and pharmacists in personal control of a registered pharmacy premises have statutory functions detailed in the Medicines Act 1968.[1] The specific professional requirements for pharmacists undertaking these statutory roles and the relationship between the two roles are explained below.

Superintendent pharmacists

Standards

As a superintendent pharmacist you are required to manage the keeping, preparing, dispensing and sale or supply of medicinal products by a registered retail pharmacy business owned by a body corporate. You have a responsibility to set the overarching standards and policies for the pharmaceutical aspects of the business. You must ensure that all legal and professional requirements are adhered to and must respond appropriately to any systems failures or concerns that may arise.

The role of superintendent pharmacist is a key position carrying full time responsibility and accountability within a company. You must be satisfied that you have sufficient resources, authority and influence within your organisation to comply with your legal and professional responsibilities. You must also make sure that the members of the board of the body corporate are aware of and understand your responsibilities. As superintendent pharmacist, you retain overall professional accountability for the pharmaceutical aspects of the business even if you are employed for fewer hours than the pharmacy business operates. If you are employed as a superintendent pharmacist on a part time basis, or are not resident in the UK it is very unlikely that you will be able to comply adequately with the legal and professional responsibilities of this role.

Pharmacist in personal control

Standards

As a pharmacist in personal control of a registered pharmacy premises you have responsibility for the sale of all medicinal products from that pharmacy while you are in control. Where a pharmacy premises is owned by a body corporate, the superintendent pharmacist is required to set the overarching standards and policies for the pharmacy business. As the pharmacist in personal control of a particular pharmacy at any given time, you must ensure the safe and effective running of that pharmacy for the sale and supply of medicinal products.

---

[1] When the changes made to the Medicines Act 1968 by the Health Act 2006 are brought into force, the requirement for each pharmacy to be under the personal control of a pharmacist will be replaced with a requirement for each pharmacy to have a responsible pharmacist in charge of the pharmacy who is responsible for the safe and effective running of the pharmacy business. These changes will clearly set out in legislation the duties of the pharmacist responsible for the day-to-day running of a registered pharmacy. The responsibilities of the superintendent pharmacist will not change as a result of the Health Act 2006. This document will be updated once the new regulatory requirements are finalised.

You are responsible for ensuring appropriate procedures for the pharmacy while you are in control. Where model procedures have been agreed by the pharmacy owner or superintendent pharmacist you must ensure that they are implemented and adapted where necessary within the pharmacy you are assuming responsibility for. Changes to existing pharmacy procedures must be justifiable, for example, in response to patient safety issues or staffing changes, and should normally be made in conjunction with the pharmacy owner or superintendent pharmacist.

11. Bodies corporate

Standards

Where a body corporate owns a pharmacy business, a superintendent pharmacist must be appointed to manage the pharmaceutical aspects of the business. The Society expects members of the board of a body corporate to consider and act on the advice of the superintendent pharmacist when dealing with the requirements of the pharmaceutical parts of the business. The superintendent pharmacist needs to be provided with the necessary support and resources to carry out his or her legal and professional obligations as detailed in this document.

The Society must be notified in writing of any changes to the address or ownership of a registered pharmacy premises, or superintendent pharmacist of a body corporate.

Guidance that supports this document

We have produced documents or guidance bulletins on the following which should be considered in conjunction with these standards:
- Code of ethics for pharmacists and pharmacy technicians
- Professional standards and guidance for the sale and supply of medicines
- Professional standards and guidance for patient confidentiality
- Raising concerns - guidance for pharmacists and registered pharmacy technicians
- Rest breaks (*Law and Ethics Bulletin*)

You can download these documents and more copies of this document from our website (*www.rpsgb.org*) or you can telephone us on 020 7735 9141.

Professional Standards and Guidance for Patient Consent

About this document

The Code of Ethics sets out seven principles of ethical practice that you must follow as a pharmacist or pharmacy technician. It is your responsibility to apply the principles to your daily work, using your judgement in light of the principles.

The Code of Ethics says that you must **'Show respect for others'**. In meeting this principle you are expected to:

- Respect and protect the dignity and privacy of others.
- Obtain consent for the professional services, treatment or care you provide and the patient information you use.

You have both a professional and a legal duty to obtain a patient's consent for the professional services, treatment or care you provide, or patient information you use. This document expands on the principles of the Code of Ethics to explain your professional responsibilities when obtaining consent. It is designed to meet the Society's obligations under the Pharmacists and Pharmacy Technicians Order 2007 and other relevant legislation.

This document does not give detailed guidance on legal requirements, but you must ensure you comply with relevant legislative requirements and with any NHS policies that may apply to your work. The law relating to consent is complex and differs across the United Kingdom. If you are in doubt about your responsibilities, you should seek legal or specialist advice.

1. Consent

Standards
The Oxford English Dictionary defines consent as 'permission or agreement'. Consent is a person's agreement to receive a professional service or treatment appropriate for them and will be based on both their preferences and values and the information with which they have been provided. Patients have a basic right to be involved in decisions about their healthcare and the process of obtaining consent is fundamental for patient autonomy.

The consent you obtain must be valid. For consent to be valid the person must be:

- capable of making that particular decision,
- acting voluntarily, that is, they must not be under pressure from you or anyone else to make a particular decision,
- provided with sufficient information to enable them to make the decision,
- capable of using and weighing up the information provided during the decision-making process.

Obtaining consent is an on-going process not a single event. You must seek a patient's consent on each occasion that it is necessary, for example due to a change in circumstances, rather than simply at the beginning of a process.

2. Obtaining consent

2.1 Providing sufficient information

Standards
To provide valid consent patients must be given sufficient information to enable them to make an informed decision. Information must be clear, accurate and presented in a way that patients can easily understand. The information you provide may vary depending on the purpose for which consent is being obtained, the complexity of the information being provided and the needs of the individual patient. You must give consideration to the type of information patients are likely to want and need. This may be influenced by their personal beliefs.

Information the patient is likely to want includes:

- the service or activity they are being asked to consent to.
- the benefits to themselves of providing consent.
- the risks involved in providing consent.
- the implications of not providing consent.
- the alternatives that may be available to them.

You must provide information on the potential risks associated with the patient's decision, particularly serious adverse outcomes, even if the likelihood of them happening is very small. If you provide insufficient information the patient's consent may not be valid.

2.2 Presenting information to patients

Standards
You must communicate information in a manner that is appropriate for the individual patient. Before speaking to the patient you need to consider whether the patient suffers from a disability (e.g. poor sight or hearing) or whether there is a language barrier. To ensure that patients are able to provide valid consent these must be overcome. You must consider whether patients need time to absorb the information they have been given and offer them an opportunity to come back later with questions.

Good Practice Guidance

- **Use of visual aids, written material or the assistance of a translator or patient representative may assist you in ensuring that the patient understands the information they are being given.**

2.3 Responding to questions

Standards
Part of the patient's decision-making process may involve asking questions and the patient must be given the opportunity to do so. You must respond to questions and concerns openly and honestly, and must not mislead the patient in order to obtain consent.

2.4 Confirming patients' understanding

Standards
You must be satisfied that patients have understood the information provided to them, and that patients are fully aware of what they are consenting or refusing consent to.

Good Practice Guidance

- **Asking the patient a few simple questions is one way you could satisfy yourself that the patient has understood the information.**

2.5 Who obtains consent?

Standards
Generally, the person treating the patient, or providing a professional service for them should obtain consent. You must use your professional judgement to decide whether it is appropriate to delegate the task to another member of staff.

There may be occasions when you judge this to be acceptable, for example, when a patient is providing consent to be part of a prescription collection service. Alternatively, if you are a pharmacist prescriber, it is more likely to be appropriate to obtain consent yourself.

Where the task of obtaining consent is delegated to a member of staff you still have overall responsibility for it. You must be satisfied that the member of staff is suitably trained and competent. Failure to do so may cause patients to lack confidence in the information with which they are being provided.

2.6 Patients' right to change their mind

Standards
Patients are entitled to change the decision they have made with regard to providing consent. You must not assume that because patients have consented to a particular treatment or service in the past they will consent to it again. This may work both ways and patients could decide to give consent where they have initially refused. Patient choice must be respected. Patients must not be placed under pressure to make a decision, nor must they be pressured into accepting the advice provided by you or anyone else.

2.7 Standard operating procedures

Standards
The process of obtaining consent must be taken into account when developing standard operating procedures for pharmacy services. Procedures must cover:

- which activities within the pharmacy require patient consent.
- which activities require the pharmacist to obtain consent.
- which members of staff may obtain consent on your behalf.
- the information that should be provided.
- the type of consent required, e.g. implied, written or verbal. (See Section 3 of this document)

2.8 Presence of a third person

Standards
Where you would like a third person to observe your practice, for example a pre-registration trainee listening to a private consultation, you must seek the consent of the patient. You must inform the patient who the third person is, in what capacity they are working and what activities they will be undertaking, for example, observing or taking notes. You must give the patient the opportunity to refuse the presence of a third person. Where a third person is privy to confidential information they must be made aware that they are under the same duty of confidentiality as you are. This must also be made clear to the patient.

Good Practice Guidance

- **If a patient requests that a third person of their choice is present, you should be clear about the information they are content to discuss in the third person's presence.**

3. Forms of consent

Standards

Consent may be obtained in the following ways:

• Explicit consent

- verbally – the patient orally indicates their consent, e.g. by saying yes or no.

- in writing – the patient signs a document stating they provide consent e.g. signing a declaration to receive a collection and delivery service, or a medicines use review.

• Implied Consent - the patient indicates their consent without writing or speaking, for example, a patient who brings their prescriptions to you for dispensing.

You must use your professional judgement when deciding which method you use to obtain consent; this may vary depending on the activity for which consent is being sought. You must be careful about relying on a patient's apparent compliance as an indication of his or her understanding or agreement.

Obtaining the signature of the patient provides evidence that consent was given, however it does not prove that the patient gave valid consent as the signature does not prove that they made an informed decision. It is the validity of the consent that is critical and even a signed consent form can be subject to dispute.

Good Practice Guidance

• **Written consent should be obtained when you are providing services that require physical examination or diagnostic testing.**

4. Capacity

4.1 Assessing capacity to provide consent

Standards

As part of your assessment of capacity for both adults and children to provide consent, you must consider whether the patient:

• is able to retain the information you provided;
• has understood the information you provided;
• has understood the implications of their decision;
• is able to communicate their decision to you.

If you are unsure about a patient's capacity to make a decision you must seek specialist advice from another colleague or healthcare professional with relevant experience. If the patient's capacity remains in doubt you must seek legal advice.

4.2 Adults with capacity

Standards

You must assume that every adult has the capacity to provide consent unless they have demonstrated otherwise.

In order for a patient to be considered capable of providing consent they must be able to understand and retain the information being given.

You must not assume that a patient who asks questions lacks capacity. Additionally patients do not lack capacity simply because they do not accept professional recommendations.

As part of the process of providing consent requires the patient to understand and retain the information they are being given, a patient may be considered capable of making some decisions but not others.

You must remember that a patient's capacity to provide consent may be temporarily affected by other external or associated factors e.g. the information they are being given may cause them to become anxious or agitated therefore temporarily influencing their ability to provide consent. However, anxiety on its own is not evidence that a patient lacks capacity.

4.3 Adults without capacity

Standards

You must use your professional judgement, taking into account relevant legislation, such as those parts of the Mental Capacity Act 2005 that are now in force and the Adults with Incapacity (Scotland) Act 2000, when determining whether a patient is considered to have the capacity to provide consent.

There are provisions in certain circumstances for third parties to provide consent on behalf of an adult without capacity, as outlined in the Mental Capacity Act: *http://www.dca.gov.uk/menincap/legis.htm.*

Arrangements also exist in the Adults with Incapacity (Scotland) Act 2000 for proxy consent to be given where the person lacking capacity will benefit from the treatment.

Where you consider a patient lacks capacity to provide consent, you must record the discussions that have taken place and the reasons for your conclusion.

4.4 Children with capacity

4.4.1 Children aged 16 and over

Standards

Children aged 16 or over are considered to have the capacity to provide consent unless they have demonstrated otherwise. Therefore, in many respects they must be treated as adults.

The standards as set out above for adults with capacity apply equally to children aged 16 and over (also see Section 5.2 of this standard).

4.4.2 Children under 16

Standards

England and Wales

There is no set age at which a person under the age of 16 has the capacity to provide consent.

Children under the age of 16 must be assessed to determine whether they are capable of making decisions about their healthcare and therefore provide consent. The courts have stated that a person under the age of 16 can give consent if he or she has 'sufficient understanding and intelligence to enable him or her to understand fully what is proposed'. (Gillick v West Norfolk and Wisbech Area Health Authority [1985] 3 All ER 402 (HL))

Where a child with capacity under the age of 16 provides consent to medical services this cannot be over-ridden by a person with parental responsibility.

Scotland

Where a qualified medical practitioner attending a child under the age of 16 is of the opinion that the child is capable of understanding the nature and possible consequences of the procedure, the child can provide consent. Parental consent to treatment will only be relevant if the medical practitioner feels that the child does not have sufficient understanding.

Good Practice Guidance

• **It is good practice for you to encourage children to involve their parents in the decisions they make about their healthcare, but where the young person has capacity parental authority is not needed. Indeed, the young person can reasonably expect that their discussion with you will be kept confidential.**

• **The Society has produced guidance on child protection which outlines when you should consider speaking with other professionals who are involved in the child's care, for example, their doctor.**

4.5 Children without capacity

Standards
Where a child lacks capacity, any person holding parental rights and responsibilities can give or refuse consent. Where there is no such person, a person who has the care and control of the child for the time being can give consent provided this person does not already know that the child's parent would refuse to do so.

5. Refusal of consent

5.1 Adults

Standards
An adult with capacity may refuse treatment even if that refusal results in harm. The exception to this is where a person is being treated under mental health legislation or the Public Health Act

You must respect a patient's decision to refuse treatment, even when you think their decision is wrong.

If a patient without capacity has clearly indicated in the past, while capable, that they would refuse treatment in certain circumstances (an 'advance refusal/directive'), and those circumstances arise, you must abide by that refusal.

Where a patient refuses to provide consent a record of this must be made together with a record of the discussions that have taken place.

5.2 Children

Standards
In England and Wales, where children under 16 years and young people aged 16 and 17 refuse to give consent their decision may, exceptionally, be over-ridden by a person with parental responsibility or alternatively the courts, where this is considered to be in the child or young person's best interests. Where a person with parental responsibility refuses to give consent on a child's behalf the courts may intervene.

However, in Scotland the decision of a young person aged 16 or 17 cannot be overridden either by parents or by a court. Legislation also supports the right of a young person under the age of 16 with capacity to refuse consent to medical treatment on their own behalf.

6. Emergencies

Standards
Treatment may be provided without patient consent in an emergency when necessary to save a life or prevent deterioration in the patient's condition. The exception to this is where an advance refusal exists that you know about or is drawn to your attention. The Mental Capacity Act Code of Practice must be consulted for further information.

An example of when this may arise is where a patient suffers from anaphylactic shock and an Epipen is administered for the purpose of saving a life.

Good Practice Guidance

• **Emergency situations may be more prevalent within the hospital setting and you should ensure that you have read any relevant policy regarding patient consent.**

Guidance that supports this document

We have produced documents or guidance bulletins on the following which should be considered in conjunction with these standards:

• Code of ethics for pharmacists and pharmacy technicians
• Professional standards and guidance for patient confidentiality
• Child protection
• Protection of vulnerable adults

You can download these documents and more copies of this document from our website (*www.rpsgb.org*) or you can telephone us on 020 7735 9141.

Other useful sources of information:

• Mental Capacity Act:
  http://www.dca.gov.uk/menincap/legis.htm
• Mental Capacity Act Code of Practice:
  http://www.dca.gov.uk/menincap/legis.htm
• Department of Health:
  www.dh.gov.uk
• A Good Practice Guide on Consent for Health Professionals in NHS Scotland:
  http://www.sehd.scot.nhs.uk/mels/HDL2006_34.pdf
• Adults with Incapacity (Scotland) Act 2000:
  http://www.opsi.gov.uk/acts.htm

Professional Standards and Guidance for Patient Confidentiality

About this document

The Code of Ethics sets out seven principles of ethical practice that you must follow as a pharmacist or pharmacy technician. It is your responsibility to apply the principles to your daily work, using your professional judgement in light of the principles.

The Code of Ethics says that you must **'Show respect for others'**. In meeting this principle you are expected to:

- Respect and protect the dignity and privacy of others. Take all reasonable steps to prevent accidental disclosure or unauthorised access to confidential information and ensure that you do not disclose confidential information without consent, apart from where permitted to do so by the law or in exceptional circumstances.
- Use information obtained in the course of professional practice only for the purposes for which it was given, or where otherwise lawful.

You have both a professional and a legal duty to keep patient information confidential. This document expands on the principles of the Code of Ethics to explain your professional responsibilities around protecting the confidentiality of patient information. It is designed to meet the Society's obligations under the Pharmacists and Pharmacy Technicians Order 2007 and other relevant legislation.

This document does not detail specific legal requirements, but you must ensure you comply with relevant legislative requirements set out in the Data Protection Act and associated legislation, as well complying with common law principles and with any NHS or employment policies that may apply to your work.

1. Duty of confidentiality

Standards
Patients have the right to expect that information you obtain about them is kept confidential and is used only for the purposes for which it was given. This duty of confidentiality applies to all information obtained about a patient during the course of professional practice and extends to all members of the pharmacy team. Maintaining a patient's confidentiality is fundamental to the partnership between yourself and the patient. A patient may be reluctant to seek advice from you in your capacity as a healthcare professional where he/she has concerns that you will not maintain confidentiality.

Confidential information includes:

- personal details (including information that is not directly relevant to a patient's medical history)
- information about a patient's medication (both prescribed and non-prescribed) and
- other information about a patient's medical history, treatment or care.

2. Keeping information confidential

2.1 Preventing information being released accidentally

Standards
Accidental disclosure of information still constitutes a breach of confidentiality. You must take all reasonable steps to prevent accidental disclosure or unauthorised access to confidential information. Robust procedures must be in place to protect the confidentiality of information you receive, store, send or destroy. Patient identifiable information includes the patient's name, postal address, date of birth, NHS number, video footage, and anything else that can identify a patient either directly or indirectly.

All records, registers, prescriptions and other sources of confidential information must be stored securely and be kept out of sight of patients, members of the public and any other person who should not have access to them. Security measures must be appropriate to the location where the confidential information is being stored.

You must also take all reasonable steps to ensure appropriate levels of privacy for patient consultations so that confidential information is not overheard or accessed by others.

2.2 Disposal of patient identifiable information

Standards
In order to maintain a patient's confidentiality, sources of patient identifiable information must be disposed of in a manner that prevents the information being seen by, or available to, unauthorised persons.

Good Practice Guidance

- **Disposing of patient indentifiable information may involve shredding documentation, or alternatively placing it in confidential waste or deleting the information by way of a permanent marker.**

2.3 Computer records

Standards
Patients have the right to expect that any computer records about them are held securely. You must be satisfied that any system used is capable of restricting access. Suitable passwords, Personal Identification Number (PIN) or other restricted access systems must be in place. Any information stored about a patient must be pertinent, accurate and up-to-date. Computers must be situated so that data cannot be seen intentionally, or by accident, by those who are not authorised to have access to it.

Good Practice Guidance

- **PIN numbers or passwords should be changed at regular intervals (for example if a member of staff terminates employment at the pharmacy).**

- **The level of access that various members of the pharmacy team have to a patient's records should be appropriate to their duties. For example, a member of staff who is responsible only for ordering stock will not need access to patient medication records.**

2.4 Notification to the Information Commissioner's Office

Standards
The processing of personal data, including the pharmacy patient medication record system, must be notified to the Information Commissioner's Office and records must be kept in accordance with relevant legislation. Unnecessary access to patient specific data must be prevented whether data is held electronically or in hard copy format.

2.5 Pharmacy staff

Standards
You must ensure that all members of the pharmacy team are aware and demonstrate an understanding of their duty to maintain and respect a patient's right to confidentiality.

<u>Good Practice Guidance</u>

- **Members of staff, where necessary, should read this document and comply with the guidance contained in it.**

2.6 Standard operating procedures

Standards
The way in which confidential information is handled must be taken into account when developing and reviewing standard operating procedures. Procedures must cover:

- who has access to confidential information and in what circumstances.
- how confidential information will be processed, used and stored.
- disclosure of information.
- maintenance of appropriate records of requests for disclosure and details of the information disclosed.

3. Disclosure of information

3.1 Obtaining patient consent

Standards
Information about patients must not be disclosed without their consent other than in exceptional circumstances, or where required or permitted to by law, or by order of a Court (See section 4 of this document).
   Where patients allow you to share information about them you must make sure that they understand:

- what information you will be releasing;
- the circumstances in which the information will be released and who it will be released to; and
- the likely consequences of releasing the information.

   Patients will generally expect that information you obtain in the course of your professional practice may be shared with other healthcare professionals or others who have a duty of confidentiality, where necessary for their care. However, you must ensure that patients are aware of who may have access to the personal information you hold and the extent that the information may need to be shared. You must check that they do not have an objection to this.

There may be occasions when patients refuse to consent to particular information being shared with others providing care for them, for example, their general practitioner. Other than in exceptional circumstances you must respect the patient's decision (see section 4.2 of this document). The patient must be made aware of the possible implications of not consenting to disclosure and his or her refusal to give consent must be documented.
   Further information on obtaining consent can be found in our document 'Professional standards and guidance for patient consent'.

3.2 Releasing the minimum amount of information necessary

Standards
When disclosing patient information, you must release only the minimum amount of information necessary for the purpose. You must use your professional judgement to consider the information you need to disclose, taking into account who is requesting the information and why.
   If it is not necessary for the patient to be identified, you must make sure that the patient cannot be identified from the information you release.

<u>Good Practice Guidance</u>

- **Where appropriate, consideration should be given to the use of anonymised data.**

3.3 Confidentiality and others

Standards
When you disclose confidential patient information you must ensure those you release it to are aware they are being provided with the information in confidence. These people are required to respect the patient's right to confidentiality.

3.4 Deceased patients

Standards
The records of deceased patients must be treated with the same level of confidentiality as those who are living. The Health Records Act 1990 governs access to the health records of deceased patients. Further information about the requirements of this Act can be found at *www.dh.gov.uk*.

4. Releasing information without consent

4.1 Deciding to release information without consent

Standards
Confidential information must only be disclosed without consent in exceptional circumstances or when permitted or required by law, for example, where disclosure is by an order of the court, or where the public interest overrides the need to keep the information confidential. Examples of the circumstances where information may be disclosed without consent are detailed in section 4.2 of this document. Before releasing information without consent you must, where practical or appropriate, endeavour to persuade the patient either to release the information themselves, or give you permission to release it. If you decide to reveal confidential information

without obtaining consent you must be prepared to justify your decision and any action you take.

4.2 Exceptional circumstances (including those permitted by law)

Information can be disclosed without patient consent only in the following circumstances:

4.2.1 Where the patient's parent, guardian or carer has consented to the disclosure and the patient is deemed by law to be, or appears to be, incapable of consenting.

Our document *Professional standards and guidance for patient consent* provides information on determining a patient's capacity to provide consent.

4.2.2 Where disclosure of the information is to a person or body empowered by a statute to require disclosure.

Standards
Where you are required to disclose information because of a statutory requirement you do not have to obtain consent prior to disclosure. You must ensure you release the information only to an authorised person who is requesting disclosure in the performance of their statutory duties.

Good Practice Guidance

• **All reasonable efforts should be made to tell the patient that information will be released, why it is being released and to whom it is being released.**

4.2.3 Where disclosure is directed by H.M Coroner, a judge or other presiding officer of a court, Crown Prosecution Office in England and Wales or Procurator Fiscal in Scotland.

Standards
A court may order you to release patient information without consent. If so, you must release only the minimum information needed to follow the order. In certain situations your refusal to disclose information could result in you being found in contempt of court.

Good Practice Guidance

• **You should seek further legal or specialist advice in these situations.**

4.2.4 To a police officer or NHS fraud investigation officer who provides in writing confirmation that disclosure is necessary to assist in the prevention, detection or prosecution of serious crime.

Standards
There may be occasions where obtaining patient consent prior to disclosure will be inappropriate e.g. a request for information from the police to detect a serious crime, where attempting to obtain consent may allow time for destruction of evidence. The request to disclose such information must be made in writing, stating the purpose for which the information is required.

Good Practice Guidance

• **When faced with requests from the Police or a NHS fraud investigation officer you should consider whether there are any alternative sources for the information being requested that would not cause a breach of trust between you and the patient. You should also discuss the matter with the person making the request and be satisfied that without disclosure, the investigation would be delayed or prejudiced.**

4.2.5 Where necessary to prevent serious injury or damage to the health of a patient, a third party or to public health.

For example, this situation may arise where a patient that should not be driving (possibly due to epilepsy, diabetes) continues to do so without appropriate disclosures.

Good Practice Guidance

• **You should discuss with the patient the implications of continuing to undertake the activity that may cause serious injury or damage.**

4.2.6 Where disclosure is necessary for the protection of children or vulnerable adults

Standards
Where abuse or neglect of a person is suspected, that person's wellbeing is of utmost importance and ensuring this must be your prime concern.

Good Practice Guidance

• **You should attempt to encourage the person to consent to disclosure; however in situations where they refuse you will need to use your professional judgement to determine the best course of action.**

• **You should consider speaking with other healthcare professionals who are also involved in the patient's care e.g. their doctor. We have produced guidance on 'Child protection' and 'The protection of vulnerable adults'.**

You should consult the Information Commissioner's Office where you have queries about the appropriateness of disclosure in any of the above circumstances.

4.3 Maintaining records

Standard
When you make a decision to disclose information without consent, you must keep an accurate record of:

• who the request came from.
• the reasons for releasing the information without consent.
• whether you attempted to obtain patient consent, and if not why not.
• why patient consent was refused.
• what information was disclosed.

If a patient refuses to provide consent in one situation you must not assume that they will refuse to provide consent for disclosure in the future, whether the situation is the same or the circumstances are different.

5. NHS Code of Practice on Confidentiality

Standards

In England and Wales, the NHS Code of Practice on Confidentiality was published in 2003. It is a guide to the practice required of those who work within or under contract to NHS organisations, including pharmacists and all pharmacy staff. It is concerned with issues surrounding confidentiality and patients' consent to the use of their health records. The NHS Code of Practice can be viewed at: *http://www.dh.gov.uk/assetRoot/04/06/92/54/04069254.pdf*

In Scotland, the NHS Scotland Code of Practice on Protecting Patient Confidentiality is a guide to the required practice of those who work within NHS Scotland. The NHS Scotland Code of Practice on Protecting Patient Confidentiality can be viewed at: *http://www.confidentiality. scot.nhs.uk/publications/6074NHSCode.pdf*

These, and other relevant standards or guidance on patient confidentiality, must be adhered to unless you have good reason not to do so.

Guidance that supports this document

We have produced documents or guidance bulletins on the following which should be considered in conjunction with these standards:

* Code of ethics for pharmacists and pharmacy technicians
* Professional standards and guidance for patient consent
* Child protection
* Protection of vulnerable adults
* Fact sheet 12: Confidentiality and the Data Protection Act 1998 and disclosure of information
* Guidance on the NHS Code of Practice on confidentiality

You can download these documents and more copies of this document from our website (*www.rpsgb.org*) or you can telephone us on 020 7735 9141.

Other useful sources of information:

* NHS Scotland Code of Practice on Protecting Patient Confidentiality: *http://www.confidentiality.scot.nhs.uk/publications/6074NHSCode.pdf*
* NHS Scotland Confidentiality website: *http://www.confidentiality.scot.nhs.uk/*
* Confidentiality NHS Code of Practice (England and Wales): *http://www.dh.gov.uk/assetRoot/04/06/92/54/04069254.pdf*

Professional Standards and Guidance for the Sale and Supply of Medicines

About this document

The Code of Ethics sets out seven principles of ethical practice that you must follow as a pharmacist or pharmacy technician. It is your responsibility to apply the principles to your daily work, using your judgement in light of the principles.

The Code of Ethics says that you must '**Make the care of patients your first concern**'. In meeting this principle you are expected to:

* Provide a proper standard of practice and care to those for whom you provide professional services.
* Seek all relevant information required to assess an individual's needs and provide appropriate treatment and care. Where necessary, refer patients to other health or social care professionals or other relevant organisations.
* Seek to ensure safe and timely access to medicines and take steps to be satisfied of the clinical appropriateness of medicines supplied to individual patients.
* Encourage the effective use of medicines and be satisfied that patients, or those who care for them, know how to use their medicines.
* Be satisfied as to the integrity and quality of products to be supplied to patients.
* Ensure that you have access to the facilities, equipment and materials necessary to provide services to professionally accepted standards.

This document expands on the principles of the Code of Ethics to set out your professional responsibilities if you are involved in the sale and supply of medicines. It is designed to meet the Society's obligations under the Pharmacists and Pharmacy Technicians Order 2007 and other relevant legislation.

This document does not detail legislative requirements, but when selling or supplying medicines you must comply with relevant legislative and contractual requirements, including NHS terms of service.

1. Pharmaceutical stock

Standards

Patients, members of the public and other healthcare professionals are entitled to expect that medicines sold or supplied within the course of professional pharmacy practice are obtained from a reputable source and fit for the intended purpose. You must ensure that:

1.1 if you suspect you have been offered or supplied a counterfeit or defective medicine, this is reported to the Medicines and Healthcare products Regulatory Agency, the Royal Pharmaceutical Society, the Veterinary Medicines Directorate or the marketing authorisation holder as appropriate to the individual situation. Any such stock must be segregated from other pharmacy stock and must not be sold or supplied for the treatment of any person(s).

1.2 pharmaceutical stock is stored under suitable conditions, taking into consideration the stability of the drug.

1.3 particular attention is paid to protection of pharmaceutical stock from contamination, sunlight, atmospheric moisture and adverse temperatures. You must ensure that where you have concerns about the stability of a medicine, it is segregated from the rest of the stock and not sold or supplied for patient use.

1.4 refrigerators used for pharmaceutical stock are capable of storing products between 2C and 8C. They must be equipped with a maximum/minimum thermometer, or other suitable alternative, which is checked on each day the pharmacy is open and the maximum and minimum temperatures recorded. Steps must be taken to rectify discrepancies in temperatures.

1.5 all stocks of medicines in the pharmacy have batch and expiry details. Medicines must be removed from blister or foil packs only at the time of dispensing to assist an individual patient.

1.6 date expired stock is segregated from the rest of the pharmacy stock and appropriately disposed of. Procedures must be in place to reduce the risk of short dated or out-of-date stock being accidentally supplied to a patient or member of the public. In the event of a pandemic flu, Level 6, date expired medicines may be supplied to patients, where this is in line with guidance issued by the Government and/or the RPSGB.

1.7 products that may be injurious to a person's health, for example tobacco products, alcoholic beverages and products intended to mask the signs of alcohol or drug consumption are not sold or supplied from registered pharmacy premises.

1.8 medicines returned to the pharmacy from a patient's home, a care home or a similar institution are not supplied to another patient. While awaiting disposal, these medicines must be clearly marked and segregated from other stock.[1] In the event of a pandemic flu, Level 6, patient returned medicines may be supplied to patients, where this is in line with guidance by the Government and/or the RPSGB.

1.9 within the hospital setting, all medicines returned to the pharmacy department from a ward or other hospital department are examined under the direction of a pharmacist to assess their suitability for being returned to stock. Patients' own drugs brought into hospital with them must not be returned to pharmacy stock or be supplied to another patient.[1]

2. Supply of over the counter (OTC) medicines

Standards

When purchasing medicines from pharmacies patients expect to be provided with high quality, relevant information in a manner they can easily understand. You must ensure that:

2.1 procedures for sales of OTC medicines enable intervention and professional advice to be given whenever this can assist the safe and effective use of medicines. Pharmacy medicines must not be accessible to the public by self-selection.

2.2 when a patient or their carer requests advice on treatment, sufficient information is obtained to enable an assessment to be made of whether self-care is appropriate, and to enable a suitable product(s) to be recommended.

2.3 if a sale is not considered suitable, the reasons for this are explained to the patient and they are referred to another healthcare professional where appropriate.

2.4 when an OTC medicine is supplied, sufficient advice to ensure the safe and effective use of the medicine is provided. You must take into account any other specific information such as safe storage, or short expiry dates that the patient may need to be counselled on.

2.5 all staff involved in the sale or supply of an OTC medicine are trained, or are undertaking the training required for their duties, and are aware of situations where referral to the pharmacist or other registered healthcare professional may be necessary. Consideration must be given to the types of OTC medicines that may require the personal intervention of a pharmacist e.g. those that have recently become available without prescription, those that may be subject to abuse or misuse, or where the marketing authorisation for non-prescription use is restricted to certain conditions and circumstances.

2.6 all persons involved in the sale of OTC products are aware of the abuse potential of certain OTC medicines and other products. You must be alert to requests for large quantities and abnormally frequent requests and refuse to make a supply where there are reasonable grounds for suspecting misuse.

2.7 particular care is exercised when supplying products for children, the elderly and other special groups or individuals, or where the product is for animal use.

2.8 requests for certain medicines such as emergency hormonal contraception are handled sensitively and the patient's right to privacy and confidentiality is respected.

2.9 any information provided about OTC medicines is up to date, accurate and reliable.

2.10 you keep up to date with developments regarding new products and policies for health promotion and are aware of local and major national and topical health promotion initiatives.

3. Supply of prescribed medicines

Standards

Patients are entitled to expect the dispensing service provided to be accurate, accessible and reasonably prompt. Appropriate standard operating procedures must be in place for the dispensing services you provide, or are responsible for and you must ensure that:

3.1 you seek to maintain adequate stock holdings.

3.2 every prescription is clinically assessed by a pharmacist to determine its suitability for the patient.

3.3 the patient receives sufficient information and advice to enable the safe and effective use of the prescribed medicine.

3.4 appropriate records of clinical interventions are maintained.

3.5 patients or their carers are informed if you are unable to dispense their prescription in its entirety and given the opportunity to take their prescription to another pharmacy.

3.6 when medication is outstanding, the patient, carer or their representative is provided with a legible note detailing the name and quantity of medicine outstanding and, where possible, informed when the balance will be available for collection. A record of the medicine owed must be kept in the pharmacy.

3.7 a product with a marketing authorisation is supplied where such a product exists in a suitable formulation and is available, in preference to an unlicensed product or food supplement.[2]

---

[1] The Society is currently considering its policy on the re-use of patient returned medicines. Until such time that this has been given full consideration 1.8 and 1.9 must be complied with. Any change in policy will be notified via the pharmacy press.

---

[2] except where methadone mixture is prepared extemporaneously in accordance with Appendix 1

3.8 except in an emergency, a specifically named product is not substituted for any other product without the approval of the patient or carer and the prescriber, a hospital drug and therapeutics committee, or other similar locally agreed protocols.

3.9 when providing services for drug misusers you do not deviate from the instructions given on the prescription. Sugar and/or colour-free products have a greater potential for abuse than syrup based and coloured products and must not be dispensed unless specifically prescribed.

3.10 all solid dose and all oral and external liquid preparations are dispensed in suitable reclosable child resistant containers unless:
- the medicine is in an original pack or patient pack such as to make this inadvisable;
- the patient has difficulty in opening a child resistant container;
- a specific request is made by the patient, their carer or representative that the product is not dispensed in a child resistant container;
- no suitable child resistant container exists for a particular liquid preparation, or
- the patient has been assessed as requiring a compliance aid.

3.11 labelling of dispensed products is clear and legible and where appropriate includes any cautionary and advisory labelling recommended by the current British National Formulary.

3.12 appropriate systems and procedures are in place if you prepare monitored dosage systems.

3.13 reimbursement claims for NHS or other professional services are honest and accurate.

3.14 procedures are in place to minimise the risk of dispensing errors or contamination of medicines. A record of errors or near miss incidents must be made and practices reviewed in light of such incidents.

Good Practice Guidance

• Where verbal information is provided about a prescribed medicine necessary records of this should be maintained, when clinically appropriate.

4. Extemporaneous preparation or compounding

Standards
This standard is not intended to cover the reconstitution of dry powders with water or other diluents.

Patients are entitled to expect that products extemporaneously prepared in a pharmacy are prepared accurately and are suitable for use. If you wish to be involved in extemporaneous preparation you must ensure that:

4.1 a product is extemporaneously prepared only when there is no product with a marketing authorisation available[3] and where you are able to prepare the product in compliance with accepted standards.

4.2 you and any other staff involved are competent to undertake the tasks to be performed.

4.3 the requisite facilities and equipment are available. Equipment must be maintained in good order to ensure

---

[3] except where methadone mixture is prepared extemporaneously in accordance with Appendix 1

that performance is unimpaired, and must be fit for the intended purpose.

4.4 you are satisfied as to the safety and appropriateness of the formula of the product.

4.5 ingredients are sourced from recognised pharmaceutical manufacturers and are of a quality accepted for use in the preparation and manufacture of pharmaceutical products. Where appropriate, relevant legislation must be complied with.

4.6 particular attention and care is paid to substances which may be hazardous and require special handling techniques.

4.7 the product is labelled with the necessary particulars, including an expiry date and any special requirements for the safe handling or storage of the product.

4.8 if you are undertaking large scale preparation of medicinal products, all relevant standards and guidance are adhered to.

4.9 records are kept for a minimum of two years. The records must include:

- the formula,
- the ingredients,
- the quantities used,
- their source,
- the batch number,
- the expiry date,
- where the preparation is dispensed in response to a prescription, the patient's and prescription details and the date of dispensing,
- the personnel involved, including the identity of the pharmacist taking overall responsibility.

Good Practice Guidance

• Where possible, all calculations and measurements should be double checked by a second appropriately trained member of staff.

5. Repeat medication services

Standards
A repeat medication service is a service operated in co-operation with local prescribers, in which pharmacists will provide professional support to assist in the rational, safe, effective and economic use of medicines. In order to provide a repeat medication service, you must:

5.1 ensure the pharmacy operates a patient medication record system notified to the Information Commissioner's Office.

5.2 ensure that an audit trail exists to identify each request and supply.

5.3 establish, at the time of each request, which items the patient or carer considers are required and ensure that unnecessary supplies are not made. At this stage pharmacists must also use their professional judgement to decide whether concordance or other problems encountered by the patient may require early reference to the prescriber.

5.4 not request a repeat prescription from a surgery before obtaining the patient's or carer's consent. You may however institute a patient reminder system.

5.5 record all interventions in order to be able to deal with any queries that may arise.

6. Delivery services

Standards
A delivery service is where the medicine is handed to the patient or their carer other than on registered pharmacy premises. When providing medicines via a delivery service you still have a professional responsibility to ensure that patients or their carers know how to use the medication safely, effectively and appropriately and check that they are not experiencing adverse effects or compliance difficulties. You must ensure that:

6.1 on each occasion a delivery service is provided you use your professional judgement to determine whether direct face-to-face contact with the patient or their carer is necessary.

6.2 you obtain consent from the patient or their carer to provide the delivery service on a single occasion or for a set period of time.

6.3 delivery to a person other than the patient or carer is undertaken only where they have been specifically designated by the patient or their carer.

6.4 you maintain appropriate records of requests for the service.

6.5 the delivery mechanism used:

- enables the medicine to be delivered securely and promptly to the intended recipient with any necessary information to enable safe and effective use of their medicine;
- caters for any special security/storage requirements of the medicine;
- incorporates a verifiable audit trail for the medicine from the point at which it leaves the pharmacy to the point at which it is handed to the patient, their carer or other designated person, or returned to the pharmacy in the event of a delivery failure;
- safeguards confidential information about the medication that a patient is taking.

Good Practice Guidance

• Wherever possible a signature should be obtained to indicate safe receipt of the medicines.

• Systems should be in place to inform a patient who is not at home that delivery was attempted.

7. Prescription collection service

Standards
A prescription collection service encompasses any scheme where a pharmacy receives prescriptions other than directly from the patient, their carer or their representative. When providing such a service you must:

7.1 obtain consent to receive patients' prescriptions. The request for the ongoing service must be from the patient or their carer and procedures must exist for maintaining records of the initial request for the service.

7.2 explain fully to patients, or their carers, what the service involves, including the time period required to collect/receive and dispense their prescription.

7.3 ensure that any members of staff who collect prescriptions are acting in accordance with your directions.

7.4 take all reasonable steps to ensure patient confidentiality and the security of prescriptions.

7.5 make sure that requests for repeat prescriptions are initiated by the patient or their carer. A reminder system may be instituted but a prescription must not be requested from a surgery before obtaining the patient's or their carer's consent.

7.6 on receipt of prescriptions, including electronic prescriptions, be satisfied that you are authorised to receive and dispense them. Any prescription received for which you do not have the authority, must be returned to the surgery for collection by the patient or carer, or be directed to the pharmacy authorised to receive it.

8. Complementary therapies and medicines

Standards
You must ensure that you are competent in any area in which you offer advice on treatment or medicines. If you sell or supply homoeopathic or herbal medicines, or other complementary therapies, you must:

8.1 assist patients in making informed decisions by providing them with necessary and relevant information.

8.2 ensure any stock is obtained from a reputable source.

8.3 recommend a remedy only where you can be satisfied of its safety and quality, taking into account the Medicines and Healthcare products Regulatory Agency registration schemes for homoeopathic and herbal remedies.

9. Emergencies

Standards
There may be occasions when you are required to assist members of the public or patients in an emergency. In such situations you must:

9.1 where appropriate, consider using the exemption in legislation that allows pharmacists to make an emergency supply of medicines if a patient has an urgent need for them. You must consider the medical consequences, if any, of not making the supply and be satisfied that your decision will not lead to patient care being compromised.

9.2 advise the patient on how to obtain essential medical care where you do not consider an emergency supply to be appropriate.

9.3 assist persons in need of emergency first aid or medical treatment whether by administering first aid within your competence or by summoning assistance.

10. Patient group directions

Standards
If you are involved in the supply and/or administration of a medicine under a patient group direction (PGD) you must:

10.1 be satisfied that the PGD is legally valid and that it has been approved by the relevant authorising body.

10.2 ensure that when supplies are made the agreed protocol is followed and the information specified in the PGD is recorded. These records must include the identity of the pharmacist assuming responsibility for each supply.

10.3 ensure you have up-to-date knowledge relating to the clinical situation covered by the PGD, the medicine and its use for the indications specified.

10.4 ensure that you have undertaken any training required for operation of the PGD.

If you are involved in writing and/or approving patient group directions (PGD) you are accountable for their content and must ensure that:

10.5 you are familiar with your role and responsibilities and the government advice set out in relevant guidance.

10.6 only PGDs which comply with legal requirements are approved.

10.7 the staff training specified will enable safe operation of the PGD.

10.8 the appropriate people have been involved in the drafting, approval and signing of the PGD.

10.9 you have up-to-date knowledge relating to the clinical situation being covered by the PGD, the medicine and its use for indications specified in the PGD.

Guidance that supports this document

We have produced documents or guidance bulletins on the following which should be considered in conjunction with these standards:

- Code of ethics for pharmacists and pharmacy technicians
- Professional standards and guidance for patient consent
- Professional standards and guidance for patient confidentiality
- Emergency first aid; guidance for pharmacists
- Patient group directions: a resource pack for pharmacists
- The safe and secure handling of medicines: a team approach (The Duthie Report)
- Emergency supplies guidance (Law and Ethics Bulletin)
- Safe storage of medicines in patients homes (Law and Ethics Bulletin)

You can download these documents and more copies of this document from our website (_www.rpsgb.org_) or you can telephone us on 020 7735 9141.

Appendix 1: Extemporaneous preparation of methadone mixture

You must supply a product with a marketing authorisation, where such a product exists in a suitable formulation and is available, in preference to an unlicensed product or food supplement. You must only prepare a product extemporaneously if there is no product with a marketing authorisation available and where you are able to prepare the product in compliance with accepted standards.

An exception to these requirements, to permit the extemporaneous preparation of methadone mixture in circumstances where a licensed product is available, will be granted provided the following requirements are adhered to:

Standards

(a) If a licensed product is available, methadone mixture may only be prepared extemporaneously if the quantity of methadone dispensed on a regular basis is large enough to preclude storage of sufficient quantities of the licensed product within the pharmacy, in accordance with the safe custody requirements of the Misuse of Drugs legislation.

(b) In addition to the standard operating procedures (SOPs) required for dispensing, a SOP must be in place for the extemporaneous preparation of methadone. The SOP must ensure safe systems and provide a verifiable audit trail. Adherence to the SOP must be ensured.

(c) Extemporaneous preparation must only be carried out by persons who are appropriately trained and competent to do so.

(d) All quantities of methadone powder and diluent, and any colourings, flavourings and stabilisers, must be accurately measured. You must not rely on the accuracy of the quantities of powder, diluent etc stated on the manufacturers packs.

(e) The equipment used to measure and prepare extemporaneous methadone products must be appropriate and be maintained in good order to ensure that performance is unimpaired.

(f) Equipment must be properly cleaned between each batch of extemporaneously prepared product to ensure that no residue from previous batches remains.

(g) Visual checks must be made to ensure the methadone powder has fully dissolved in the diluent.

(h) Stock bottles must not be reused.

(i) The product must be labelled with the necessary particulars, including:
- The name and strength of the product
- The quantity of medicinal product in the container
- Any special handling and storage requirements (eg, store in safe custody)
- The batch expiry date
- A batch reference number

(j) For each batch of extemporaneous methadone mixture prepared a record must be maintained for a minimum of two years of:
- The formula
- The ingredients and quantities used
- The source, batch number and expiry date of the ingredients
- The batch number and expiry date of the extemporaneously prepared mixture
- The persons involved in preparing the product, including the identity of the pharmacist assuming overall responsibility

(k) Extemporaneously prepared methadone mixture must be stored in a cabinet, cupboard or room that meets the requirements of the Misuse of Drugs (Safe Custody) Regulations 1973.

(l) Extemporaneous preparation of methadone mixture, when a licensed product is available, carries increased liability and must be covered by indemnity insurance arrangements.

Good Practice Guidance

- **Running balances of methadone powder and the resulting extemporaneously prepared methadone mixture should be maintained.**

- **The prescriber and the patient should be informed that the methadone product being supplied does not have a marketing authorisation.**

- **Wherever possible all measurements should be checked by a second person.**

Professional Standards and Guidance for Advertising Medicines and Professional Services

About this document

The Code of Ethics sets out seven principles of ethical practice that you must follow as a pharmacist or pharmacy technician. It is your responsibility to apply the principles to your daily work, using your judgement in light of the principles.

The Code of Ethics says that you must **'Be honest and trustworthy'**. In meeting this principle you are expected to:

- Ensure you do not abuse your professional position or exploit the vulnerability or lack of knowledge of others.
- Be accurate and impartial when teaching others and when providing or publishing information to ensure that you do not mislead others, or make claims that cannot be justified.

This document expands on the principles of the Code of Ethics to set out your professional responsibilities when advertising medicines and services to patients. It is designed to meet the Society's obligations under the Pharmacists and Pharmacy Technicians Order 2007 and other relevant legislation.

This document does not detail legislative requirements, but when advertising medicines or professional services, you must comply with legislative requirements and with other relevant codes of practice and guidelines.

1. Background

It is in the public interest to publish information about pharmacy opening hours and pharmaceutical services. All information or publicity material regarding pharmacy services must be honest and accurate and reflect the professional nature of pharmacy. Promotional material and advertisements come in various formats including:
- TV, radio and internet advertisements
- Newspaper and magazine articles
- Posters
- Leaflets
- Emails and other forms of electronic messaging

Legislation prohibits the advertising of Prescription Only Medicines (POM) for human use to members of the public. However, there are exemptions to allow information such as price lists and reference materials, for example Summary of Product Characteristics, to be made available. The advertising and promotion of General Sales List (GSL) and Pharmacy (P) medicines are permitted, but you must adhere to the standards in this document and other relevant documents as listed in 'Other useful sources of information' at the end of this document.

There are specific restrictions on the advertising of veterinary medicines set out in the current Veterinary Medicines Regulations. Further guidance on these requirements can be found in the Society's guidance 'Guidance on the sale and supply of veterinary medicines' (*www.rpsgb.org*).

The Association of the British Pharmaceutical Industry Code of Practice sets out the requirements for the promotion of medicines by the pharmaceutical industry. It covers the promotion of medicines to health professionals and appropriate administrative staff. The advertising and promotion of non-prescription medicines is regulated by the Proprietary Association of Great Britain through its Codes of Advertising Practice. These self-regulatory codes reflect and extend beyond UK legislative requirements.

2. Information and publicity

Standards
All information and publicity for goods and professional pharmacy services, including publicity issued by a third party on your behalf, must:

2.1 be accurate, legal, decent and truthful.
2.2 not bring the profession into disrepute.
2.3 be presented and distributed in a way that allows the recipient to decide independently whether or not to use a service. Information held in a patient's patient medication record must not be abused.
2.4 not abuse the trust or exploit the lack of knowledge of the public.
2.5 be compatible with the role of pharmacy professionals as skilled and informed advisors about medicines, common ailments, general health care and well being.
2.6 be presented in a manner that does not disparage the service of other pharmacies or pharmacy professionals.

Good Practice Guidance

- **Consideration should be given to what creates a professional image in the eyes of the general public. The style, presentation and content of the advertisement need to be considered.**

- **Care should be taken to ensure that the public are not misled as to the specific services being offered at the pharmacy and their availability. For example: 'Pharmacist is available at all times for consultation'- Is this always the case?**

- **The use of the article 'The' is accepted in proposed pharmacy business names.**

- **Advertisements dealing with both professional and non professional services are generally accepted, but the two types of service should be detailed separately.**

- **Leaflets, or other similar materials, can be left in GP practices for self-selection by patients of the surgery; however, you should not seek exclusive deals in this respect.**

- **Particular care should be exercised when preparing advertisements for inclusion in newspapers or other forms of media. It is advisable to check the final proof of the article or advertisment before going to print.**

3. Promotion of medicines

Standards
Pharmacies may advertise the prices at which they sell medicines (subject to any legal restrictions) including any discounts offered. However, medicines are not ordinary items of commerce and there is a professional responsibility to ensure that promotions emphasise the special nature of medicines

and do not encourage inappropriate or excessive consumption or use of them. Pharmacy owners and superintendent pharmacists have a responsibility to ensure that medicines promotions are professionally acceptable. Individual pharmacists and pharmacy technicians must be able to justify decisions to supply medicines to a particular purchaser. Promotions for medicines aimed at the public must:

3.1 comply with relevant legislation and codes of practice.

3.2 be carried out with respect to the special nature of medicines.

3.3 not make any medicinal claim that is not capable of substantiation.

3.4 be consistent with the summary of product characteristics approved by the Medicines and Healthcare products Regulatory Agency (MHRA) as part of the licensing procedures. Where the product is an herbal or homeopathic remedy, promotions must be consistent with the MHRA registration scheme.

3.5 not promote a medicine by way of endorsement by a pharmacist or pharmacy technician. You may recommend a product only in response to a request for advice from an individual patient, or their representative.

3.6 not promote inappropriate or excessive consumption or use of medicines, or promote their misuse, injudicious or unsafe use which may be injurious to health.

3.7 not seek to persuade patients to obtain medicines that are not needed, or quantities substantially in excess of those needed.

Good Practice Guidance

- **The Blue Guide - Advertising and promotion of medicines in the UK, published by the Medicines and Healthcare Regulatory Agency, contains specific advice regarding 'multiple purchase promotions for analgesics' and advertising medicines via the internet, which you should comply with.**

- **Promotions involving Pharmacy (P) medicines need to be considered on their merits. Consideration should be given to the product, the pack size, the condition to be treated and the intended recipient. You have to make a professional judgement in deciding where to draw the line. For instance, a 3 for 2 promotion on Kaolin and Morphine is unlikely to be justifiable, but a similar promotion on an antihistamine product, where the pack size is small and the patient is likely to need the medicine for an extended period of time, may well be acceptable provided that you are able to justify your decision.**

4. The Green Cross

Standards
The faceted Green Cross is a symbol over which the Society holds intellectual property rights in order to restrict its use. The Green Cross can be used to identify pharmacy premises and any material or qualified pharmacy professional associated with pharmacy premises, for example on notepaper, labels, visiting cards and compliments slips. The Green Cross can also be used to identify the profession of pharmacy as an entity as opposed to in connection with an individual pharmacy company. When using the Green Cross on promotional material you must comply with the conditions of use of the logo.

Further information on the Green Cross can be obtained from the Society's Legal and Ethical Advisory Service (tel: 020 7572 2308; e-mail: *leadvice@rpsgb.org*).

5. Society Crest

Standards
The use of the Society's coat of arms by third parties, for whatever purpose, is not permitted. Its use is restricted to publications (both printed and electronic) generated directly by the Society.

Guidance that supports this document

We have produced documents or guidance bulletins on the following which should be considered in conjunction with these standards:
- Code of ethics for pharmacists and pharmacy technicians
- Guidance on the sale and supply of veterinary medicines

You can download these documents and more copies of this document from our website (*www.rpsgb.org*) or you can telephone us on 020 7735 9141.

Other useful sources of information:

- The Blue Guide – Advertising and Promotion of Medicines in the UK: *www.mhra.gsi.gov.uk*
- Association of British Pharmaceutical Industry Code of Practice: *www.abpi.org.uk*
- Proprietary Association of Great Britain Codes of Advertising Practice: *www.pagb.co.uk*

Professional Standards and Guidance for Internet Pharmacy Services

About this document

The Code of Ethics sets out seven principles of ethical practice that you must follow as a pharmacist or pharmacy technician. It is your responsibility to apply the principles to your daily work, using your judgement in light of the principles.

The Code of Ethics says that you must '**Make the care of patients your first concern**'. In meeting this principle you are expected to:

- Provide a proper standard of practice and care to those for whom you provide professional services.
- Seek all relevant information required to assess an individual's needs and provide appropriate treatment and care. Where necessary, refer patients to other health or social care professionals or other relevant organisations.
- Seek to ensure safe and timely access to medicines and take steps to be satisfied of the clinical appropriateness of medicines supplied to individual patients.
- Encourage the effective use of medicines and be satisfied that patients, or those who care for them, know how to use their medicines.
- Be satisfied as to the integrity and quality of products to be supplied to patients.
- Ensure you have access to the facilities, equipment and materials necessary to provide services to professionally accepted standards.

This document expands on the principles of the Code of Ethics to set out your professional responsibilities if you are involved in the sale and supply of medicines via the internet. It is designed to meet the Society's obligations under the Pharmacists and Pharmacy Technicians Order 2007 and other relevant legislation.

This document does not detail legislative requirements, but when selling or supplying medicines via the internet, you must comply with relevant legislative and contractual requirements, including NHS terms of service.

1. Background

Pharmaceutical services provided to the public via the internet include amongst other things, the dispensing of prescriptions, the sale of medicines and the provision of information on web site pages. For the purpose of this document, the Society defines internet pharmacy as:

'A registered pharmacy which offers to sell or supply medicines (or other pharmaceutical products) and/or provides other professional services over the internet, or makes arrangements for the supply of such products or provision of such services over the internet.'

The sale and supply of general sale list, pharmacy and prescription only medicines (POM) for human use via the internet must be made in accordance with the Medicines Act 1968.

This requires that:

1.1 the pharmacy premises from where the sale or supply of a pharmacy and prescription only medicine takes place must be registered with the Society.

1.2 the pharmacy must be under the personal control[1] of a pharmacist and supervision requirements for pharmacy and prescription only medicine sales must be met.

1.3 prescription only medicines must be supplied only in accordance with a legally valid prescription or patient group direction, by way of an emergency supply or by way of wholesale.

England, Scotland and Wales have different NHS Pharmaceutical Services Regulations and contractual arrangements. You must comply with the NHS regulations and contractual arrangements for internet pharmacy services that apply in the country or countries in which you operate.

The sale of veterinary medicines via the internet must be made in accordance with the current Veterinary Medicines Regulations. Further guidance on these requirements can be found in the Society's guidance 'Guidance on the sale and supply of veterinary medicines' (*www.rpsgb.org*).

2. Website requirements

Standards
Patients must be readily able to identify who is operating an internet site from a registered pharmacy premises. Pharmacy websites must clearly display:[2]

2.1 the name of the owner of the business.

2.2 the address of the pharmacy at which the business is conducted.

2.3 where applicable, the name of the superintendent pharmacist.

2.4 information about how to confirm the registration status of the pharmacy and pharmacist.

2.5 details of how to make a complaint about the on-line services provided.

3. Security and confidentiality

Standards
Patients are entitled to expect pharmacists and pharmacy staff to respect and protect the confidentiality of information acquired in the course of their professional duties. When providing internet pharmacy services you must be satisfied that:

3.1 the confidentiality and integrity of all patient information is protected to the standard specified by the International Organisation for Standardisation (ISO) in ISO/IEC 27001:2005: *www.bsi-global.com*.

3.2 all patient data transmissions are encrypted to prevent the possibility of the internet service provider or any other unauthorised party accessing patient information either accidentally or deliberately.

4. Protecting patient choice

Standards
Co-operation and close working between health professionals is encouraged, but patients must be free to choose where and how they obtain their pharmaceutical services. When providing internet pharmacy services, you must:

4.1 not participate in any agreement with a prescriber or other person that limits patient choice.

4.2 ensure that patients are able to identify which pharmacy is providing pharmaceutical services to them and be satisfied that they have consented to this.

4.3 take all reasonable steps to ensure that direction of prescriptions has not occurred.

5. Supplying medicines

Standards
Patients are entitled to expect the same quality of pharmaceutical care irrespective of whether the service is provided on-line or face to face on the pharmacy premises.

5.1 Supply of non-prescription medicines and supplements

Standards
When selling or supplying non-prescription medicines via the internet, you must:

---

[1] When the changes made to the Medicines Act 1968 by the Health Act 2006 are brought into force, the requirement for each pharmacy to be under the personal control of a pharmacist will be replaced with a requirement for each pharmacy to have a responsible pharmacist in charge of the pharmacy who is responsible for the safe and effective running of the pharmacy business.

[2] The Society has been piloting the use of an internet pharmacy logo to aid members of the public in identifying registered pharmacy premises operating internet sites. Once widely rolled out it is intended that all registered pharmacy internet sites will be required to display the logo. Further information will be issued in 2010.

5.1.1 ensure advice is available to all prospective purchasers of over-the-counter (OTC) medicines and vitamin and mineral supplements.

5.1.2 establish whether the intended user is the person requesting the product.

5.1.3 assess the suitability of the product for the intended user. Sufficient information about the patient and the condition(s) being treated must be obtained.

5.1.4 provide appropriate counselling or advice on the safe and effective use of the product to be supplied.

5.1.5 be aware of the abuse potential of some OTC medicines and other products. You must be alert to requests for large quantities of a product, or abnormally frequent requests, and refuse to make a supply where there are reasonable grounds for suspecting misuse and/or abuse.

5.1.6 advise the patient to consult a local pharmacy or other appropriate healthcare professional whenever a request for a medicine or the symptoms described indicate that their best interests would be served by a face-to-face consultation.

5.1.7 inform patients of the identity of the pharmacist assuming professional responsibility for the supply of medicines.

5.2 Supply of medicines against prescriptions

Standards

Apart from limited exceptions (for example, emergency supplies and patient group directions), POMs must be supplied only in accordance with a legally valid prescription. When supplying medicines against prescriptions you must:

5.2.1 ensure that patients have consented to the pharmacy dispensing their prescription.

5.2.2 have systems in place to prevent the unlawful sale or supply of POMs. You must be satisfied that the prescriber and prescription are genuine.

5.2.3 ensure a pharmacist assesses the clinical appropriateness of the prescription for the patient.

5.2.4 ensure the patient, or their carer, receives sufficient information to enable the safe and effective use of the medicine and is aware how further information can be obtained.

5.2.5 advise the patient to consult a local pharmacy whenever a prescription indicates that their interests would be better served by a face-to-face consultation.

Good Practice Guidance

• **An e-mail of prescription details from the prescriber to the pharmacy does not meet the legal requirements for electronic prescribing. It does not confirm that a legally valid prescription exists and supplies should not be made against information which a prescriber or patient has sent by e-mail until the original prescription has been received.**

• **You should be alert to potential indicators that an adequate clinical assessment of a patient has not been undertaken; for example, where a prescriber is issuing, or countersigning a high volume of prescriptions for overseas patients, or where a commercial company has employed/contracted a prescriber to issue prescriptions for patients who access its site. In such circumstances you should use your professional judgement to assess the appropriateness of making the supply to the patient.**

6. Information and advice

Standards

Patients and the public recognise the expertise that pharmacy professionals have in relation to medicines and expect to be provided with high quality, relevant information in a manner they can easily understand. When providing internet pharmacy services you must ensure that:

6.1 generic healthcare advice (i.e. not specific to a patient) provided on pharmacy websites is accurate, up-to-date and of a high professional standard.

6.2 all information relating to specific products complies with the marketing authorisation, the patient information leaflet and relevant legislative requirements.

6.3 information relating to medicines includes all relevant details of contra-indications and side effects.

6.4 product recommendations are given only in respect of individual patients.

6.5 any advertising or publicity complies with relevant legislation. Promotional material you authorise or are responsible for must be accurate and honest and must not abuse the trust or exploit the lack of knowledge of the public.

7. Posting and delivering medicines

Standards

Your responsibility towards your patients extends to the delivery of medicines. Medicines must be delivered safely and with appropriate instructions. When delivering medicines to a patient, whether by post or other means, you must:

7.1 obtain consent from the patient or their carer to provide the delivery service on a single occasion or for a set period of time.

7.2 ensure that delivery to a person other than the patient or carer is undertaken only where they have been specifically designated by the patient or their carer.

7.3 take adequate steps to ensure that the delivery mechanism used is secure and that medicines are delivered to the patient, their carer or other designated person promptly, safely and in a condition appropriate for use.

7.4 ensure that medicines are packed, transported and delivered in such a way that their integrity, quality and effectiveness are preserved. Care must be exercised with thermolabile products.

7.5 ensure the delivery mechanism used provides a verifiable audit trail for the medicine from the point at which it leaves the pharmacy to the point at which it is handed to the patient, carer or other designated person, or returned to the pharmacy in the event of a delivery failure.

7.6 ensure that delivery mechanisms safeguard confidential information about the medication a patient is taking.

Good Practice Guidance

• **Wherever possible a signature should be obtained to indicate safe receipt of the medicines.**

• **Systems should be in place to inform a patient who is not at home that delivery was attempted.**

8. Overseas prescriptions

Standards

Supplying medicines to patients overseas carries particular risk. There may be differences in a product's licensed name, indications for use or the recommended dosage regimen. Prior to supplying a prescription only medicine to an overseas patient, you must ensure that:

8.1 the prescription is legally valid.

8.2 due consideration is given to any differences in the licensed indications and/or legal classification of the prescribed medicine in the UK and the patient's country of residence and that, where necessary, these are explained to the patient.

8.3 appropriate information and advice is provided to the patient.

8.4 legal requirements for export are met.

8.5 medicines will be delivered safely, securely and in accordance with standard 7.

8.6 professional indemnity insurance arrangements adequately cover the supply of medicines and provision of other pharmaceutical services to overseas patients.

Good Practice Guidance

• **While a prescription issued, or countersigned, by a UK registered prescriber for an overseas patient may be legally valid, the General Medical Council advises that doctors prescribe drugs or treatment (including repeat prescriptions) only when they have adequate knowledge of a patient's health and medical needs. Given this, you also need to be satisfied of the appropriateness of dispensing such a prescription. You should consider contacting the prescriber to ascertain their reasons for prescribing for a patient abroad and satisfy yourself that there has been an appropriate clinical assessment of the patient.**

• **The Misuse of Drugs Regulations prohibits a prescription for a Schedule 2 or 3 Controlled Drug from being signed by a prescriber whose address is not within the UK.**

9. Record keeping

Standards

Records about on-line consultations and medicines supplies sufficient to guard against risks of abuse or misuse must be maintained. A verifiable audit trail from the initial request for a medicine through to its delivery to the patient must exist. If you provide internet pharmacy services you must maintain records of:

9.1 the identity of customers who have been supplied with medicines via the internet.

9.2 details of the medicines requested and supplied.

9.3 the information upon which decisions to supply were made.

9.4 the identity of the pharmacist who has assumed profesional responsibility for supply of a medicine following an e-mail/ on-line request to purchase.

Guidance that supports this document

We have produced documents or guidance bulletins on the following which should be considered in conjunction with these standards:

• Code of ethics for pharmacists and pharmacy technicians
• Professional standards and guidance for the sale and supply of medicines
• Professional standards and guidance for patient consent
• Professional standards and guidance for patient confidentiality
• Factsheet 4: Export of medicines
• Raising concerns – guidance for pharmacists and registered pharmacy technicians
• Guidance on the sale and supply of veterinary medicines
• Dispensing overseas prescriptions (Law and Ethics Bulletin)

You can download these documents and more copies of this document from our website (*www.rpsgb.org*) or you can telephone us on 020 7735 9141.

Professional Standards and Guidance for Pharmacist Prescribers

About this document

The Code of Ethics sets out seven principles of ethical practice that you must follow as a pharmacist. It is your responsibility to apply the principles to your daily work, using your professional judgement in light of the principles.

This document expands on the principles of the Code of Ethics to explain your responsibilities as a supplementary or independent pharmacist prescriber. It is designed to meet the Society's obligations under the Pharmacists and Pharmacy technicians Order 2007 and other relevant legislation.

This document applies to all settings in which a pharmacist may prescribe, both within and outside the NHS, including primary care, secondary care, private sector, armed forces and the prison service. It should be read alongside other relevant documents from the Department of Health (England), Welsh Assembly Government and Scottish Executive Health Department. The standards in this document aim to be consistent with those in place for other prescribing professions. A list of useful websites and supporting guidance can be found at the end of this document.

1. Background

The main legislation that enables pharmacists to prescribe medicinal products for human use is the Prescription Only Medicines (Human Use) Order 1997 as amended and the Medicines (Pharmacy and General Sale – Exemption) Order 1980 as amended. Pharmacists gained the ability to achieve supplementary prescribing status in 2003 and independent prescribing status in 2006.

1.1. Types of pharmacist prescribing

There are currently two types of prescribing which you may undertake as a pharmacist prescriber: supplementary and independent prescribing. Some pharmacists will be qualified as both, others as only a supplementary prescriber. A pharmacist independent prescriber can practise as either a pharmacist independent prescriber or pharmacist supplementary prescriber. The mode of prescribing practice will depend on your personal choice and practice circumstances. You may practise solely in one practice mode or move between modes according to patient or practice circumstances.

Definition of supplementary prescribing

A voluntary partnership between an independent prescriber (doctor or dentist) and a supplementary prescriber to implement an agreed patient–specific clinical management plan (CMP) with the patient's agreement.

Definition of independent prescribing

Prescribing by a practitioner (e.g. doctor, registered nurse, pharmacist) who is responsible and accountable for the assessment of patients with undiagnosed or diagnosed conditions and for decisions about the clinical management required, including prescribing.

Good Practice Guidance

• **Other methods for supplying and administering medicines include the use of patient group directions, patient specific directions and minor ailment schemes. Some of the standards and guidance outlined in this document will also apply to these situations.**

1.2. Working within requirements

As a pharmacist prescriber you must comply with the relevant legislation and frameworks and should always be able to justify your actions.

Legal requirements for pharmacist prescribers

• You may prescribe only once you have successfully completed a Society accredited programme and your name in the Society's practising register for pharmacists has been annotated to reflect this.
• You may prescribe only in relation to your prescribing status (independent or supplementary) and must comply with statutory requirements applicable to your prescribing practice.
• You are legally accountable for your prescribing decisions, including actions and omissions, and cannot delegate this accountability to any other person. (You are solely accountable as an independent prescriber and jointly accountable as a supplementary prescriber in that as a supplementary prescriber the joint responsibility is for the content of the clinical management plan, but you are still solely responsible for your decision to prescribe).
    Prescribing outside the legal parameters of either supplementary or independent prescribing is a criminal offence.

Clinical governance framework

The Society has produced a clinical governance framework for pharmacist prescribers. The framework includes recommendations for NHS organisations, employers and individual prescribers. It also includes indicators and examples of good practice. It is available at:
http://www.rpsgb.org/pdfs/clincgovframeworkpharm.pdf.

Competencies

You must attain and maintain competencies specific to your role as a prescriber. The main competencies required are outlined in the National Prescribing Centre document – 'Maintaining Competency in Prescribing: An outline framework to help pharmacist prescribers'. These competencies have been incorporated into the training courses for pharmacist prescribers. They are a useful tool as part of personal development plans and can help identify gaps and needs. The NPC document can be found at: *http://www.npc.co.uk/pdf/ pharmacist_comp_framework_Oct06.pdf.*

Private practice

All pharmacists who prescribe privately must also follow the standards and guidance outlined in this document. It is up to individuals to ensure that arrangements for good governance are in place.

Liability and indemnity arrangements

The Society requires that all activities pharmacists undertake be covered by professional indemnity arrangements. You must ensure that you have professional indemnity arrangements in place which cover the scope of your prescribing practice regardless of whether you prescribe within or outside the NHS.
    For the purposes of indemnity within the NHS (and similarly for other organisations) you need to ensure, along with your manager, that the trust has approved pharmacist prescribing at an appropriate level within the organisation e.g. Trust Board or Clinical Governance meeting, and that this has been recorded in the minutes of that meeting.

Veterinary prescriptions

Existing legislation permits pharmacists to dispense veterinary prescriptions and to sell certain classes of veterinary medicinal product over-the-counter. Pharmacists can also prescribe veterinary medicinal products classified as POM-VPS in accordance with the current Veterinary Medicines Regulations.

2. Standards and guidance for pharmacist prescribers

The mandatory professional standards and good practice guidance have been laid out under the seven principles of the Code of Ethics.

The seven principles are:

• Make the care of patients your first concern
• Exercise your professional judgement in the interest of patients and the public
• Show respect for others
• Encourage patients to participate in decisions about their care

- Develop your professional knowledge and competence
- Be honest and trustworthy
- Take responsibility for your working practices

2.1 Make the care of patients your first concern

Standards

2.1.1 In order to prescribe for a patient you must satisfy yourself that you have undertaken an adequate assessment of the patient by taking a history, performing an appropriate examination and/or by accessing the appropriate parts of their clinical records.

2.1.2 You are accountable for your decision to prescribe and must prescribe only where you have relevant knowledge of the patient's health and medical history and of the medicines required for treating their condition(s).

2.1.3 You must ensure relevant physical examinations of the patient are carried out where appropriate or necessary, including any diagnostic tests in order to exclude contra-indications, clarify doses or treatment cautions.

2.1.4 You must prescribe only where there is a genuine, identifiable clinical need for treatment and not based solely on the demands of a patient. Consider non-pharmacological treatments where appropriate.

2.1.5 Independent pharmacist prescribers can prescribe both where a diagnosis has been made previously and also where no working diagnosis of the patient's condition has been made. If you are unable to reach a working diagnosis of a patient's condition you must refer them to an appropriate medical practitioner or other health professional.

2.1.6 If you are carrying out a diagnosis of a patient's condition you must have the appropriate facilities and equipment to do this. Any equipment used must undergo appropriate regular quality assurance checks.

2.1.7 You must ensure that an adequate risk assessment has been undertaken in respect of the patient's current medicines or their medical condition(s) and include any risk of potential for confusion or interaction with other medicines.

2.1.8 When prescribing unlicensed medicines or medicines outside their licensed indications ('off-label') you must be satisfied that it would better serve the patient's needs than a licensed alternative and ensure that the patient, or their representative, is aware that it is unlicensed or outside of licence. In the case of unlicensed medicines patient consent must be obtained (see section 3.3 and 3.4 of this document).

2.1.9 You must provide clear dosage administration instructions to the patient or carer to avoid uncertainty for the patient, or any other health professional.

2.1.10 A retrievable audit trail of your prescribing actions must be maintained e.g. keeping records of your prescribing in the patient's notes.

2.1.11 You must refer the patient to another prescriber where prescribing for the patient is outside your competency.

Good Practice Guidance

• **Whenever possible, when prescribing for a patient you should have concurrent access to the patient's full health records.**

• **The maximum time allowed between writing the prescription and entering the details into the contemporaneous patient record should not exceed 48 hours, unless there are exceptional circumstances.**

• **You should review the patient's medication each time you prescribe for them and consider stopping any unsuitable or unnecessary medicines. In certain circumstances it may be in the patient's best interest not to prescribe medicines for them.**

• **Ideally the dosage instructions should be on the prescription itself, or otherwise in an appropriate format.**

2.2 Exercise your professional judgement in the interest of patients and the public

Standards

2.2.1 Your prescribing practice must, wherever possible, be evidence-based and be in accordance with relevant national and local guidance. Deviations from these policies must be justifiable and be in the best interest of the patient.

Good Practice Guidance

• **You should be familiar with current guidance published in the British National Formulary (including the use, side effects and contra-indications of the medicines that you prescribe) as well as having access to a wider range of information. Where local policy varies from current national guidelines, you should seek guidance through clinical governance structures in respect of your vicarious liability within your employing organisations (NHS trust, primary care organisation, Local Health Board in Wales, Health Boards in Scotland, head office of a multiple, pharmacy company etc).**

• **In some cases you may be working at the emerging or leading edge of practice, or in an area where the available evidence base is poor. In these circumstances there may not be any evidence available for the medicines prescribed and decisions should be based on current thinking and peer opinion.**

2.3 Show respect for others

Standards

2.3.1 You must explain your role as a non-medical prescriber to the patient or their representative.

2.3.2 You must be aware of cultural and religious differences in so far as they apply to prescribing.

2.3.3 You must obtain the patient's consent for the prescribing process and for any physical examinations or diagnostic testing undertaken. This can be verbal or written consent.

2.3.4 You must gain patients' consent to share information about them with other health and social care professionals. Only where there is real danger of harm to the patient or anyone else must information be shared without patient consent.

2.3.5 If a patient's consent to share information is not forthcoming you must offer an explanation of the risks of not doing so. If the patient continues to refuse to give consent this must be documented in their records.

2.3.6 You must inform anyone else who may be in a position to prescribe for that patient of your actions, where relevant and possible, and where consent to do this has been obtained. This is most likely to be the patient's general medical practitioner but may also include other non-medical prescribers and other health / social care professionals. The main way to do this is to enter your interventions and actions in the common prescribing record.

For more information on consent refer to the Society's 'Professional standards and guidance for patient consent' and refer to DH guidance at: *http://www.dh.gov.uk/en/ Policyandguidance/Healthandsocialcaretopics/Consent/index.htm.*

2.4 Encourage patients to participate in decisions about their care

Standards

2.4.1 When prescribing, you must take the views of the patient into account in order to create an environment where shared-decision making is the norm. This will include taking into account the patient's personal views and beliefs and discussing treatments in relation to these.

Good Practice Guidance

• **There will be occasions when the patient's views cannot be fully accommodated. In these circumstances, to be sure that the patient complies with the treatment, you should explain to them why you consider a particular choice is the best choice for them.**

2.5 Develop your professional knowledge and competence

Standards

2.5.1 You must prescribe only within your level of expertise and competence and not outside your clinical knowledge of either the condition, or the medicines required to treat that condition.

2.5.2 You must refer the patient to an appropriate prescriber if you are not competent to prescribe in disease areas with which the patient may present.

2.5.3 If you move to another area of practice (a different sector of pharmacy, a different therapeutic area or a different geographical area) you must consider the requirements of your new role and prescribe only within your level of expertise and competence. You may require the approval of your employer for this new role and may need to undertake additional training to ensure you are competent, in addition to the educational course which allows you to prescribe. This may also affect your professional indemnity arrangements.

2.5.4 It is your responsibility to remain up to date with the knowledge and skills to enable you to prescribe competently and safely within your area of expertise.

2.5.5 As a pharmacist who is recorded on the register as being a prescriber, you must ensure that part of your continuing professional development (CPD) directly addresses your role as a prescriber. This includes keeping up to date with relevant changes in the law as well as the therapeutic areas in which you prescribe.

Good Practice Guidance

• **Employers have a responsibility to ensure that prescribers are competent to carry out their duties as prescribers.**

• **While you are legally able to prescribe from the whole of the British National Formulary and British National Formulary for Children, you can prescribe only within your competence. You are not expected to be competent in all disease areas. You may also be able to prescribe only within parameters agreed with your employer.**

2.6 Be honest and trustworthy

Standards

2.6.1 You must inform anyone who needs to know about any restrictions placed on your prescribing practice. In particular, other practitioners with dispensing responsibilities need to know about this. For example, you must inform your primary care organisation (PCO) if you had restrictions placed upon your prescribing. They would inform the relevant people using the systems they have developed for this purpose.

2.6.2 You cannot both prescribe and dispense medicines except in exceptional circumstances e.g. where the need for the medicine is urgent and not to dispense would compromise patient care. You must have robust procedures in place to demonstrate the separation of prescribing and dispensing.

2.6.3 Where you are involved in both prescribing and dispensing a patient's medication, a second suitably competent person must be involved in checking the accuracy of the medicines provided, and wherever possible, carrying out a clinical check.

2.6.4 You must make your choice of medicinal product for the patient based on clinical suitability and clinical and cost effectiveness. The decision must not be based on potentially biased information, fraud or commercial gain.

2.6.5 You must maintain a declaration of interest, which you must produce on request if required for audit purposes. You must adhere to local policy when maintaining this.

2.6.6 You must not prescribe for yourself.

2.6.7 You must not prescribe for anyone with whom you have a close personal or emotional relationship, except in exceptional circumstances such as:

• No other person with the legal right to prescribe is available and only then if that treatment is necessary to:

  ○ Save a life,
  ○ Avoid serious deterioration in the patient's health, or
  ○ Alleviate otherwise uncontrollable pain.

2.6.8 You must be able to justify your actions and must document your relationship and the exceptional circumstances that required you to prescribe for someone close to you.

2.6.9 If you have concerns about the competence, behaviour or conduct of a professional colleague, which impacts on patient safety, you must take appropriate action to raise this as a concern.

<u>**Good Practice Guidance**</u>

• **The Medicines (Advertising) Regulations 1994 govern the supply, offer or promise of gifts to healthcare professionals, including pharmacists, by drug manufacturers and distributors. Pharmacists accepting items such as gift vouchers, bonus points, discount holidays, sports equipment etc, would be in breach of Regulation 21 of the Medicines (Advertising) Regulations 1994.**

• **It is good practice to carry out a self-audit of your prescribing practice at regular intervals, at least on an annual basis.**

• **If it is clinically appropriate to alter another prescriber's prescription, it should be clearly documented on the prescription who made the change. The change needs to be agreed with the original prescriber.**

2.7 Take responsibility for your working practices

Standards

2.7.1   You have a responsibility to communicate effectively with other practitioners involved in the care of the patient, provided patient consent is given.

2.7.2   You must ensure that the records you make are accurate, comprehensive and contemporaneous.

2.7.3   You must ensure that you have professional indemnity arrangements which cover the scope of your prescribing practice regardless of whether you prescribe within, or outside the NHS.

<u>**Good Practice Guidance**</u>

• **A written agreement which outlines your scope of practice, should be in place between yourself and the employing organisation (e.g. PCO, NHS Trust, Care Home, Phamacy). This 'scope of practice agreement' should outline the areas in which you will prescribe and should determine the methods that are to be used to communicate effectively with other health professionals involved in the patient's care.**

3. Additional information

3.1 Guidance on writing prescriptions:

The legal requirements for writing a prescription are outlined in the Society's Medicines, Ethics and Practice Guide.

3.1.1 Prescriptions should always be signed and dated immediately and should never be left blank if they have been signed.

3.1.2 Computer-generated prescriptions should be used, providing the necessary software is available. However, you still need to be competent to write a prescription by hand.

3.1.3 You are responsible for the safety of your prescription pad. You should take all reasonable precautions to prevent loss or inappropriate use. You should use only one prescription pad at a time. You should keep a record of the first and last serial number of prescriptions in pads issued to you.

3.1.4 It is good practice to record the serial number of the first and last remaining prescription form of an in-use pad at the beginning and end of each working day. This would help to identify any forms lost or stolen overnight. If a prescription pad is lost, mislaid or stolen this should be reported immediately to your employer or contractor and local policy should be followed.

3.1.5 You should ensure that it is your prescriber details on the prescription.

For computer generated prescriptions, you need to ensure you are registered with the relevant NHS Business Authority (NHS Business Services Authority for England, NHS National Services Scotland for Scotland and Health Solutions Wales for Wales) in order to be able to prescribe from a medical practice's system. This will prevent incorrect allocation of prescribing budgets and incorrect ePACT / PRISMS data.

For further guidance on writing a prescription, see 'Prescription writing' in the BNF.

3.2 Guidance on prescribing Controlled Drugs (CDs)

3.2.1 You may prescribe CDs only where you are legally entitled to do so.

3.2.2 It is strongly recommended, as good practice, that the quantity of any CDs prescribed, excluding those in Schedule 5, should not exceed 30 days of clinical need per prescription. If more than 30 days supply is made, the reason for this should be noted in the patient's notes.

3.2.3 You may use computer-generated prescriptions for all CDs, providing the necessary software is in place and there is an audit trail of your prescribing practice.

3.2.4 All CD prescriptions for Schedule 2, 3 and 4 CDs are only valid for 28 days from the date of signing or appropriate start date specified in the prescription.

The Department of Health website has the most up to date information on the management and use of controlled drugs and it can be accessed at: *http://www.dh.gov.uk/en/ Policyandguidance/Medicinespharmacyandindustry/ Prescriptions/ControlledDrugs/DH_4131301.*

Please refer to the most up to date guidance to ensure you are abreast of all the relevant legislative requirements.

3.3 Guidance on prescribing unlicensed medicines

Unlicensed medicines are those medicines without a current marketing authorisation. Independent pharmacist prescribers are not legally permitted to prescribe unlicensed medicines.

You may prescribe an unlicensed medicine as a supplementary prescriber as part of a CMP providing:

- The doctor or dentist and you, acting as a supplementary prescriber, have agreed the plan with the patient in a voluntary relationship.
- You are satisfied an alternative licensed medicine would not meet the patient's needs.
- You are satisfied there is a sufficient evidence base and / or experience to demonstrate the medicine's safety and efficacy for that particular patient.
- The doctor / dentist and yourself are prepared to take the responsibility for prescribing the unlicensed medicine and have agreed the patient's CMP to that effect.
- The patient agrees to a prescription in the knowledge that the medicine is unlicensed and understands the implications of this.
- The medication chosen and the reason for choosing it is documented in the CMP/ clinical records.

3.4 Guidance on prescribing medicines for use outside the terms of their licence (off-label)

Off-label prescribing is where a licensed medicine is prescribed outside the terms of its licence.

It is possible, under current legislation, for pharmacist prescribers (both independent and supplementary) to prescribe off-label. However, in order to do so you should ensure the following conditions are met:

- You are satisfied that there is a sufficient evidence base and/or experience of using the medicine to demonstrate its safety and efficacy in these circumstances. Where the manufacturer's information is of limited help, the necessary information should be sought from another source.
- You have explained to the patient or parent or carer in broad terms, the reasons why medicines are not licensed for their proposed use.
- You make a clear, accurate and legible record of all medicines prescribed and the reasons for prescribing a medicine off-label.
- You may also, as a supplementary prescriber, prescribe a medicine for use outside the terms of its licence providing:
  - ᴍ There is a CMP in place, written in conjunction with a doctor or dentist and in voluntary partnership with the patient or parent or carer.
  - ᴍ A doctor or dentist and you take responsibility for prescribing the medicine and you jointly oversee the patient's care, monitor the situation or outcome and ensure any follow up treatment is given as required.

Any verbal information given to patients or their representative should be supported by written information provided by the pharmacist prescriber.

3.5 Guidance on repeat prescribing

Repeat prescribing is where a prescription is issued authorising several supplies to be made without further consultation with the prescriber.

3.5.1 As a pharmacist prescriber you may issue a repeat prescription.
3.5.2 Before signing a repeat prescription you need to be satisfied that it is safe and appropriate to do so and that secure procedures are in place to ensure that:

- The patient is issued with the correct prescription.
- Each prescription is regularly reviewed and is re-issued only to meet clinical need.
- A review takes place following a maximum of six prescriptions or six months elapsing, whichever comes first. In certain circumstances this review period may be longer provided the prescriber is satisfied the patient is stable and knowledgeable about their own condition.
- The correct dose and quantity is prescribed.
- Suitable provision for monitoring each patient's condition is in place to ensure that patients who need a further examination or assessment do not receive repeat prescriptions without being seen by an appropriate prescriber.

3.6 Guidance on remote prescribing via telephone, email, fax, video-link or website

From time to time it may be appropriate to use a telephone or other non face to face medium to prescribe medicines and treatments for patients. Such situations may occur where:

- You have responsibility for the care of the patient.
- You are providing out of hours or urgent care services.
- You are working in remote and/or rural areas.
- You have prior knowledge and understanding of the patient's condition and medical history.
- You have authority to access the patient's records and you are working as a supplementary prescriber, but the doctor or dentist required to authorise the CMP works at a distance.

You should carry out an adequate risk assessment for each individual case of remote prescribing. Records of remote prescribing, including the reasons for prescribing in this manner, should be made.

If remote prescribing is necessary, clear protocols for operating remote prescribing need to be agreed with employers.

You should not give directions to other professionals to administer medicines verbally. The Nursing and Midwifery Council guidelines for the administration of medicines has useful information on this subject:
http://www.nmc-uk.org/aFrameDisplay.aspx? DocumentID=221.

3.7 Guidance on reporting adverse reactions

The same guidance on reporting adverse reactions applies to pharmacist prescribers as to pharmacists generally.

- If a patient experiences an adverse reaction to a medication they have been prescribed you should record this in the patient's notes, notify the prescriber if you did not prescribe the medicine and notify via the Yellow Card Scheme immediately, where appropriate. Yellow cards are found in the back of the British National Formulary or online at: *www.yellowcard.gov.uk.*
- In addition you have a duty to inform the patient that they may also report an adverse reaction independently under the Yellow Card Scheme.
- You can also report adverse reactions via the Medicines and Healthcare products Regulatory Agency website at *www.mhra.gov.uk.*

- Any untoward incidents should be reported to the National Reporting and Learning System which is the reporting system of the National Patient Safety Agency directly, or through your own organisation's reporting mechanism; *http://www.npsa.nhs.uk/health/reporting.*
- Local reporting schemes may be in place.

Guidance that supports this document

We have produced documents or guidance bulletins on the following which should be considered in conjunction with these standards:
- Code of ethics for pharmacists and pharmacy technicians
- Professional standards and guidance for the sale and supply of medicines
- Professional standards and guidance for patient consent
- Professional standards and guidance for patient confidentiality
- Pharmacist prescribing pack
- Clinical governance framework for pharmacist prescribers and organisations commissioning or participating in pharmacist prescribing
- Protection of vulnerable adults

You can download these documents and more copies of this document from our website (*www.rpsgb.org*) or you can telephone us on 020 7735 9141.

Additional resources:

The resources listed here are not applicable in all three countries of Great Britain but are valuable resources for those undertaking pharmacist prescribing:

- Department of Health information on non-medical prescribing
http://www.dh.gov.uk/en/Policyandguidance/Medicinespharmac yandindustry/Prescriptions/TheNon-MedicalPrescribingProgramme/index.htm
- Drugs and Therapeutics Bulletin on non-medical prescribing
www.npc.co.uk
- Maintaining competency in prescribing: an outline framework for pharmacist prescribers
http://www.npc.co.uk/pdf/pharmacist_comp_framework_Oct06. pdf
- Medicines Matters DOH July 06 – A guide to mechanisms for the prescribing, supply and administration of medicines
http://www.dh.gov.uk/en/Publicationsandstatistics/Publications/ PublicationsPolicyAndGuidance/DH_064325
- National Prescribing Centre: A guide to good practice in the management of controlled drugs in primary care (England) - Second Edition
http://www.npc.co.uk/controlled_drugs/cdpublications.htm
- NHS Scotland National Education Scotland: Supplementary prescribing for pharmacists in Scotland
http://www.nes.scot.nhs.uk/pharmacy/prescribing/

- Nursing and Midwifery Council Guidelines for the administration of medicines
http://www.nmcuk.org/aFrameDisplay.aspx?DocumentID=221
- Nursing and Midwifery Council prescribing standards
http://www.nmcuk.org/aFrameDisplay.aspx?DocumentID=1645
- Patient Group Directions: A guide to good practice
http://www.npc.co.uk/publications/pgd/pgd.htm
- Saving time, helping patients: a good practice guide to quality repeat prescribing
http://www.npc.co.uk/repeat_prescribing/repeat_presc.htm
- Scottish Executive Health Department HDL 2004 35: Implementation of supplementary prescribing for pharmacists *http://www.scotland.gov.uk/ Publications/2004/06/19514/39164*

Useful websites:

- Clinical Management Plan Library Online
http://www.cmponline.info
- Centre for Postgraduate Pharmacy Education
http://www.cppe.manchester.ac.uk/
- Department of Health
http://www.dh.gov.uk/PolicyAndGuidance/MedicinesPharmacy AndIndustry/Prescriptions/NonmedicalPrescribing/fs/en
- Eguidelines
http://www.eguidelines.co.uk/
- Faculty of Prescribing and Medicines Management
http://fpmm.collpharm.co.uk/
- Medicines and Healthcare products Regulatory Agency
http://www.mhra.gov.uk
- National Electronic Library for Medicines: (now includes druginfozone)
http://www.nelm.nhs.uk/home/default.aspx
- National Prescribing Centre
http://www.npc.co.uk/non_medical.htm
- NHS Education for Scotland
http://www.nes.scot.nhs.uk/
- Nurse Practitioner website
http://www.nursepractitioner.org.uk/
- Nurse Prescriber website
http://www.nurse-prescriber.co.uk
- Patient Group Directions website
http://www.pgd.nhs.uk/
- Prodigy
http://www.prodigy.nhs.uk/indexMain.asp
- Royal Pharmaceutical Society of Great Britain
http://www.rpsgb.org/worldofpharmacy/currentdevelopmentsin-pharmacy/pharmacistprescribing/index.html
- Scottish Executive
http://www.scotland.gov.uk/Home
- Scottish Intercollegiate Guideline Network (SIGN)
http://www.sign.ac.uk
- Welsh Assembly
http://www.wales.gov.uk/index.htm
- Welsh Centre for Postgraduate Pharmacy Education
http://www.cf.ac.uk/phrmy/WCPPE/index.html

Professional Standards and Guidance for Continuing Professional Development

About this document

The Code of Ethics sets out seven principles of ethical practice that you must follow as a pharmacist or pharmacy technician. It is your responsibility to apply the principles to your daily work, using your professional judgement in light of the principles.

The Code of Ethics says that you must '**Develop your professional knowledge and competence**'. In meeting this principle you are expected to:

- Undertake and maintain up-to-date evidence of continuing professional development relevant to your field of pratice.

This document expands on the principles of the Code of Ethics to explain your professional responsibilities in respect of CPD. It is designed to meet the Society's obligations under the Pharmacists and Pharmacy Technicians Order 2007.

The CPD requirements apply equally to all practitioners. They are not changed by factors such as part-time employment, or working in positions of authority. You are expected to cover the full scope of your practice in your CPD record, including responsibilities such as superintendent or pharmacist prescriber and roles in different settings such as industry and community pharmacy.

Standards
Patients, the public and government expect that every practising pharmacist and registered pharmacy technician maintains their professional capability throughout their career. Keeping a record of your continuing professional development (CPD) enables you to confirm that you are meeting these expectations. It also helps you to retain and build your confidence as a professional and it will provide evidence that you meet the Society's CPD requirement. In order to comply with the requirements of the Code of Ethics, you must:

1.1. Keep a record of your CPD that is legible; either electronically online at the Society's website *www.uptodate.org.uk*, on another computer or as hardcopy on paper and in a format published or approved by the Society and carrying the RPSGB CPD approved logo.
1.2. Make a minimum of nine CPD entries per year which reflect the context and scope of your practice as a pharmacist or pharmacy technician.
1.3. Keep a CPD record that complies with the good practice criteria for CPD recording published in Plan and Record by the Society.
1.4 Record how your CPD has contributed to the quality or development of your practice using the Society's CPD framework.
1.5 Submit your CPD record to the Society on request.

Good Practice Guidance

- **You should maintain a learning portfolio with records of attendance and key learning points from continuing education and notes of other learning e.g. through work. This will provide a useful resource for reference. (The learning portfolio is a personal record of professional development that can provide evidence for your CPD record).**

- **You are likely to learn more than you need to meet the Society's CPD requirement through working as a pharmacists or pharmacy technician. You should aim to complete more than the minimum number of CPD entries each year and reflect on your practice at least once per month.**

- **You should make some CPD entries that start at reflection.**

- **You should ensure that your CPD record is up to date.**

- **You should take part in and record CPD that results from a range of learning activities that is relevant to your practice as a pharmacist or pharmacy technician and is, overall, relevant to pharmacy.**

There is no defined activity requirement, however as a guide, the following activities may lead to learning that could be included in a CPD record.

a) learning knowledge and skills on conferences and courses;
b) practice-based learning including feedback from patients and audit;
c) analysis and review of critical incidents;
d) self directed learning, including reading, writing and undertaking research;
e) learning with others including peer review;
f) interactions with other healthcare professionals;
g) giving lectures and writing publications and the design and delivery of training courses; and other activities that result in learning relevant to practice.

Guidance that supports this document

We have produced documents or guidance bulletins on the following which should be considered in conjunction with these standards:
- Code of ethics for pharmacists and pharmacy technicians
- CPD for Pharmacists and Pharmacy Technicians in Great Britain.
  - Plan and Record for Pharmacists
  - Plan and Record for Pharmacy Technicians
  - Other CPD materials

You can download these documents and more copies of this document from our website (*www.rpsgb.org*), the CPD website (*www.uptodate.org.uk*) or you can telephone us on 020 7735 9141.

Other sources of Society advice

Further information and advice on CPD recording is available from the Society's CPD team on 020 7572 2540 or by e-mail *cpd@rpsgb.org*

Technical support is available from the CPD Technical Help desk on 01225 383663 or e-mail: *helpdesk@coacs.com*

Further information or advice on the professional or legal obligations of the pharmacy profession can be obtained by contacting the Society's legal and ethical advisory service on 020 7572 2308 or by e-mail *leadvice@rpsgb.org*.

Professional Standards and Guidance for Responsible Pharmacists (*Effective 1 October 2009*)

About this document

The Code of Ethics sets out seven principles of ethical practice that you must follow as a pharmacist. It is your responsibility to apply the principles to your daily work, using your judgement in light of the principles.

The Code of Ethics says that you must '**Make the care of patients your first concern**'. In meeting this principle you are expected to:

- Provide a proper standard of practice and care to those for whom you provide professional services.
- Be satisfied as to the integrity and quality of products to be supplied to patients.
- Maintain timely, accurate and adequate records and include all relevant information in a clear and legible form.
- Undertake regular reviews, audits and risk assessments to improve the quality of services and minimise risks to patient and public safety.

As the responsible pharmacist for a registered pharmacy, you have both a professional and a legal duty to comply with the requirements of the Medicines Act 1968 and the regulations made under the Act, The Medicines (Pharmacies) (Responsible Pharmacist) Regulations 2008. This document expands on the principles of the Code of Ethics to explain your professional responsibilities when acting in your capacity as the responsible pharmacist. It is designed to meet the Society's obligations under the Pharmacists and Pharmacy Technicians Order 2007 and other relevant legislation.

From 2010 the current regulatory responsibilities of the Royal Pharmaceutical Society will be transferred to the General Pharmaceutical Council, the arrangements for which are currently under discussion at the time of writing. The regulatory role of the Pharmaceutical Society of Northern Ireland is similarly under discussion.

This document does not give detailed guidance on the legal requirements, but you must ensure you comply with relevant legislative requirements. The UK Health Departments have produced factual guidance on the Health Act 2006 amendments to the Medicines Act 1968, and the responsible pharmacist regulations made under section 72A of the 1968 Act.

Where this document refers to 'the Act' this is the Medicines Act 1968 as amended by the Health Act 2006. Where this document refers to 'the regulations' these are The Medicines (Pharmacies) (Responsible Pharmacist) Regulations 2008. This document does not detail all the requirements of the Act or the regulations, but will reference these where appropriate.

1. The responsible pharmacist

The responsible pharmacist is the pharmacist appointed to secure the safe and effective running of the pharmacy in relation to the sale and supply of medicines. At any one time there can only be one responsible pharmacist for a registered pharmacy premises.

Standards
The Act requires each registered pharmacy premises to have a responsible pharmacist in order to operate lawfully. As the responsible pharmacist, the Act requires you to secure the safe and effective running of the pharmacy. In complying with this legal duty and exercising your professional judgement, you must:

1.1 establish the scope of your role and responsibilities and take all reasonable steps to clarify any ambiguities or uncertainties with the pharmacist in a position of authority or other delegated person
1.2 not undertake work that is outside of your competency

2. Pharmacy procedures

To comply with the Act, the responsible pharmacist is required to establish, if not already established, maintain and review pharmacy procedures. Appendix A lists the minimum information to be included in pharmacy procedures that must be in place, as required in the regulations.

Where this document refers to pharmacy procedures, these are currently known as standard operating procedures. The standards in this section apply to those procedures detailed in Appendix A.

In this section, reference to an **amendment** to a procedure is intended to mean a temporary change to the procedure due to a change in the pharmacy's circumstances, for example a member of staff is off sick or a power failure. Where amended, the procedure must revert to its original content once the change in circumstance is resolved.

In this section, a **review** is where you revaluate the content of the current procedure to ensure that it is still applicable and workable. Review must be in accordance with the standards below, or following an incident in the pharmacy which indicates that it may no longer be operating safely and effectively, for example a near miss.

Standards
The pharmacy procedures form part of the quality framework for the safe and effective running of the pharmacy. Pharmacy procedures must be fit for purpose, and reflect the day to day running of the specific pharmacy premises. The regulations set out the minimum areas information required in the pharmacy procedures that must be in place.

In addition, you must ensure that:

2.1 the procedures are being operated in the pharmacy and the requirement for amendment or review is assessed by you.
2.2 it is clear to staff on duty which procedures are in operation on the day.
2.3 adequate back ups of the content of pharmacy procedures are maintained.
2.4 pharmacy procedures must be applicable at all times under normal circumstances;

Establishing the pharmacy procedures

2.5 if you are the responsible pharmacist who is responsible for establishing the pharmacy procedure(s), these are:

2.5.1 marked with the date of preparation.
2.5.2 marked with the date it is due for review.

The amendment of pharmacy procedures

2.6 in the event that you make a temporary amendment to the pharmacy procedure, an audit trail is maintained to identify:

2.6.1 what procedures are currently in place;

2.6.2 what procedures were previously in place;

2.6.3 the responsible pharmacist who amended or reviewed the procedures and date on which any changes were made.

The review of pharmacy procedures

2.7 the procedures are reviewed at least once every two years, and at any time that an incident or event occurs which indicates that the pharmacy is not running safely and effectively

2.8 any changes to the procedures, following their review, are notified to the person in position of authority as soon as it is reasonably practicable.

2.9 an audit trail is maintained to identify:

2.9.1 what procedures are currently in place;

2.9.2 what procedures were previously in place;

2.9.3 the responsible pharmacist who reviewed the procedures and date on which any changes were made.

Good Practice Guidance

• **All members of staff involved in the sale and supply of medicines should read and comply with the pharmacy procedures**

• **Pharmacy procedures should not be dependant on the presence and ways of working of the responsible pharmacist under whose authority they were established**

• **You should record the reason for the review or amendment**

3. Pharmacy records

Standards

Failure to complete the pharmacy record, as required in the Act, is a criminal offence that could result in prosecution. Appendix B sets out the minimum information to be included in the pharmacy record, as required by the regulations. In addition, you must:

3.1 ensure the record is accurate and contemporaneous

3.2 make appropriate back-ups of an electronic record to ensure the record is available at the premises

3.3 safeguard a paper based record by initialling and dating any amendments to an entry made in the record

3.4 ensure that any alterations to the electronic record identify when and by whom the alteration was made.

4. Absence from the pharmacy

The regulations enable the pharmacy to continue to operate for the sale and supply of medicines for a maximum of two hours during the operational hours of the pharmacy between midnight and midnight without the presence of a responsible pharmacist, subject to specified conditions. The regulations require you to remain contactable with pharmacy staff where this is practical. You must also be able to return with reasonable promptness. You must return with reasonable promptness, where in your opinion this is necessary to secure the safe and effective running of the pharmacy. If you cannot remain contactable, you must arrange for another pharmacist to provide advice throughout the period of absence or for any time during that period that you are out of contact. You must exercise your professional judgment in deciding whether to be absent from the pharmacy.

Good practice guidance

• **You should record your reason for absence**

• **You should wherever possible, plan your absence in advance of leaving the pharmacy**

• **You should consider the length of time it will take for you to travel to and from the pharmacy to the alternative destination, in considering your ability to return with reasonable promptness.**

• **You should consider what would be the most appropriate means to remain contactable with the pharmacy, for example a pager or mobile telephone and any risks in being able to remain contactable, for example where travelling through areas with poor mobile phone reception.**

Appendix A

The regulations require that the pharmacy procedures must provide information on the following:

• Arrangements to ensure that medicinal products are:-
  ○ ordered
  ○ stored
  ○ prepared
  ○ sold by retail
  ○ supplied in circumstances corresponding to retail sale
  ○ delivered outside the pharmacy and
  ○ disposed of
  in a safe and effective manner

• The circumstances in which a member of pharmacy staff who is not a pharmacist may give advice about medicinal products
• The identification of members of pharmacy staff who are, in the view of the responsible pharmacist, competent to perform specified tasks relating to the pharmacy business
• The keeping of records about the matters mentioned above
• Arrangements which are to apply during the absence of the responsible pharmacist from the premises
• Steps to be taken when there is a change of responsible pharmacist at the premises
• The procedure which is followed if a complaint is made about the pharmacy business
• The procedure which is to be followed if an incident occurs which may indicate that the pharmacy business is not running in a safe and effective manner and
• The manner in which changes to the pharmacy procedures are to be notified to the staff.

Appendix B

The regulations require the following details to be included in the pharmacy record:

- The responsible pharmacist's name
- Their registration number
- The date and time at which the responsible pharmacist became the responsible pharmacist
- The date and time at which the responsible pharmacist ceased to be the responsible pharmacist
- In relation to absence from the premises by the responsible pharmacist:
  - The date of absence
  - The time at which the absence commenced
  - The time at which they returned
- If they have been responsible pharmacist for more than one premises, this fact[1]

---

[1] At this time a responsible pharmacist cannot be responsible for more than one pharmacy premises.

Guidance that supports this document

We have produced documents or on the following which should be considered in conjunction with these standards:

- Code of ethics for pharmacists and pharmacy technicians
- Professional standards and guidance for pharmacists and pharmacy technicians in positions of authority
- The Responsible Pharmacist Toolkit

You can download these documents and more copies of this document from our website (www.rpsgb.org) or you can telephone us on 020 7735 9141. The responsible pharmacist toolkit is available at www.responsiblepharmacist.org

Other sources of Society advice

Further information or advice on the professional or legal obligations of the pharmacy profession can be obtained by contacting the Society's legal and ethical advisory service on 020 7572 2308, or e-mail leadvice@rpsgb.org

3: Improving Pharmacy Practice

The key responsibilities of pharmacists are set out in the Code of Ethics and to ensure that the knowledge, skills and performance of themselves and their staff are of high quality, up to date, evidence based and relevant to their field of practice. Pharmacists must ensure that they practise safely and that the services they provide to patients and the public are of high quality, safe and effective. Pharmacists should use the tenets of clinical governance (see section 3.1.1) when developing any service specifications. Section 3 covers the following:

Improving the quality of pharmacy practice (3.1)
    Clinical governance (3.1.1)
    Continuing professional development (3.1.2)
    Pharmacy support staff (3.1.3)
    Pharmacist prescribing (3.1.4)
Practice guidance documents (3.2)
Law and Ethics fact sheets (3.3)

3.1 Improving the quality of pharmacy practice

3.1.1 Clinical governance

Clinical governance can be described as the process by which high quality services are delivered. It is the "how to" part of a broader quality improvement agenda for the National Health Service, which includes setting standards via the National Institute for Health and Clinical Excellence (NICE) and national service frameworks (NSFs) and the monitoring of standards by the Care Quality Commission and others.

Clinical governance and continuing professional development (CPD) are tools to help individual pharmacists, their managers and their employers to recognise and celebrate good professional practice and to highlight areas where there is potential for improvement. Engaging with clinical governance and CPD will help pharmacists to maintain and improve the quality of their practice.

Clinical governance involves learning not just from what worked well but also from what went wrong to prevent similar incidents happening again. For this, pharmacists need to learn from each other and to encourage a fair and open culture where they can share their experiences to promote best practice for all patients.

All pharmacists need to comply with legal obligations on data protection and confidentiality and must conform to the NHS Code of Practice on Confidentiality.

There is no single task which is clinical governance but there is a series of processes which, when undertaken individually, build up the picture that is clinical governance. These processes are:
- Accountability
- Audit
- Clinical effectiveness
- Patient and public involvement
- Remedying under performance
- Risk management
- Staff management
- Continuing professional development

Accountability

Pharmacists are accountable for the quality and standards of the services they provide within pharmacies or pharmacy departments, and for their individual professional practice. Clinical governance reinforces this accountability and reminds pharmacists that they are just as accountable for the quality and standards of clinical advice given to patients and professionals about treatment, policies and procedures as they are for the dispensing, sale and supply of medicines.

Audit

Audit involves systematic evaluation of professional work against set standards. Audit templates are available from the Society's website (www.rpsgb.org), or on CD-ROM (e-mail qualityimprovement@rpsgb.org). Every community pharmacy in England and Wales with an NHS contract must carry out at least two clinical audits annually, one practice-based audit and one primary care organisation (PCO)-determined multidisciplinary audit.

Clinical effectiveness

Pharmacists should be aware of current evidence and apply this to their practice and also be open to sharing of ideas with professional colleagues and patients. Pharmacists should ensure that they monitor patients' care, including drug interactions and adverse drug reactions, based on the information available to them at the time.

Patient and public involvement

Pharmacists need to involve patients and the public in redesigning and improving services they deliver. Community pharmacists in England and Wales with an NHS contract should undertake an annual patient satisfaction survey. Pharmacists should consider ways to promote concordance to ensure that patients become full partners in medicines taking.

Community pharmacists in England and Wales with an NHS contract will be expected to co-operate with other organisations such as PCOs, patient and public involvement forums and the Care Quality Commission on monitoring and audit of pharmacy services.

Remedying underperformance

To meet their Code of Ethics responsibilities to patients and the public, pharmacists need to ensure that they use CPD and other resources available as a means of improving in those areas of practice where they are performing less well.

Risk management

Pharmacists should ensure that they have robust risk management procedures in place. These include standard operating procedures, recording systems for interventions, a robust complaints procedure and reporting systems for errors and near misses.

Staff management

Pharmacists should ensure that all staff and locums receive an appropriate induction on undertaking employment in the pharmacy.

Continuing professional development

Continuing professional development is covered in the next section, Section 3.1.2.

3.1.2 Continuing professional development

All pharmacists and pharmacy technicians are expected to make a declaration that they are either practising or non-practising when they renew their membership of the Society each year. A person practises as a pharmacist or a pharmacy technician if, whilst acting in the capacity of or holding himself out as a pharmacist or a pharmacy technician, he undertakes any work or gives any advice in relation to the dispensing or use of medicines, the science of medicines, the practice of pharmacy or the provision of health care. Guidance on making the practising/non-practising declaration is available on the Society's website at www.rpsgb.org. The main points covered in the guidance are shown in the panel on p139.

All practising pharmacists and pharmacy technicians have a professional obligation to maintain a record of their CPD. In March 2009 the Society issued professional standards and guidance for CPD under the Code of Ethics. The Society also provides CPD support materials and facilities for recording CPD online, on paper or on a freestanding personal computer.

Non-practising registrants and pharmacists registered as overseas members of the Society are not required to maintain a CPD record. If they wish, they can keep a record of their CPD on the Society's online CPD recording facility. Log into www.uptodate.org.uk for further details and to register as a user. The remaining information given here is based on the *CPD Plan and Record*, the guidance document that is available to all practising pharmacists and pharmacy technicians. The *Plan and Record* is available on the Society's website at www.rpsgb.org

What is CPD?

Continuing professional development (CPD) is a framework for the maintenance of professional competence. The Society's framework applies equally to pharmacists and pharmacy technicians. CPD is a cyclical process of reflection, planning, action and evaluation. It includes everything that a pharmacist or pharmacy technician learns which makes her or him better able to do her or his job.

CPD standards

The professional standards and guidance for continuing professional development (p133) state that practising pharmacists and pharmacy technicians must keep a CPD record that complies with the good practice criteria for CPD recording either electronically by logging into the Society's CPD website www.uptodate.org.uk, on a PC with the desktop program, or on paper using the Society's *Plan and Record* system. They also state that practising pharmacists and pharmacy technicians must make a minimum of nine entries in a 12-month period which reflect the context and scope of their practice, and submit these to the Society on request.

The CPD cycle enables you to update, maintain and develop your capabilities by:
- Helping you identify your individual learning needs
- Recognising the learning that occurs in the workplace
- Acknowledging that we learn in a variety of ways and that you will have your own preferred approaches
- Linking your learning to your own practice and development

reflection

What do I want to learn?

evaluation

What have I learned?
Who is benefiting?
How? Why?

planning

What is the best way of
learning what I want to?

action

Doing the learning

CPD cycle

- Avoiding the need to complete a fixed number of hours of continuing education. The emphasis of your CPD should be on quality, rather than quantity.

It is important to distinguish CPD from the more familiar term continuing education (CE). CE refers to traditional methods of learning such as attending workshops, following diploma or distance learning courses, or structured reading. These activities are very useful and will inevitably form part of most pharmacists' or pharmacy technicians' CPD, but continuing professional development is much wider than CE. CE is only one type of activity within CPD. CPD covers all job-related learning. The key difference in CPD is that you focus on what you have learnt and the result of the learning on your practice as a pharmacist or pharmacy technician, for example, what you do differently or the actions that you take as a result of your new learning.

CPD also includes activities such as:
- Learning by doing
- Dealing with problems/situations in the workplace or elsewhere (including incidents outside your professional responsibilities from which you learn something that is applicable to them)
- Participating in group activities, eg, staff meetings, staff training or working groups
- Projects and professional audits
- Preparation for a presentation or teaching others
- Work shadowing ("sitting next to Nelly")
- Secondment to another department
- Research into a topic, new drug or practice area, etc

This list is not exhaustive and could include any other activities that develop your professional capabilities.

Advice on making a CPD entry

The CPD standards state that you must make a minimum of nine CPD entries per year. Individual pharmacists will find their own pattern, perhaps two every other month, for example. Evidence from the Society's pilots indicates that pharmacists and pharmacy technicians are learning all the time, and need to be selective about what they choose to enter in their CPD record. Our advice is that you work towards a balanced CPD record that complies with the Society's professional standards and guidance for CPD and that you keep this record up to date. The guidance suggests a range of learning activities that could be included in your CPD record. It also advises that you should make some CPD entries that start at Reflection.

A person practises as a pharmacist or phamacy technician if, while acting in the capacity of or holding himself out as a pharmacist or pharmacy technician, he undertakes any work, or gives any advice, in or in relation to the dispensing or use of medicines, the science of medicines or the practice of pharmacy or the provision of healthcare.

Key points to note are:

• When you consider your practising status, it may be helpful to ask yourself whether you or others feel that the work you undertake or advice you give has added value or credibility because you are a pharmacist. If so, you are practising.
• It is possible still to be practising if you are retired or not working if, for example, you continue to provide advice on pharmacy matters.
• It is a misconception that a pharmacist who is not dispensing can place themselves in the non-practising category. Even if you do not dispense, you are not automatically non-practising.
• Most working pharmacists are practising, not only those who dispense, or work or provide advice in a clinical context. It includes, for example, those working in industry, academia and administration.
• Just because you undertake work or give advice that could be provided by someone who is not a pharmacist, does not mean that you are non-practising. The fact that those you work with or advise, know you are a pharmacist adds professional credibility to your work and advice.
• If you are in doubt, the fact that something has made you question whether you are a practising pharmacist probably means that you are.
• To assume that you are practising is a good place to start. Only those pharmacists who have truly retired from work, or those who have moved on to other non-related careers, have the non-practising route open to them.

The same guidance applies to registered pharmacy technicians.

You might want to record a combination of CPD entries that demonstrate an impact on different parties (on yourself, colleagues, organisations and, particularly, on users of your products and/or services). Likewise, you may choose to illustrate the range of activities you participate in as part of your CPD (such as reading, workshops and discussion with peers).

You can also start some CPD entries at Action. This is where you have learnt something but had not initially set out to learn it. For example, in a discussion with colleagues you might discover that there is a better way of doing something, and you then try it out in your own practice. These records starting at Action are quicker to record as you only need to record the action and the evaluation. However, please note that only some of your entries can start at Action.

The Society will start to call in CPD records for review from July 2009. When your CPD record is called, you may chose which entries to submit. These may be entries that you have found to be most meaningful for you in the work you undertake as a pharmacist or pharmacy technician.

Contact:
CPD Manager
Tel: 020 7572 2667
e-mail: cpd@rpsgb.org

3.1.3 Pharmacy support staff

The Society has a range of policies covering minimum training and competence requirements for pharmacy support staff. For pharmacy technicians a regulatory framework is now in place and this became statutory on 1 July 2009.

Further information on all of these policies can be found in the Pharmacy support staff section of the Society's website *www.rpsgb.org*.

Medicines counter assistants

Since 1996 it has been a professional requirement that any assistant who is given delegated authority to sell medicines under a protocol should have undertaken, or be undertaking an accredited course relevant to their duties. The Society's requirement is that courses should cover the knowledge and understanding associated with units 2.04 and 2.05 of the Pharmacy Services S/NVQ level 2, entitled *Assist in the Sale of OTC medicines and provide information to customers on symptoms and products* and *Assist in the supply of prescribed items* (taking in a prescription and issuing prescribed items).

Medicines counter assistant courses have been accredited for the Society by the College of Pharmacy Practice since 1996. Under this arrangement the following training providers currently have their courses accredited:
- Boots the Chemist (until 7 December 2009)
- Buttercups Training (until 12 March 2009)
- CMP Information Ltd (until 12 March 2009)
- Mediapharm (until 16 February 2009)
- Tesco Stores Ltd (until 31 March 2009)

From 2006 the Society has also accredited medicines counter assistant courses. The following training providers have had their courses accredited by the Society:
- Alliance Pharmacy (until 12 June 2010)
- Buttercups Training (until 20 December 2009)
- CMP Medica (until 5 May 2012)
- Co-operative Group Pharmacy (until 28 February 2011)
- National Pharmacy Association (until 14 August 2010)

Dispensing/pharmacy assistants

From January 1 2005 pharmacists have had a professional obligation to ensure that dispensing/pharmacy assistants are competent in the areas in which they are working to a minimum standard equivalent to the Pharmacy Services Scottish/National Vocational Qualification (S/NVQ) level 2 qualification or undertaking training towards this. This policy applies to staff working in the following areas:
- Sale of over the counter medicines and the provision of information to customers on symptoms and products*
- Prescription receipt and collection*
- The assembly of prescribed items (including the generation of labels)
- Ordering, receiving and storing pharmaceutical stock

---

* Medicines counter assistants are exempt from further training in these units provided they have successfully completed an accredited MCA course or have previously been considered to have met the Society's requirements for MCAs

- The supply of pharmaceutical stock
- Preparation for the manufacture of pharmaceutical products (including aseptic products)
- Manufacture and assembly of medicinal products (including aseptic products)

The requirement can be met by completing a training programme relevant to the job role and there are four acceptable ways of doing this:
(a) Successful achievement of Pharmacy Services S/NVQ level 2
(b) Successful achievement of relevant units of the Pharmacy Services S/NVQ level 2
(c) Successful achievement of a training programme accredited to be of an equivalent level to S/NVQ level 2
(d) Successful achievement of relevant units of an accredited training programme of an equivalent level to Pharmacy Services S/NVQ level 2.

Training programmes have been accredited for the Society by the College of Pharmacy Practice since late 2004. Under this arrangement the following training providers currently have their programmes accredited:
- Tesco Stores Ltd (until 7 January 2010)

From 2006 the Society has also accredited training programmes. The following training providers have had their programmes accredited by the Society:
- Buttercups Training (until 20 December 2009)
- CMP Medica (until 5 May 2012)
- Co-operative Group Pharmacy (until 28 February 2011)
- National Pharmacy Association (until 14 August 2010)

Dispensing/pharmacy assistants and medicines counter assistants should be enrolled on a training programme within three months of commencing their role (or as soon as practical within local training arrangements) and the programme should be completed within a three-year time period.

Pharmacy technician registration

The Society opened a voluntary register of pharmacy technicians in January 2005. The voluntary register became a statutory register across Great Britain on 1 July 2009. Registration will continue to be voluntary for two years after this date. On 1 July 2011 registration will become mandatory (compulsory) and the title "pharmacy technician" will become protected in law. All those currently practising as pharmacy technicians will need to apply to register by midnight on 30 June 2011 to continue working as pharmacy technicians.

From 1 July 2011 the educational standard for entry to the register will be the Pharmacy Services S/NVQ level 3 together with an accredited underpinning knowledge programme. Until this date transitional arrangements for entry onto the register will apply (this is sometimes referred to as grandparenting) and a range of pharmacy technician qualifications will be accepted. These arrangements enable those with the responsibilities, experience and training background of pharmacy technicians (though this may have predated S/NVQs and/or been delivered through a company scheme) to apply for registration. Evidence of recent work experience under the supervision, direction or guidance of a pharmacist as a pharmacy technician or trainee pharmacy technician is also required.

Further information on pharmacy technician registration is available on the pharmacy technician page of the Society's website *www.rpsgb.org*.

Contact:
Support Staff Regulation Division
Tel: 020 7572 2610
e-mail: *supportstaff@rpsgb.org* (MCAs or D/PAs)
e-mail: *pharmacytechnician@rpsgb.org* (Pharmacy Technicians

3.1.4 Pharmacist prescribing

The policy framework for supplementary prescribing by nurses and pharmacists was completed in April 2003 when the regulations came into force. The regulations for pharmacist independent prescribing took effect in May 2006. The current Department of Health guidance on independent prescribing by pharmacists and nurses can be found on the department's website *www.dh.gov.uk*.

Prescribing by pharmacists takes two forms. Supplementary prescribing is a partnership between a medical practitioner (independent prescriber) who establishes the diagnosis and initiates treatment, a pharmacist supplementary prescriber who monitors the patient and prescribes further supplies of medication and the patient who agrees to the supplementary prescribing arrangement. For each patient, the framework for supplementary prescribing is set out in an individual clinical management plan (*see* p12) which contains details of the patient, their condition, treatment with medicines and when the patient should be referred back to the independent prescriber.

A pharmacist supplementary prescriber may prescribe all medicines, including controlled drugs and unlicensed medicines providing they are included in the clinical management plan.

A pharmacist independent prescriber is qualified to work as an independent or supplementary prescriber. They may practise solely in one practice mode or move between modes according to patient or practice circumstances. As an independent prescriber a pharmacist works as an autonomous practitioner and takes full clinical responsibility for their prescribing practice. They are responsible for the clinical assessment of a patient's condition, formulating or reviewing a diagnosis and devising an appropriate treatment plan. A pharmacist independent prescriber must also ensure that they do not miss signs of a significant clinical problem.

Pharmacist independent prescribers can prescribe for any clinical condition but they must only prescribe within their professional and clinical competence.

Unlike supplementary prescribers, pharmacist independent prescribers cannot at present prescribe Controlled Drugs or unlicensed medicines. They can, however, prescribe these groups of medicines if they choose to practise as a supplementary prescriber for specific patients or groups of patients – as long as they are included in the clinical management plan specific to that patient.

The maintenance of shared patient records in a timely fashion and effective communication with other prescribers and members of the health care team are essential features of prescribing by pharmacists.

Pharmacists who wish to become a pharmacist prescriber must complete an accredited education and training programme. The duration of study is between 25 and 27 days including attendance at classes. Students also have to complete an additional 12-14 days' learning in practice supervised by a medical practitioner.

Pharmacists who successfully complete one of the pharmacist prescriber courses accredited by the Society must register with the Society as a prescriber before they can prescribe (*see* p5). For further information see the Society's website *www.rpsgb.org*.

For a clinical governance framework for pharmacist prescribers published by the Society see *www.rpsgb.org*.

For professional standards and guidance for pharmacist prescribers published by the Society (*see also* p122), *see www.rpsgb.org*.

Contact:
Pharmacist Prescribing
Tel: 020 7572 2604
e-mail: philippa.strevens@rpsgb.org

3.2 Practice guidance documents

Practice guidance in Section 3.2 is available via the RPSGB website at *www.rpsgb.org*. Current and future guidance topics are under review by the Practice department. To enquire whether individual guidance documents are also available as hard copy, please e-mail *practice@rpsgb.org*. Brief descriptions of the contents of the documents are given below:

5 and 10 High impact changes

These documents are part of a strategy to promote the role of pharmacists to commissioners, managers, general practitioners and others in primary care. The documents seek to influence the commissioning of pharmacy services by PCTs under world class commissioning and the integration of pharmacy into practice based commissioning (PBC). They have been produced as a provider perspective on commissioning. They provide PCTs and SHAs with suggestions of how to work with pharmacists in order to maximise their contribution to the development of PBC and commissioning.

Amorolfine nail lacquer

This guidance outlines the over-the-counter indications for amorolfine nail lacquer as well as important points to consider when counter prescribing.

Atopic eczema in children: NICE quick reference sheet for community pharmacists

This guidance demonstrates how pharmacists can implement the NICE guidance on atopic eczema.

Azithromycin

This guidance outlines the over-the-counter indications for azithromycin and provides key practice points.

Best practice guidance for commissioners and providers of pharmaceutical services for drug users

This document offers best practice guidance for commissioners and providers on the development of service specifications for pharmacists providing services to drug users in England. The guidance, produced jointly by the RPSGB and NTA, was developed in collaboration with and endorsed by the PSNC.

Blood pressure/hypertension management

This guidance highlights the implications for community pharmacy of the key priorities of the NICE guidelines on the management of hypertension in adults in primary care.

Bowel cancer

This guidance on best practice for pharmacists when advising on suspected, or diagnosed, bowel cancer has been prepared in conjunction with the charity Beating Bowel Cancer.

Child protection

This guidance is intended to inform pharmacists and pharmacy staff about their responsibilities under child protection legislation and advise on further sources of information and advice. The guidance outlines the principles of child protection and provides advice about what to do if child abuse or neglect is suspected.

Chloramphenicol eye drops

This guidance outlines the over-the-counter indications for chloramphenicol eye-drops and provides key practice points.

Cholesterol testing

This guidance is aimed at community pharmacists wishing to provide a cholesterol testing service to the public. The guidance incorporates a top 10 tips panel produced by the Medicines and Healthcare products Regulatory Agency.

Clinical governance framework for pharmacist prescribers and organisations commissioning or participating in pharmacist prescribing

The Society has produced this clinical governance framework to support the development of high quality care and patient safety in this particular area of practice. This framework for pharmacist prescribing has been developed from two distinct viewpoints: both from an organisational perspective and an individual prescriber's perspective.

Clinical trials: pharmacy services

This guidance has been produced by the Institute of Clinical Research and the Royal Pharmaceutical Society of Great Britain and should be used by pharmacy staff involved with the provision of clinical trials services at policy, strategic and operational levels. It applies to all clinical trials that are regulated by the Medicines for Human Use (Clinical Trials) Regulations 2004, including commercial and non-commercial clinical trials and investigator initiated clinical research.

Clinical trials may involve medicines, biological substances, gene therapy or radiopharmaceuticals. Specific guidelines and regulations exist for the management of these products. It is the responsibility of the pharmacy staff involved to ensure compliance.

Collection and delivery services from central points

This guidance is intended as a resource for pharmacists involved in setting up collection and delivery services from a central point, or pharmacists who are planning to set up such a scheme.

Community pharmacy contract: national resources

This is a list of national resources available to support the community pharmacy contract in England and Wales.

Controlled Drugs management: changes affecting pharmacy

A number of changes to the monitoring and inspection, prescribing, dispensing, record keeping and destruction of Controlled Drugs (CDs) have been introduced as part of the ongoing programme of work to implement the recommendations of the Shipman Inquiry. These are a mixture of legislative requirements and professional good practice guidance. This guidance sets out what changes are occurring in England, Scotland and Wales, when they are expected to happen and whether they are legislative or good practice.

Guidance on the use of Controlled Drugs in secondary care is now available. This replaces Appendix 1 of *Safe and secure handling of medicines* (revised Duthie report) and can be accessed via the RPSGB website.

Controlled Drugs stock: maintaining running balances

It is now strongly recommended that pharmacists should keep a running balance of stock in the Controlled Drug register. This guidance sets out how to maintain a running balance and how to deal with discrepancies.

Cough and cold treatment for children

This guidance was issued in light of the Medicines and Healthcare products Regulatory Agency (MHRA) decision in March 2008 to review the sale and supply of cough and cold products for children less than two years of age.

Counterfeit medicines

Guidance for pharmacists providing information about counterfeit medicines - the causes and the consequences, as well as top tips for detecting counterfeits and actions that pharmacists should take if a counterfeit medicine is suspected.

Diabetes care

This guidance updates earlier guidance documents on *Care of people with diabetes* and *Early identification of diabetes by community pharmacists*, and merges them into a single document.

Diagnostic testing and screening services

This guidance outlines 10 "Principles of good practice" which should be taken into consideration when setting up and providing any NHS or private diagnostic testing/ screening service.

Dispensing EEA and Swiss prescriptions

This guidance provides information for pharmacists about what to do when they receive a prescription from the EEA or Switzerland.

Emergency hormonal contraception (EHC) as a Pharmacy medicine

This guidance is intended to support the provision of emergency hormonal contraception through pharmacy and ensure the relevant professional standards are met. It covers the process of obtaining information before the supply is made, how EHC is taken, advice to clients, terms of the marketing authorisation and guidance for pharmacists who choose not to supply EHC.

In December 2006 the Society issued a press release providing updated advice relating to advance supply of EHC (see *www.rpsgb.org/pdfs/pr061218.pdf*).

Epilepsy

These guidance documents for community pharmacists and hospital pharmacists cover the causes of epilepsy and information relating to treatment and therapeutic management.

Glaucoma

This guidance demonstrates how pharmacists can implement the NICE guidance on glaucoma.

Handling of medicines in social care

This document provides professional pharmaceutical guidance for people in every aspect of social care who are involved in handling medicines. It replaces the earlier publication *The administration and control of medicines in care homes and children's services* (2003).

Hazardous Waste (England and Wales) Regulations 2005

Guidance for community and hospital pharmacists in England and Wales. The Department of Health has also issued additional guidance to the hazardous waste regulations (*Safe Management of Healthcare Waste*), for England and Wales, which specifically covers healthcare waste including pharmaceutical waste and disposal.

Medical devices

This guidance outlines what medical devices are, how they are regulated, what information pharmacists should know and consider when supplying and stocking medical devices as well as how to deal with medical device alerts.

Medicine administration record (MAR) charts, principles of safe and appropriate production

This has been updated to enable pharmacists to adhere to good practice principles when supplying MAR charts while using their professional judgement.

Medicines adherence: NICE implementation guidance for pharmacists

This guidance demonstrates how pharmacists can implement the NICE guidance on medicines adherence.

Medicines management during patient admission to the ward

Produced by the Hospital Pharmacists Group, this document highlights the key issues for medicines management during patient admission to the ward.

Moving patients, moving medicines, moving safely: Discharge and transfer planning

This guidance aims to help multidisciplinary teams maximise good practice and minimise the risks for patients associated with their medicines, in the transfer and discharge process.

It provides practical guidance on developing systems to tackle discharge and transfer problems between different settings and is based on experiences and evidence available, including examples and paperwork from existing schemes. An accompanying workbook is intended as a practical guide to help PCOs, NHS trusts and health professionals implement successful processes for discharge and transfer planning.

NHS Code of Practice on confidentiality

This guidance outlines the NHS Code of Practice on Confidentiality and demonstrates how this relates to community pharmacy practice in England and Wales.

Obesity

This guidance provides points for pharmacists to consider when advising on obesity management.

Omeprazole

This guidance outlines the over-the-counter indications for omeprazole and provides key practice points.

Orlistat

This guidance outlines the over-the-counter indications for orlistat and provides key practice points.

Pharmacist poor performance: identifying and remedying

This interim guidance is intended to assist organisations to recognise poor performance and outline the principles which employers, including the managed care sector (NHS), should apply in identifying and remedying poor performance.

Practice based commissioning: a resource for community pharmacists in England

This guidance provides local pharmaceutical committees and community pharmacists with the knowledge to effectively engage with practice based commissioning (PBC), improving the quality of services offered and developing better access for patients.

Practice based commissioning: a resource for primary care pharmacists in England

This guidance provides primary care pharmacists with the knowledge to effectively engage with practice based commissioning (PBC), improving the quality of services offered and developing better access for patients.

Pregnancy testing in the pharmacy

Pregnancy testing is a professional service which is sometimes offered by community pharmacists. This guidance covers issues such as confidentiality, advertising, facilities, requests for a test, records and communicating results.

Prescribing pack for pharmacists

This pack provides resources and information for those who have qualified as pharmacist prescribers and want to start prescribing. It is also useful for those who are in the process of training as pharmacist prescribers as it can help with planning the implementation of prescribing.

Protection of vulnerable adults

This guidance is intended to help raise awareness of the ways in which vulnerable adults may be abused and advise what to do if abuse is suspected.

Pseudoephedrine and ephedrine

This guidance highlights what to do if you receive suspicious requests for medicines containing pseudoephedrine or ephedrine.

Raising concerns

The purpose of this guidance is to help pharmacists and registered pharmacy technicians confidently report concerns about possible dangerous, illegal or unprofessional behaviour in the workplace and advise on the legal protection and support available.

Recording interventions

This guidance provides advice on when to record an intervention, the content of records that should be made, where such records should be made, how these records could be utilised to improve efficiency and safety across the NHS and the length of time these records need to be retained for. It applies to England and Wales.

Resource tools for community pharmacists

The tools have been developed in conjuction with the Society's Inspectorate to help community pharmacists in everyday practice. They cover: Dealing with dispensing errors; Destruction of Controlled Drugs; Fridge temperature monitoring; How to use your thermometer; Near miss error log; Products with a short shelf life; Recommended procedures for date checking of pharmacy stock; Records of supplies of unlicensed medicinal products; Reducing risk and improving quality; Risk minimisation with regard to dispensing and checking; Records of supplies of extemporaneous preparations

These resource tools can be found on the Inspectorate section of the Society's website *www.rpsgb.org*

Responsible pharmacist toolkit

This practical toolkit provides pharmacists with all the information and tools they will need to undertake the role of a responsible pharmacist.

Safe and secure handling of medicines (revised Duthie report)

Comprehensive guidance on safe and secure handling of medicines was last issued to the NHS in 1988, in the report of a working group chaired by Professor RB Duthie.

There have been many changes in legislation and practice since then and the Royal Pharmaceutical Society of Great Britain has led a multidiscliplinary review to produce this updated report, in consultation with revelant stakeholders including pharmacist, medical and nursing organisations and the National Patient Safety Agency.

Self-care challenge - A strategy for pharmacists in England

This document has been produced on behalf of the Royal Pharmaceutical Society of Great Britain's self-care working group and seeks to create a call for action to engage pharmacists in increasing self-care support. The main position paper is accompanied by a list of useful resources relating to self-care, including a paper aimed at commissioners.

Service continuity planning for community pharmacists

This guidance focuses on service continuity planning within each individual pharmacy or pharmacy department. It looks at procedures required to prevent and prepare for emergencies, the response during the experience and the action required to recover a business from the situation that will affect its ability to operate and function effectively. A template to assist in structured planning is also available.

Service continuity planning for pandemic flu

This document gives guidance on continuity planning for community pharmacy services during an influenza pandemic. The guidance advises pharmacists that they should try to maintain business as usual during a pandemic situation, with the emphasis on ensuring patient safety and the supply of medicines for those with long-term conditions.

Sexual boundaries: Maintaining clear boundaries

This guidance highlights to pharmacists how they should maintain clear sexual boundaries in everyday practice.

Simvastatin

This guidance outlines the over-the-counter indications for simvastatin and provides key practice points.

Smoking: guidance to help smokers to stop

This joint guidance for pharmacists in England was produced in August 2005 with the National Institute for Health and Clinical Excellence and PharmacyHealthLink.

Smoking, stopping: role of pharmacy

This document highlights the services pharmacy can provide to those wishing to stop smoking. Pharmacists should use it to promote their role to those who have influence over developing local services.

Smoking, stopping: knowledge and resource tools

This document provides pharmacists with a list of resources to help them in the development and provision of stop smoking services.

Standard operating procedures for dispensing: development and implementation

Since January 1, 2005, the Royal Pharmaceutical Society of Great Britain requires pharmacists to put in place and operate written standard operating procedures (SOPs) within individual pharmacies covering the dispensing process, including the transfer of prescribed items to patients. The requirement applies to both the hospital and community sectors and covers all of the activities which occur from the time that prescriptions are received in the pharmacy or by a pharmacist until medicines or other prescribed items have been collected or transferred to the patient.

This guidance sets out the areas of the dispensing process for which SOPs are required and provides guidance on how to write them.

Standards checklist for registered pharmacy premises

This document has been produced as guidance on the basic standards that the Society's inspector will be looking for during a routine pharmacy visit.

Substances of misuse

This updated document is intended to alert pharmacists to the classes of substances that might be subject to misuse.

Sumatriptan

This guidance outlines the over-the-counter indications for sumatriptan and provides key practice points.

Veterinary medicines: sale and supply

This document advises on both the legislation and best practice guidance when selling or supplying a veterinary medicine from a pharmacy.

Visits to pharmacies by external monitoring bodies

The pharmacy contract and the associated Terms of Service allow several external bodies to visit pharmacies in England and Wales. This guidance outlines who can visit, what the pharmacist needs to do, the content of visits and potential feedback mechanisms.

Working with the pharmaceutical industry

This guidance assists pharmacists whose work brings them into regular contact with the pharmaceutical industry. It is not intended to apply to pharmacists who are employed by, or carrying out remunerated work for, the pharmaceutical industry. The guidance promotes best practice and offers general advice to pharmacists who are likely to liaise with pharmaceutical companies in product-specific or business-orientated discussions.

3.3 Law and Ethics fact sheets

The Royal Pharmaceutical Society of Great Britain produces a series of fact sheets for pharmacists, covering areas of practice that are frequently the subject of queries to the Legal and Ethical Advisory Service.

The fact sheets are available on the Society's website, *www.rpsgb.org* under Legal and Ethical Advisory Service. For paper copies please write to the Legal and Ethical Advisory Service with a stamped (value of 72p for one fact sheet; £1.04 for all), self-addressed C4 envelope, including the number(s) of the required fact sheet(s). No telephone requests will be taken.

The titles of the fact sheets are:

1. Controlled Drugs and community pharmacy
2. Controlled Drugs and hospital pharmacy (see *Safer management of Controlled Drugs: a guide to good practice in secondary care [England, Scotland]*, which the RPSGB helped develop)
3. The Medicines for Human Use (Marketing Authorisations Etc.) Regulations 1994, and the effect thereof
4. The export of medicines
5. The use of unlicensed medicines in pharmacy
6. Monitored dosage systems and compliance aids
7. Patient group directions: A resource pack for pharmacists
8. Dealing with dispensing errors
9. Confidentiality, the Data Protection Act 1998 and the disclosure of information (superseded by *Professional standards and guidance for patient confidentiality*; see p114)
10. Employing a locum/Working as a locum
11. Poisons

Patients in police custody Guidance on dealing with prescriptions written by forensic physicians for patients in police custody can be obtained from the Legal and Ethical Advisory Service.

Warning/treatment cards and booklets

Steroid cards

Steroid treatment cards can be purchased from:
England and Wales: 3MSPSL, Gorse Street, Chadderton, Oldham OL9 9QH. Tel 0845 610 1112; Fax: 0161 683 2188; e-mail *nhsforms@spsl.uk.com*
Scotland: R.R. Donnelley Global Document Solutions, 8 South Gyle, Crescent Lane, Edinburgh EH12 9EG. Tel: 0131 334 1229; Fax: 0131 334 5946; e-mail *ian.fruish@rrd.com*

MAOI cards

The monoamine oxidase inhibitor card, which was a joint publication of the British Medical Association, the Royal Pharmaceutical Society and the Department of Health, has been discontinued and will not be reprinted. The Department's view is that a great deal of the information contained on the card will be incorporated in patient information leaflets, so that the card is no longer needed. The Society is unable to respond to requests for MAOI cards.

Lithium cards

Lithium treatment cards can be purchased from the National Pharmacy Association, 38-42 St. Peter's Street, St Albans, Herts AL1 3NP. Tel: 01727 858687; Fax 01727 795904; e-mail *sales@npa.co.uk*

Anticoagulant booklets

Anticoagulant treatment booklets are held by primary care organisations for distribution to local healthcare professionals. They can also be obtained from:
England and Wales: 3MSPSL, Gorse Street, Chadderton, Oldham OL9 9QH. Tel 0845 610 1112; Fax: 0161 683 2188; e-mail *nhsforms@spsl.uk.com*
Scotland: R.R. Donnelley Global Document Solutions, 8 South Gyle, Crescent Lane, Edinburgh EH12 9EG. Tel: 0131 334 1229; Fax: 0131 334 5946; e-mail *ian.fruish@rrd.com*

4: References

4.1 Council Members and National Pharmacy Boards Members 2009-2010

Council

President
Mr Steve Churton

Vice-President
Mr Martin Astbury

Treasurer
Mr John Gentle

Mr Steve Acres
Ms Seema Agha
Mr Gerald Alexander
Mrs Margaret Allan
Professor Nicholas Barber
Mrs Kay Blair
Mrs Cathryn Brown
Mr David Carter
Dr Catherine Duggan
Mrs Dorothy Drury
Dr Phillida Entwistle
Mr Graeme Hall
Mrs Sylvia Hikins
Mrs Lorna Jacobs
Mr Raymond Jobling
Mr John Jolley
Mr Alan Kershaw
Mrs Sue Kilby
Dr Tristan Learoyd
Miss Yvonne Liddell
Professor Alistair Michell
Mrs Alison Moore
Ms Jane Ramsey
Ms Marcia Saunders
Mr David Thomson
Mrs Valerie Turner
Professor Keith Wilson

English Pharmacy Board

Chairman
Dr Brian Curwain

Vice-Chairman
Mr Richard Daniszewski

Ms Seema Agha
Mr Martin Astbury
Mr Jonathan Buisson
Mrs Gail Curphey
Mr Sid Dajani
Dr Catherine Duggan
Mrs Lindsey Gilpin
Miss Rachael Lemon
Mr David Miller
Professor David Mottram
Mr Graham Phillips
Mrs Beth Taylor
Mr Steve Wicks

Scottish Pharmacy Board

Chairman
Mrs Sandra Melville

Vice-Chairman
Mr Alistair Jack

Mr Ewan Black
Dr Anne Boyter
Mr Stuart Johnstone
Mrs Alpana Mair
Mr Frank Owens
Dr Rose Marie Parr
Dr Derek Stewart
Mr Charles Tait
Mr William Templeton
Ms Angela Timoney

Welsh Pharmacy Board

Chairman
Mr Marc Donovan

Vice-Chairman
Mr Peter Jones

Mrs Mair Davies
Miss Jodine Evans
Mr Richard Evans
Mr Brian Hawkins
Ms Diane Heath
Mr Carwyn Jones
Mrs Rowena McArtney
Mr Phillip Parry
Mrs Fiona Price
Dr David Temple

4.2 Support for pharmacists

Pharmacist Support is an organisation working for pharmacists and their families in times of need.

Our support services include a variety of programmes developed in consultation with pharmacists to offer a helping hand to colleagues who find themselves confronted by difficult circumstances for whatever reason. Our services include:

- Listening Friends
- Specialist advice services
- Pharmacists Health Support Programme
- Grants and financial assistance
- Signposting

Many of the services are delivered directly by volunteer pharmacists located throughout the United Kingdom. Because there is a shared professional background, our volunteers are uniquely able to understand the specific pressures affecting pharmacists and their families.

If you are currently affected by any issues, please do not hesitate to contact us by ringing our freephone number on 0808 168 2233. Your enquiry will be dealt with promptly and in complete confidence.

More information about our range of services

Listening Friends offers free listening services to pharmacists suffering from stress. The service is entirely confidential and anonymous, and provides the opportunity to talk to a pharmacist trained to offer support regarding the particular pressures that apply to the pharmacy profession. The service is not restricted to work related problems, but offers support for all causes of stress such as ill-health, family issues, and bereavement.
To access the Listening Friends service call 0808 168 5133

Specialist advice services in the areas of benefits, debt and employment law are provided completely free of charge and are confidential. Specially trained advisers will help you by offering a range of advice in response to your particular problem. Examples of this support include 'benefit checks' to ensure you are receiving the correct amount of benefits and tax credits, preparation of financial statements, rescheduling of payments to creditors if you have multiple debts, and advice in connection with your employment.
To access the specialist advice services call 0808 168 2233

The Pharmacists Health Support Programme exists to help pharmacists who experience problems with alcohol, drug or other types of dependency. If you have an alcohol or drug problem, or other type of dependency, or you know of a friend or colleague with a problem, you can contact the Pharmacists Health Support Programme for advice on how we can help.
To access the Pharmacists Health Support Programme call 0808 168 5132

Grants and financial assistance are offered to cover a range of circumstances:

Health and wellbeing grants are provided to pharmacists and their families to support mental or physical quality of life. Typical funding examples include grants for respite care for a family member, for counselling and therapies, for convalescence after an illness or accident, for home help during convalescence, for purchasing a particular disability aid, or for contributions towards nursing or residential care fees.

One-off grants are provided for those who cannot meet a specific cost and require temporary assistance. Often applicants for these grants have been affected by an unforeseen loss of work due to redundancy or ill-health, or are living on a very low income and can't afford to pay an unexpected bill. Examples of one-off grants include financial assistance to purchase a washing machine, essential car or household repairs, or to pay winter fuel bills.

Regular grants provide a 'top-up' for people who have a very low income and are finding it difficult to make ends meet without getting into debt. Applicants are often widows/widowers or retired pharmacists, and these grants can help them to maintain a quality of life which they would otherwise lose.

Student hardship grants can be made available to students who are bearing particular hardship. We realise that most students leave university with significant debt. However, some students face particular hardship due to unforeseen circumstances such as family issues, ill-health or bereavement.
To find out more about the grants and financial assistance programme call our freephone number on 0808 168 2233

Signposting We will always try to support pharmacists and their families by providing a helping hand ourselves. However, if we can't address a specific problem, we may know someone else who can. Our experienced staff will point you in the direction of an individual, agency or initiative that will be able to provide support or advice to meet your needs.
To access our Signposting service call 0808 168 2233, or see our online directory at www.pharmacistsupport.org

Who is eligible?

If you are a pharmacist, a widow or widower of a pharmacist, a retired pharmacist, a pharmacy student, or a preregistration trainee you are eligible to apply for support; as long as you or your partner have been on the register at some point. We may also be able to help any member of your family who is dependent on you for financial support. If you have a friend who is a pharmacist, or a colleague who needs support, please contact us, and you can be sure of complete confidentiality in making your enquiry.

Listening Friends, the Pharmacists Health Support Programme, and the specialist advice services are made automatically available to pharmacists and their dependents, retired pharmacists, pharmacy students and preregistration trainees.

Grants and financial assistance applications are granted on a case-by-case basis, and eligibility is assessed based on the level of income against the level of outgoings; therefore, your income need not be exceptionally low to apply, and you may still be eligible if you have savings. As a rule, most people who receive means tested benefits, including pension credit, are automatically eligible for consideration.

Contact us

For more information on Pharmacist Support and our services, contact a member of the support team on 0808 168 2233. Alternatively, you can visit our website *www.pharmacistsupport.org* where you will find a number of useful factsheets and a directory listing the details of a wide range of organisations that can give help, advice and support in a number of different subject areas.

Pharmacist Support is a registered charity, Number 221438, and is funded by donations from pharmacists.

4.3 Headquarters telephone enquiries guide

Following the publication in 2007 of the Government White Paper *Trust, Assurance and Safety - The Regulation of Health Professionals in the 21st Century*, the Society is working towards the demerger of its regulatory and professional roles. This will see the establishment of a new General Pharmaceutical Council and a new professional body for pharmacy in 2010.

In preparation for its demerger into two organisations the Society is undergoing internal restructuring. For up to date information on the Society's staff contact details please go to *www.rpsgb.org*.

A list of direct dial telephone numbers correct at 1 July 2009 is given below. If you are not sure who you wish to speak to please dial the Society's main switchboard number

020 7735 9141

so that your call can be routed to the appropriate person. The e-mail address for general enquiries is:

<enquiries@rpsgb.org>

Chief Executive and Registrar Jeremy Holmes	020 7572 2201
Director of Professional Services (Vacancy)	020 7572 2208
Managing Director, RPS Publishing Bob Bolick	020 7572 2273
Director of Policy and Communications David Pruce	020 7572 2338
Director of Finance and Resources Bernard Kelly	020 7572 2245
Deputy Registrar and Director of Regulation Wendy Harris	020 7572 2267
Director for Scotland Lyndon Braddick	0131 556 4386
Director for England Howard Duff	020 7572 2519
Director for Wales Paul Gimson (from 1 August 2009)	029 2073 0310

Advertising (PJ Publications)	020 7572 2222
Branches and regions	020 7572 2333
British National Formulary (editorial)	020 7572 2282
British Pharmaceutical Conference	020 7572 2332
Byelaws and Regulations	020 7572 2206
Careers	020 7572 2330
Code of conduct (Society employees)	020 7572 2543
Complaints:	
About a pharmacist/pharmacy	020 7572 2308
About services/Society staff	020 7572 2463
Continuing professional development	020 7572 2540
Council business	020 7572 2446
Disciplinary Committee	020 7572 2623
Dispensing/pharmacy assistants	020 7572 2610
Education:	
General information/Accreditation	020 7572 2215
Undergraduate pharmacy courses	020 7572 2215

English Pharmacy Board business	020 7572 2446
Ethics	020 7572 2481
Events	020 7572 2261
Fellows	020 7572 2201
Finance	020 7572 2230
Fitness to Practise	020 7572 2308
Governance:	
Clinical	020 7572 2208
Corporate	020 7572 2206
Health Committee	020 7572 2623
Human resources	020 7572 2246
Information services:	
Information pharmacists	020 7572 2302
Legal and ethical advisory service	020 7572 2308
Library	020 7572 2300
Museum	020 7572 2210

Inspectors:
Chief Inspector: Mrs Sarah Billington 020 7572 2666/2312

Northern Region:

Lynsey Cleland (Regional Lead Inspector)	020 7572 2661
Stan Brandwood	020 7572 2550
Paula Gardner	020 7572 2577
Sheena Greig	020 7572 2555
Alison Hopkins	020 7572 2557
Helen Jackson	020 7572 2558
John Russ Liddell	020 7572 2561
Stewart Waugh	020 7572 2570
David Young	020 7572 2573

Central Region

Jill Williams (Regional Lead Inspector)	020 7572 2572
Richard Chapman	020 7572 2522
Barry Cohen	020 7572 2551
Steven Gascoigne	020 7572 2554
Akhtar Malik	020 7572 2574
Noor Mohamed	020 7572 2533

Southern Region

Tim Snewin (Regional Lead Inspector)	020 7572 2568
Monika Chowdhury	020 7572 2516
Simon Denton	020 7572 2565
Peter Gibbs	020 7572 2559
Susan Melvin	020 7572 2562
Sharon Monks	020 7572 2515
Martin Packham	020 7572 2569
Jacqueline Riley	020 7572 2566
Eilean Robson	020 7572 2552
Andrew Smith	020 7572 2408

For details of the Inspector covering your area, see the Society's website *www.rpsgb.org*

Investigating Committee	020 7572 2623
Marketing	020 7572 2688
Martindale (editorial)	020 7572 2390
Medicines counter assistants	020 7572 2610

Medicines, Ethics and Practice:		Policy development	020 7572 2218
Content Part 1 (Legal sections)	020 7572 2308	Practice:	
Content Part 2 (Code of Ethics)	020 7572 2481	Guidance documents	020 7572 2409
Content Part 3 (Pharmacy practice)	020 7572 2612	Policy	020 7572 2602
Distribution, pharmacists and		Preregistration training	020 7572 2370
pharmacy technicians	020 7572 2229	Professional leadership	0115 939 6465
Distribution, other*	0203 318 3141	Public relations and press office	020 7572 2335/6
Membership services	020 7572 2330		
		Quality improvement	020 7572 2602
The Pharmaceutical Journal:			
Editor and Editorial Director	020 7572 2429	Records management	020 7572 2212
Editorial content	020 7572 2414	Registration:	
Distribution, pharmacists and		General	020 7572 2322
pharmacy technicians	020 7572 2229	Overseas pharmacists	020 7572 2317
Distribution, other*	0203 318 3141	UK pharmacists wishing to work overseas	020 7572 2322
Pharmaceutical Press:		Registration Appeals Committee	020 7572 2623
Customer services*	0203 318 3141	Research and development	020 7572 2278
Editorial	020 7572 2273		
Sales and marketing	020 7572 2342		
		Secretariat (Corporate)	020 7572 2204
Pharmacist prescribing		Science	020 7572 2603
(accreditation of supplementary and		Scottish Pharmacy Board business	0131 556 4386
independent prescribing courses)	020 7572 2604	Statutory Committees	020 7572 2623
Annotation of register	020 7572 2322	Support staff regulation	020 7572 2610
Pharmacist Support	0808 168 2233		
Listening Friends Scheme	0808 168 5133		
Pharmacists Health Support Programme	0808 168 5132	Website	020 7572 2288
Pharmacy technicians	020 7572 2610	Welsh Pharmacy Board business	029 2073 0310
* from 1 August 2009		Your Society	020 7572 2335

Emergency connection to ex-directory telephone numbers

Community pharmacists can be connected to ex-directory, no-connection telephone numbers if they need to contact patients in a real emergency.

This privilege, which is also available to doctors, hospitals and emergency authorities, was granted to pharmacists by British Telecom in February 1998 as a result of representation to BT by the then National Pharmaceutical Association.

It is important that pharmacists use the privilege appropriately and only exercise their right of access when stricly necessary. The following guidelines must be adhered to:

Pharmacists should only consider asking for conection to an ex-directory, no-connection number in a "life and death" situation. This can be interpreted as an emergency which is likely to pose a very serious threat to the health of the patient if information cannot be passed on immediately and when the patient's telephone number cannot be found from another source (eg, the GP's surgery).

A pharmacist needing to contact an ex-directory, no-connection number should dial 100, explain the situation and request connection to the ex-directory number.

The pharmacist will only be connected when the following criteria are met:

- the pharmacist must be calling from community pharmacy premises
- the pharmacist must explain the reason for the emergency connection request and advise the operator that it is a life and death situation (the operator will not judge the nature of the emergency but will accept the word of the pharmacist)
- the pharmacist must give his or her name and the name of the pharmacy premises from which he or she is calling.

BT will monitor all requests for emergency connection. If the privilege is abused it is likely that this important facility for community pharmacists will be withdrawn.

Index

A

Accountable Officer 3, 38
  authorising persons as authorised
    witnesses 38
  definition of 3
  and destruction of CDs 39
  and CD SOPS 38

Addicts *see* Drug misusers

Additional supply optometrist
  definition of 3
  signed order for patient supply 20

Administration (of medicines)
  ambulance paramedics 22
  by operators 11
  chiropodists 19
  Controlled Drugs in hospitals 32
  midwives 18
  prescription-only drugs *see*
    Prescription-only medicines (POM)

Advanced electronic signature 12

Adverse drug reactions
  veterinary 95

Advertising
  acceptance of gifts/inducements to
    prescribe or supply 27
  chemicals 84-85
  medicines and professional services,
    professional standards
    and guidance 122
  veterinary medicines 95
  see also Promotion/
    promotional material

Advice services for pharmacists 148

Agriculture, storage of poisons for 77

Aircraft operators/commanders, exempted
  sales 22

Alcohol
  denatured 87-90

Aloxiprin
  labelling of general sale list medicines
    24
  non-effervescent 10
  not on general sale to children 7
  warning on labels of products 24-25

Ambulance paramedics, administration by
  22

Amorolfine nail lacquer 142

Anabolic steroids 29

Animal feedingstuffs, medicated (MFS) 95
  prescriptions 95

Antibiotics, emergency supply 15-16

Anticoagulant booklets 146

Antihistamines, warning on labels of
  products 25

Antimicrobial preservative, quantity in
  products 4

Appropriate date, definition 4

Appropriate date for CD prescriptions 33

Appropriate non-proprietary name,
  definition 4

Appropriate practitioner, for prescription-
  only medicines 4, 11

Appropriate quantitative particulars,
  definition 4

Approved wording for CD prescriptions 34

Arsenite, sale 77

Aspirin
  labelling of general sale list medicines
    24
  legal status (table) 45
  non-effervescent 10
  not on general sale to children 7
  warning on labels of products 24-25

Assembled medicines, labelling 23

Assembly 23
  licence 23

Assistants *see* Pharmacy assistants

Asthma
  emergency supply of medicines 15-16
  warning on labels of pharmacy
    medicines 24-25

Atopic eczema in children, guidance 142

Audit 138

Authorisation
  marketing *see* Marketing authorisation

Authority, pharmacists and pharmacy technicians in positions of, professional standards for 106

Azithromycin, OTC supply, guidance 142

B

Bed cards 13, 32

Benzodiazepines 29

Bisacodyl 8

Blood pressure, monitoring, guidance 142

Bottles, fluted
exceptions 26-27
use 26

Bowel cancer, guidance 142

British Red Cross Society, exempted supplies 21

British Standards Institution, exempted sales 22

C

Calcium cyanide, sale 77

Cannabis 28

Capsules 8

Care home service
definition 4
waste 27-28

Care homes
definition 4
waste 27-28
see also Nursing homes

Care of patients 104

Care, social, handling of medicines in 143

Cascade, prescribing 93

CD Anab (Controlled Drugs, Schedule 4 Part II) 29, 40, 41, 43
CD Benz (Controlled Drugs, Schedule 4 Part I) 29, 40, 41, 43
CD Inv. (Controlled Drugs, Schedule 5) 29, 40, 41, 43
CD Lic (Controlled Drugs Schedule 1) 28, 43
CD No Register (Controlled Drugs, Schedule 3) 29, 40, 41, 43
CD POM (Controlled Drugs, Schedule 2) 28, 40, 41, 43

CE marking, medical devices 27

Certificate, purchase of poisons 76

Cetirizine hydrochloride 8

Chemicals 82-86

Chemicals (Hazard Information and Packaging for Supply) Regulations 2002 (CHIP) 82

Chemists' nostrums 23
labelling 23-24

Child protection 142

Children
cough and cold treatments 143
formulations, labelling (GSL products) 24
products not on general sale for 7

Child-resistant containers
for chemicals 84

CHIP see Chemicals (Hazard Information and Packaging for Supply) Regulations 2002 (CHIP)

Chiropodists
exempted sales 18
parenteral administration of drugs 19
registered, definition 6

Chloramphenicol eye drops, OTC supply, guidance 142

Chloroform, sale and supply 27

Cholesterol testing, guidance 142

Classification, Labelling and Packaging of Substances and Mixtures (CLP) 82

Clinical effectiveness 138

Clinical governance 137-138
defined 137
framework for prescribing 142

Clinical management plan 4, 14
including a Controlled Drug 37

Clinical trials 142

Clotrimazole 8

Code of Ethics for Pharmacists and Pharmacy Technicians 103-106

Collection
of medicines from central points 9
practice guidance 142
of prescriptions see Prescription collection services

of Schedule 2 and 3 Controlled Drugs 35-36

Common name, definition 4

Community pharmacies see Pharmacies; Premises

Community practitioner nurse prescriber, definition 4
range of medicines prescribable 14

Competence see Professional competence

Completely denatured alcohol (CDA) 87

Compliance aids, law and ethics fact sheet 146

Concerns, raising, guidance 144

Confidentiality
Controlled Drug possession 28
NHS Code of Practice 144
patient, professional standards and guidance on 114

Consent, patient, professional standards and guidance on 110

Contact lenses, plano (zero powered) 27

Containers
bulk, labelling of assembled medicines 20
chemists' nostrums, labelling 23-24
child-resistant see Child-resistant containers
for Controlled Drugs, marking 39
definition 4
fluted bottles see Fluted bottles
labelling of medicinal products 23
multiple, labelling requirements 23
poisons 76
relevant medicinal products, labelling 24

Continuing education 139

Continuing professional development (CPD) 138
as component of clinical governance 138
cycle 139
definition 138
record entry, advice 139
professional standards and guidance 133
Society's programme 138

Contraception see Emergency hormonal contraception (EHC)

Contract, community pharmacy, resources supporting 142

Contracts, pharmacist in personal control and 8-9

Controlled Drugs 28-42
    changes in the management of 142
    stock, maintaining running balances 143

Cosmetics
    definition 4
    general sale list medicines 7

Cough and cold treatments for children 143

Council Members, list 147

Counter assistants 140

Counterfeit medicines 143

Cyanide, sale 77

Cyanogenetic substances 10

D

Daily dose, maximum (mdd), definition 5

Data protection legislation
    fact sheet 146

Data sheets, chemicals 82-83, 85-86

Date, appropriate
    definition 4
    on a CD prescription 33
    start date on a CD prescription 33

Definitions (Medicines Act 1968) 3-6

Denatured alcohol 87-90

Denatured ethanol B (DEB) 87

Dental practitioners
    exempted sales 18
    prescription for prescription-only medicines 11

Dental Practitioners' Formulary 12

Dental prescription 11-12
    validity 11-12

Dental schemes, exempted sales 22

Destruction of medicines
    destruction of Controlled Drugs 37-42
    see also Disposal of waste

Devices, medical 27, 143

Diabetes mellitus
    guidance on care of people with 143

Diagnostic testing
    and screening services 143
    blood pressure management 142
    cholesterol testing 142
    pregnancy testing 144

Diamorphine, prescribing for drug misusers 34

Diazepam, administration by ambulance paramedics 22

Dietitian, registered, definition 6

Dipipanone, prescribing for drug misusers 34

Discharge and transfer planning 143

Dispensed medicinal products
    definition 4, 23
    labelling 23
        veterinary drugs 93

Dispensing
    errors, law and ethics fact sheet 146
    standard operating procedures see
        Standard operating procedures (SOPs)
    supply of medicines see
        Supply of medicines

Dispensing/pharmacy assistants 140

Disposal of waste
    chemicals 86
    Controlled Drugs 39-42

Dosage units
    definition 4

Drug misusers
    Controlled Drugs prescriptions 32-34
    Controlled Drugs supply 34-36
    guidance for providers of services 142
    instalment prescribing 34-35
    prescriptions 32-34
        Controlled Drugs 32-34

Drug treatment services, exempted supplies 20

Drugs (substances of misuse)
    forged prescriptions 12
    practice guidance 145

Duthie report, revised 144

Duty free spirits 90

E

Ecstasy-type substances 28

Eczema, atopic, in children, guidance 142

Education
    continuing see Continuing education
    see also Continuing professional development (CPD)

EEA
    and Swiss healthcare professionals 11
    and Swiss prescriptions 11, 143
    and Swiss doctor or patient, emergency supply request by 15
    healthcare professional, definition 4

Effervescent, definition 4

Effervescent tablets 8

Electronic records 14
    CD register 36
    prescription records 14
    prescription transfer 12

Electronic signature 12

Electronic transfer of prescriptions 12

Emergencies
    involving chemicals 85
    parenteral prescription-only medicines 10

Emergency connection to ex-directory telephone numbers 150

Emergency hormonal contraception (EHC), guidance 143

Emergency supply
    of Controlled Drugs 15-16
    Controlled Drug stock 30
    entry in prescription-only register 15-16
    of prescription-only medicines 15-16
        conditions applicable 15-16
        request of doctor/prescribers 15
        request of EEA or Swiss doctor or patient 15
        request of patients 15-16
    signed orders for poisons 76

English Pharmacy Board, list 147

Ephedrine, sale 10, 144

Epilepsy drugs, emergency supply 15-16

Epilepsy, guidance 143

Ergometrine maleate, administration by ambulance paramedics 22

Ether 90

Ethics
    see Code of Ethics for Pharmacists and Pharmacy Technicians

Ethyl ether 90

European Directives
    labelling 23
    medical devices 27

Ex-directory telephone numbers, emergency
    connection to 150

Exemptions
    poisons sales 77
    prescription-only medicines status 10
    sales of medicines to exempted
        organisations, healthcare
        professionals or other persons 17-23
    to medicines legislation in the event of
        a pandemic 13

Expiry date, medicines
    definition 5

Export of medicines
    law and ethics fact sheet 146

External use, definition 5

F

Facsimile transmission, prescription 12

Fact sheets, law and ethics 146

Famotidine 8

Faxes, prescription 12

Fire fighting, chemical hazards 85

First aid
    chemical exposures 85
    offshore installations, exempted
        supplies 22
    organisations 21

Flu pandemic, service continuity planning
    for 145

Fluoroacetamide, sale 77

Fluoroacetic acid, sale 77

Fluted bottles
    exceptions 26-27
    use 26

Food
    definition 5
    general sale list medicines 7

Forestry, storage of poisons for 77

Forged prescriptions 12

Formulary, Dental Practitioners' 12

G

General Dental Council 11

General Medical Council 11

General sale list medicine(s) 7
    for children, labelling 24-25
    definition 5, 7
    exemptions from controls on retail sale
        17-23
    labelling 24-25
    retail sale 7
    sales/supply by optometrists 19-20

General sale list Order 7

Gifts and inducements, to prescribe/
    supply 27

Glaucoma, guidance 143

Globally Harmonised System of
    Classification and Labelling of
    Chemicals (GHS) 82

Governance, clinical 137-138

Grants and financial assistance for
    pharmacists 148

Granules 8

Group authorities and licences, exempted
    sales 22

GSL see General sale list medicine(s)

Guidance, practice 142-145

H

Hallucinogenic drugs 28

Handling of medicines, safe and secure 144

Handling of medicines in social care 143

Handling of waste medicines 27

Hazardous substances
    chemicals 82

Hazardous Waste Regulations 143

Hazards, identification, chemicals 85

Headquarters, telephone enquiries guide
    149

Health and Safety Executive
    labels for chemicals 82
    safety data sheets for chemicals 82-83,
        85-86

Health centres, exempted sales 17

Health prescription
    definition 5
    validity criteria 11

Health records
    access 14
    supplementary prescribers' access 14

Help, for pharmacists in difficulty 148

Heparinoid 8

Hexachlorophane, warning on labels of
    products 25

Home Office approved wording for CD pre-
    scriptions 34

Homes see Care homes; Nursing homes

Honesty 105

Hormonal contraception, emergency see
    Emergency hormonal contraception
    (EHC)

Horticulture, storage of poisons for 77

Hospital pharmacies
    records of medicine supply 15

Hospitals
    administration of prescription-only
        medicines, policies 11
    Bed cards 13, 32
    Controlled Drugs 32, 146
    exempted sales/supply 17
    prescription-only medicine
        administration 11
    written directions to supply
        prescription-only medicines 13

Human use, medicines for 7-42
    list 43-74

Hypertension see Blood pressure

I

Ibuprofen 8

Identification of purchasers, of poisons 75

Independent prescribing 14, 141

Importing, Controlled Drugs 30

Improving the quality of pharmacy practice
    137-141

Inducements to prescribe/supply 27

Industrial methylated spirits (IMS) 87

Industrial denatured alcohol (IDA) 87

Industry see Pharmaceutical industry

Instalment prescriptions, Controlled Drugs 34

Insulin, emergency supply 15-16

Internet pharmacy services 123

Interventions, recording 144

Intravenous infusions, administration by ambulance paramedics 22

Ionising Radiation (Medical Exposure) Regulations 2000 11

IRME practitioner
    definition 5

Isopropyl alcohol 90

K

Keep out of the reach of children 23

Keep out of the reach and sight of children 23

L

Labelling
    chemicals 83
    of containers for Controlled Drugs 39
    monitored dosage systems, fact sheet 146
    poisons 76

Labelling of medicinal products 23-26
    assembled (prepacked) medicines 23
    chemists' nostrums 23
    dispensed products 23
    general sale list (GSL) products 24
    multiple containers 23
    particulars to be included 23
    pharmacy medicines (P) 25
    prescription-only medicines (POM) 25-26
    relevant medicinal products 23
    veterinary medicines 93
    warnings and special requirements 24

Law and ethics fact sheets 146

Listening Friends Scheme 148

Lithium cards 146

Locums
    fact sheet 146

Loperamide hydrochloride 8

Loratidine 8

M

Manufacturers' licence holders, exempted sales 22

MAOI cards 146

Marketing authorisation
    prescription-only medicines 9
    products without 10

Masters of ships
    exempted supplies 20
    requisitions for Controlled Drugs 31

Maximum daily dose (mdd), definition 5
Maximum dose (md), definition 5
Maximum strength (ms), definition 5

Medical devices 27, 143

Medical Devices Regulations 27

Medicated animal feedingstuffs (MFS) 95
    prescriptions 95

Medicinal product(s) 7-42
    administration see Administration (of medicines)
    assembled (prepacked), labelling 23
    CHIP exemption 82
    classes 7
    collection see Collection
    definition 5
    dispensed, labelling see Labelling of medicinal products
    disposal see Disposal of waste
    dosage units 4
    emergency supplies 15-16
    external use, definition 5
    general sale list see General sale list medicine(s)
    for human use 7-42
        list 43-74
    labelling see Labelling of medicinal products
    liquid, in fluted bottles 26
    medicines, safe and secure handling, guidance 144
    not general sale list medicines 7
    pharmacy medicines see Pharmacy medicines (P)
    prescription-only see Prescription-only medicines (POM)

relevant
    definition 6
    labelling 24
    retail sale see Retail sale
    safe and secure handling, guidance 144
    sales of medicines to exempted organisations, healthcare professionals or other persons 17-23
    strength, definition 6
    supply, see Supply of medicines
    waste, disposal see Disposal of waste
    wholesale dealing see Wholesale dealing

Medicinal purpose, definition 5

Medicine administration record (MAR) charts, guidance 143

Medicine sales see Sale of medicines

Medicines Act 1968 3
    classes of products 7
    definitions 3-6
    principles/coverage 3
    wholesale dealing 16-17

Medicines adherence, guidance 143

Medicines (Administration of Radioactive Substances) Regulations 1978 11

Medicines counter assistants 140

Medicines legislation, exemptions in the event of a pandemic 13

Medicines management during patient admission to the ward 143

Mepyramine maleate 8

Messengers, collection of Controlled Drugs 31

Midazolam 29
    and PGDs 38
    safe custody 30

Midwives
    Controlled Drugs and 37
    exempted sales/supply 18
    parenteral administration 18
    registered, definition 6

Missed instalment collection days 34

Mineralised methylated spirits (MMS) 87

Misuse of Drugs Act 1971 28, 30
    classification 28
    Secretary of State prohibitions and 30

Moles, strychnine for killing 77

Monitored dosage systems
  labelling, law and ethics fact sheet 146

Monoamine oxidase inhibitor (MAOI) card
  146

N

National Health Service
  drug testing, exempted sales 22
  prescriptions of Controlled Drugs for
    misusers 34

National Proficiency Test Council (NPTC)
  94

Non-medicinal poisons see Poisons

Non-prescribed medicines, sales 8
  see also Pharmacy medicines (P)

Non-proprietary name, appropriate,
  definition 4

Nurse independent prescribers, definition 5
  range of medicines prescribable by 14
  Controlled Drugs and 37

Nurse, registered, definition 6

Nursing and Midwifery Council 5

Nursing homes
  requisitions for Controlled Drugs 30

O

Obesity, guidance 144

Occupational health schemes
  definition 21
  exempted supplies 22

Occupational therapist, registered,
  definition 6

OPD see Operating department practitioner

Offshore installations
  first aid personnel, exempted supplies
    22
  requisitions for Controlled Drugs 30

Omeprazole, OTC supply, guidance 144

Operating department practitioner
  definition 5
  CDs 37

Optometrists
  additional supply, definition 3
    exempted sales/supply 20

independent prescriber, definition 5
  registered, definition 6
    exempted sales/supply 19
  signed order for patient supply 16

Organophosphorus sheep dips 94

Orlistat, OTC supply, guidance 144

Orthoptist, registered, definition 6

Orthotist and prosthetist, registered,
  definition 6

Owners of ships
  exempted supplies 20
  requisitions for Controlled Drugs 31

P

Packaging
  chemicals 84
  relevant medicinal products, labelling
    24

Pandemic, exemptions to medicines legislation in 13

Pandemic flu, service continuity planning
  for 145

Paracetamol
  labelling of general sale list medicines
    24
  legal status (tables) 65, 66
  non-effervescent 10
  warning on labels of products 24

Paramedics
  ambulance, administration by 22
  registered, definition 6

Parenteral administration
  by ambulance paramedics 22
  by chiropodists 19
  definition 5
  medicinal products for 10
  by midwives 18
  prescription-only drugs, in emergencies
    10
  restrictions 10

Patient confidentiality, professional standards and guidance 114

Patient consent, professional standards and
  guidance 110

Patient group directions (PGD) 13, 38
  approval by NHS/authorities 14
  Controlled Drugs 38

definition 14
  law and ethics fact sheet 138
  resource pack 14
  types 14

Patient information leaflets (PILs) 26

Patient notes, written directions to supply
  prescription-only medicines 13

Patient participation 105

Patient returned CDs
  destruction 29
  record keeping 38, 40

Patients
  bed cards 13, 32
  involvement, pharmacy practice 138
  request for emergency supplies of
    prescription-only medicines 15

Patients' own drugs
  Controlled Drugs 30

Pentazocine, professional possession by
  midwives 37

Person collecting CDs
  misuser's representative 35
  collecting Schedule 2 CD 31, 35, 36, 41

Personal control
  definition 8
  sale of pharmacy medicines 8-9

Personnel protection, from chemicals 86

Pest control, poisons 77

Pethidine, professional possession by midwives 37

Pharmaceutical industry
  guidance for pharmacists on working
    with 145

Pharmacies
  registered, definition 6
  standards checklist 145
  visits by external bodies 145
  without pharmacist in personal control
    8-9

Pharmacist independent prescriber 14, 141
  and CDs 37
  definition 5

Pharmacist prescribers 14, 141
  and CDs 32
  clinical governance framework 141
  prescribing pack 144
  professional standards and guidance for
    126

Pharmacist, responsible 9
    professional standards and guidance
        134
    toolkit 144

Pharmacist supplementary prescribers 14,
    141

Pharmacist Support 148

Pharmacists
    accountability 137
    patient/public involvement 138
    personal control 8-9
    poor performance, remedying 138, 144
    resource tools 144
    service continuity planning 145

Pharmacists Health Support Programme
    148

Pharmacy assistants 140
    see also Counter assistants
    see also Pharmacy support staff

Pharmacy facilities
    standards checklist 145

Pharmacy medicines (P) 7, 8
    definition 8
    labelling 25
    multiple packs for onward sales 17
    preparation in pharmacy 7
    products included 8
    retail sale 8
    sales see Sale of medicines
    sales of medicines to exempted
        organisations, healthcare professionals
        or other persons 17-23
    substances of misuse 145
    warnings 25
    wholesale dealing 16-17

Pharmacy-only (PO) medicine
    definition 7
    requirements for sale of 7

Pharmacy practice, improving quality
    137-141

Pharmacy premises see Premises

Pharmacy, registered, definition 6

Pharmacy support staff 140

Pharmacy technicians 140

Phenobarbitone 29
    emergency supply 15, 16, 40
    safe custody 29, 30 40

Phosphide, zinc 77

Physiotherapist, registered, definition 6

Plano (zero powered) contact lenses 27

Podiatrists See Chiropodists

Poisons 75-78
    alphabetical list 79-81

Poisons Act 1972 3, 75, 77

Poisons book 76
    duration of retention 76

Poisons Rules 75, 76

Police, Controlled Drug destruction 28

Police custody, patients in 146

POM see Prescription-only medicines (POM)

Poor performance, remedying 138, 144

Potassium arsenite, sale 77

Potassium cyanide, sale 77

Powders 8

Practice based commissioning 142, 144

Practice guidance documents 142-145

Practice, improving quality of 137-141

Practitioners, exempted sales/supply and 18

Pregnancy testing, guidance 144

Premises, standards checklist 145

Prepacking of medicines 23

Prescriber identification number 33, 41
    definition 5

Prescribers
    contacting, forged prescriptions 11-12
    nurse see Nurse prescribers
    signature
        checking 11-12
    supplementary see Supplementary
    prescriber

Prescribing
    acceptance of gifts and inducements for
        27
    private, definition 5

Prescribing cascade 93

Prescription(s)
    collection see Prescription collection
        services
    Controlled Drugs 32-35
    date 4
    dental 12
    for drug misusers 35
    EEA and Swiss 11, 143
    electronic records 14
    electronic signature 12
    expiry 12
    facsimile (fax) transmission 12
    forged 12
    health 5, 14
    information included 11-12
    medicated feedingstuffs (MFS) 95
    for prescription-only medicines 11
    private (dental) 12
        for Controlled Drugs 32-35
        records 14
    records 14
        exemptions 14
        particulars to be recorded 15
    repeatable, validity 12
    retention at dispensing pharmacy 12
    for substances of misuse 34-35
    treatment of misusers 35
    validity criteria 11-12
    veterinary medicines 91

Prescription collection services
    from central points 9

Prescription forms, Controlled Drugs
    prescriptions for misusers 34

Prescription-only medicines (POM) 7, 9-16
    administration 10-11
        in emergencies 10
        in hospital 11
        written directions (hospitals) 11
    classes 9
    definition 5
    emergency supplies 15-16
        see also Emergency supply
    exemptions from status of 10
    labelling 25
    misuse 145
    parenteral administration 10-11
    patient group directions 13
    prescriptions for 11-12
        see also Prescription(s)
    records of supply/sales 14-15
        to exempted persons 18
        see also Prescription(s), records
    sales of medicines to exempted
        organisations, healthcare professionals
        or other persons 17-23
    supplementary prescriber 10, 14
    supply by optometrists 19
    supply in occupational health schemes
        21
    wholesale dealing 16-17

written directions to supply (in hospitals) 13

Prescription-only register, emergency supply 15-16

Prison
private prescriptions 33
PGDs 13

Private prescribing, definition 5
for Controlled Drugs 33, 41

Private prescriptions (dental) 12
records 14

Products, not on general sale 7

Professional competence 105

Professional judgement 104

Professional knowledge and competence 105

Professional register, definition 5

Professional registration number, definition 5

Professional standards and guidance documents 106-136

Promotion/promotional material
of medicines 24
see also Advertising

Pseudoephedrine, sale 10, 144

Public analysts, exempted sales 22

Public involvement, pharmacy practice 138

Q

Quality of pharmacy practice, improving 137-141

Quantitative particulars, appropriate, definition 4

R

Radiation emission 11

Radioactive medicinal product
administration 11
definition 6
see also Radiopharmaceutical

Radiographer, registered, definition 6

Radiopharmaceutical
definition 6

Raising concerns, guidance 144

Ranitidine hydrochloride 8

Records
Controlled Drug Registers 36-37, 41
electronic prescription only register 14
electronic CD register 36-37
emergency supplies 15, 16
interventions 144
patient returned CDs 38
poisons 76
prescription see Prescription(s), records
prescription-only medicines 14
veterinary medicines 93
wholesale transactions 17

Registered chiropodist, definition 6
Registered dietitian, definition 6
Registered midwife, definition 6
Registered nurse, definition 6
Registered occupational therapist, definition 6
Registered optometrist, definition 6
Registered orthoptist, definition 6
Registered orthotist and prosthetist, definition 6
Registered paramedic, definition 6
Registered pharmacy, definition 6
Registered physiotherapist, definition 6
Registered radiographer, definition 6
Registered speech and language therapist, definition 6

Registers
Controlled Drugs 36-37
in hospitals 32
electronic prescription-only medicines 14
electronic CD registers 36
emergency supplies 15-16

Registration, Evaluation, Authorisation and restriction of Chemicals (REACH) 85

Registration number, professional, definition 5

Regulation, pharmacy technicians 140

Relevant medicinal product
definition 6
labelling 24-26

Repeatable prescription
definition 6
validity 12

Representative collecting CDs
for misusers 35
for Schedule 2 CDs 35, 36, 41
recording requirements 35, 41

Requisitions, for Controlled Drugs 30-31
marking of 31, 41
sending away of 31, 41
veterinary 6, 31
Respect 104

Responsibility 105

Responsible pharmacist 9
professional standards and guidance 134
toolkit 144

Retail pharmacy business
definition 6
sale of pharmacy medicines 8

Retail sale
definition 7
general sale list medicines 7
of medicines to exempted organisations, healthcare professionals or other persons 17-23
pharmacy medicines 8
see also Sale of medicines

Risk management 138

Rodenticide 77

Royal National Lifeboat Institution, exempted supplies 21

Royal Pharmaceutical Society
headquarters telephone enquiries 149

S

Safe and secure handling of medicines, guidance 144

Safe custody, Controlled Drugs 30

Safety data sheets, chemicals 85

Sale of chemicals 82

Sale of medicines 8
non-prescribed medicines, requirements 8
pharmacy medicines 8
involvement of pharmacists 8
professional standards and guidance 117
see also Retail sale

Sale of poisons see Poisons

Sampling officers, exempted sales 22

Schedule 2 and 3 Controlled Drugs,
    collection 35

Scottish Pharmacy Board, list 147

Screening
    blood pressure monitoring 142
    cholesterol testing 142
    Diagnostic testing and screening
        services 143

Secretary of State prohibitions, Controlled
    Drugs 30

Self-care strategy 145

Sending private CD prescriptions 31, 41

Sexual boundaries, guidance 145

Sheep dips 94

Ships, owners/masters
    exempted supplies 20
    requisitions for Controlled Drugs 30-31

Signed orders
    Controlled Drugs 30-31
    for poisons 76

Simvastatin, OTC supply, guidance 145

Small Animal Exemption Scheme 95

Smallpox vaccine, administration 10

Smoking, stopping, guidance 145

Social care, handling of medicines in 143

Sodium arsenite, sale 77

Sodium cyanide, sale 77

Sodium picosulphate 8

Special labelling requirements 24

Specified publication, definition 6

Speech and language therapist, registered,
    definition 6

Staff
    induction 138
    pharmacy support staff 140
    training requirements 8

Standard operating procedures (SOPs)
    for Controlled Drugs 38
    for dispensing 145

Standards, checklist 145

Start date
    appropriate date 33
    CD prescriptions 33

Steroid cards 146

Stock
    see Medicinal product(s)
Storage
    chemicals 84
    Controlled Drugs 30
    poisons 76

Strengths
    definition 6
    relevant medicinal product 24

Strychnine
    authority for purchase 77
    sales/supply 77

Substances of misuse 145
    forged prescriptions 12
    see also Drug misusers

Substances of Very High Concern (SVHC)
    85

Sumatriptan, OTC supply, guidance 145

Supervision
    personal control and 8-9
    for sale of medicines 8

Supplementary prescriber 6, 14
    clinical management plan 14
    Controlled Drugs 14, 37
    definition 6
    health records, access 14
    prescription-only medicines (POM) 14
        emergency supply 15
        prescription for 11-12
        supply 14
    regulatory body 10

Supplementary prescribing 14, 141

Supply of medicines
    Controlled Drugs to misusers 34, 35
    emergency 15-16
        see also Emergency supply

Support for pharmacists 148

Support staff 140

Suspected adverse drug reactions, veterinary
    medicines 96

Swiss see EEA

T

Tables
    Aspirin legal status 45
    Controlled Drugs legal requirements
        40, 41
    Paracetamol legal status 65, 66
    Veterinary medicinal products 92

Tablets 8

Technical errors, Controlled Drug prescrip-
    tions 34
Technicians
    regulation 140

Telephone
    enquiries, Royal Pharmaceutical Society
        headquarters 149
    ex-directory numbers, emergency
        connection to 150

Temazepam
    prescribing 32
    private prescriber's identification number
        33, 41
    private prescription form requirements
        33, 41

Testing in pharmacies
    blood pressure 142
    cholesterol 142
    diagnostic testing and screening
        services 143
    pregnancy, guidance 144

Thallium salts, sale 77

Thallium sulphate 77

Topical use 8

Toxicology, chemical safety data sheets 86

Trade specific denatured alcohol (TSDA) 87

Training
    requirements for staff 8
    see also Continuing education

Transport, of chemicals 86

Transposition of written directions in hospi-
    tals 13

U

Unit preparation, definition 6

Universities, exempted sales 22

Unlicensed medicines use,
    law and ethics fact sheet 146

Unorthodox practitioners, exempted sales
    22

V

Veterinary medicinal product, definition 6

Veterinary medicines 91-96
    alphabetical list 97-102
    advertising 95
    classification table 92
    labelling 93
    medicated animal feedingstuffs 95
    prescribing cascade 93
    prescriptions 91, 95
    records 93
    requisition
            definition 6, 30-31
            for CD 32
    sale and supply, guidance 145
    sheep dips 94

suspected adverse drug reactions 96
wholesale dealing 94

Vitamin A products 7

Vitamin D products 7

Vulnerable adults protection 144

W

Warning cards 146

Warnings
    keep out of the reach of children 23, 24
    keep out of the reach and sight of chil-
        dren 23
    labelling 24
    pharmacy medicines 25

Waste
    hazardous, regulations 143
    medicines, handling 27

Welsh Pharmacy Board, list 147

Wholesale dealer, Controlled Drugs 30

Wholesale dealer's licence 16

Wholesale dealing 7, 16-17
    definition 7
    poisons 77
    to purchasers/organisations 16-17
    veterinary medicinal products 94

Wording approved for CD prescriptions
    34-35

Written directions
    to supply prescription-only medicines in
        hospitals 13
    transposition of 13

Z

Zinc phosphide, sale 77